CLINICAL MANAGEMENT OF EARLY PREGNANCY

CLINICAL MANAGEMENT OF EARLY PREGNANCY

Edited by

Walter Prendiville

Department of Obstetrics and Gynaecology
Royal College of Surgeons in Ireland
Dublin, Ireland

and

James R. Scott

Department of Obstetrics and Gynecology
University of Utah School of Medicine
Salt Lake City, Utah, USA

A member of the Hodder Headline Group
LONDON · SYDNEY · AUCKLAND
Co-published in the United States of America by
Oxford University Press Inc., New York

First published in Great Britain in 1999 by
Arnold, a member of the Hodder Headline Group,
338 Euston Road, London NW1 3BH

http://www.arnoldpublishers.com

Co-published in the United States of America by
Oxford University Press Inc.,
198 Madison Avenue, New York, NY10016
Oxford is a registered trademark of Oxford University Press

Whilst the advice and information in this book are believed to be true and
accurate at the date of going to press, neither the authors nor the publisher
can accept any legal responsibility or liability for any errors or omissions
that may be made. In particular (but without limiting the generality of the
preceding disclaimer) every effort has been made to check drug dosages;
however, it is still possible that errors have been missed. Furthermore,
dosage schedules are constantly being revised and new side-effects
recognized. For these reasons the reader is strongly urged to consult the
drug companies' printed instructions before administering any of the
drugs recommended in this book.

British Library Cataloguing in Publication Data
A catalogue record for this book is available from the British Library

Library of Congress Cataloging-in-Publication Data
A catalog record for this book is available from the Library of Congress

ISBN 0 340 74100 7

1 2 3 4 5 6 7 8 9 10

Composition by Type Study, Scarborough, North Yorkshire
Printed and bound in Great Britain by The Bath Press, Bath

What do you think about this book? Or any other Arnold title?
Please send your comments to feedback.arnold@hodder.co.uk

CONTENTS

CONTRIBUTORS

Dr D.W. Branch
Professor
Department of Obstetrics and Gynecology
University of Utah School of Medicine
Salt Lake City, Utah 84132, USA

Dr J.A. Coulter
Lecturer in Obstetrics and Gynaecology
Royal College of Surgeons in Ireland
Coombe Women's Hospital
Dublin 8, Ireland

Dr C.M. Craven
Research Associate
University of Utah Department of Obstetrics
and Gynecology
University of Utah School of Medicine
Salt Lake City, Utah 84132, USA

Dr P. Crowley
TCD Department of Obstetrics
and Gynaecology
Coombe Women's Hospital
Dublin 8, Ireland

Dr S. Daly
Lecturer in Obstetrics and Gynaecology
Royal College of Surgeons in Ireland
Coombe Women's Hospital
Dublin 8, Ireland

Professor A.H. DeCherney
Professor and Chairman
Department of Obstetrics and Gynecology
University of California at Los Angeles
Los Angeles, CA, USA

Dr D. Dizon-Townson
Assistant Professor
Department of Obstetrics and Gynecology
University of Utah School of Medicine
Salt Lake City, Utah 84132, USA

Dr D.J. Dudley
Associate Professor
Department of Obstetrics and Gynecology
University of Utah School of Medicine
Salt Lake City, Utah 84132, USA

Dr J.A. Hill
Director, Division of Reproductive Medicine
Department of Obstetrics, Gynaecology and
Reproductive Biology
Brigham and Women's Hospital
Harvard Medical School
Boston, MA 02115, USA

Mr K. Hinshaw
Consultant Obstetrician and Gynaecologist
Sunderland Royal Hospital
Kayll Road
Sunderland
Tyne and Wear SR4 7TP, UK

Dr J.C. Jennings
Associate Professor of Clinical Pharmacy
Department of Pharmacy Practice
College of Pharmacy
University of Utah School of Medicine
Salt Lake City, Utah 84132, USA

Dr F.D. Malone
Consultant Perinatologist
Assistant Professor of Obstetrics and
Gynecology

Tufts University School of Medicine
Division of Maternal–Fetal Medicine
New England Medical Center
Boston, MA 02111, USA

L.P. Martinez
Program Manager
Pregnancy RiskLine
Utah Department of Health
University of Utah
Division of Medical Genetics
Salt Lake City, Utah, USA

Dr H.M. McGee
Professor and Director
Health Services Research Centre
Department of Psychology
Royal College of Surgeons in Ireland
Mercer Street Lr
Dublin 2, Ireland

Dr C.M. Paterson
Consultant in Community Gynaecology and
Reproductive Health Care
St Mary's Hospital NHS Trust
Praed Street
London W2 1NY, UK

Dr W. Prendiville
Associate Professor
Royal College of Surgeons in Ireland
Department of Obstetrics
and Gynaecology
Coombe Women's Hospital
Dublin 8, Ireland

Dr J.R. Scott
Professor
Department of Obstetrics and Gynecology
University of Utah School of Medicine
Salt Lake City, Utah 84132, USA

Dr B.T. Stuart
Consultant Obstetrician and Gynaecologist
Coombe Women's Hospital and St James's
Hospital
Dublin 8, Ireland

Dr K. Ward
Professor
Department of Obstetrics and Gynecology
University of Utah School of Medicine
Salt Lake City, Utah 84132, USA

PREFACE

The volume of research in obstetrics and gynaecology which has been published has increased exponentially during the last 20 years. This is true for both clinical practice and basic science endeavours. Almost every aspect of the two disciplines has been subject to rigorous evaluation and in-depth scrutiny.

Late pregnancy problems have long been the subject of intensive investigation. Despite the fact that early pregnancy loss is the most common complication of pregnancy, the first trimester has received relatively little attention until recently. For example, measures to prevent miscarriage and to assess the effectiveness of diagnostic tests and treatment regimens were previously poorly investigated and controversial. However, the molecular events responsible for successful implantation and growth of the conceptus, along with modern sonographic techniques, have renewed interest in early pregnancy. With this book, we wish to focus the attention of scientists, epidemiologists and clinicians on normal and abnormal events of importance in the first third of pregnancy

The authors of each chapter have been chosen because of their expertise in the field. We appreciate the time and effort they have put into this project, and we are pleased with the results. We hope the reader will find this book to be an informative and stimulating source for the clinical management of early pregnancy.

W. Prendiville
J.R. Scott

PREPREGNANCY CARE

1

P. Crowley

Antenatal care is regarded by enthusiasts as preventive medicine at its best, yet evidence to support its impact on most adverse perinatal outcomes is poor. It was inevitable that this exercise in screening and intervention would be extended backwards to the period before conception, in pursuit of greater benefits. The concept of prepregnancy care became popular in the 1980s and was expounded by medical[1], non-medical[2] and political groups[3]. Prepregnancy care can be roughly divided into provision of information, screening, intervention and behavior modification. Each of these components has the potential to do good, to make no difference to outcome, or to do harm. Evaluation of the effectiveness of prepregnancy care is bedeviled by all the problems associated with assessing antenatal care. There are no randomized trials of the effects of providing or withholding information from couples planning pregnancy. Few prepregnancy programs of screening and intervention have been evaluated by randomized controlled trials, with non-medical and medical enthusiasts alike falling into the trap of comparing pregnancy outcome before and after prepregnancy care[4,5] or by using women who do not attend for prepregnancy care as a control group[6]. Evaluation of the effects of prepregnancy care is also hampered by the diversity of interventions involved, the effect of the population prevalence on the productivity of screening programs and the low incidence of most adverse pregnancy outcomes.

PREPREGNANCY CARE FOR WOMEN WITH UNDERLYING DISEASE

DIABETES MELLITUS

Women with insulin dependent diabetes mellitus are par excellence a group who might benefit from prepregnancy care. They are a readily identifiable population, are at high risk of specific adverse pregnancy outcomes, are readily accessible to either general practitioners or diabetic clinics and accustomed to a high level of medical intervention.

Prepregnancy clinics for women with diabetes can potentially offer three types of intervention – general prepregnancy care of the type that might be offered to all women, accurate information on the specific risks of pregnancy in women with diabetes and on the arduous regimen imposed on the pregnant diabetic, and measures to achieve periconceptional euglycemia in order to reduce the incidence of congenital malformation. General prepregnancy care will be discussed later. The value of informing women of the extent and nature of the risks of pregnancy to the mother and baby has not been proven. Hunter[7] states that this information is sometimes withheld on the basis that it provokes anxiety. However, assuming diabetic women are similar to other

Clinical Management of Early Pregnancy. Edited by Walter Prendiville and James R. Scott.
Published in 1999 by Arnold, ISBN 0 340 74100 7

pregnant women, adequate information may reduce anxiety[8]. Advance knowledge of the potential social disruption associated with tight control of blood sugar levels before and during pregnancy may result in a woman postponing or even abandoning plans for pregnancy. Such outcomes need not be regarded as failures, provided decisions are made on the basis of an accurate grasp of the evidence.

The major thrust of prepregnancy care for women with diabetes has been the attempt to reduce the incidence of fetal anomalies by tight control of blood glucose levels at conception and during organogenesis. There is persuasive observational evidence to support the concept that poor control of blood glucose in very early pregnancy is associated with an increased risk of malformation[9,10]. In response to this, many centers have recruited women with diabetes who are planning to conceive to prepregnancy clinics and instituted a regimen of tight control of blood sugars. There have been no randomized controlled trials of this type of intervention. Reports from a number of clinics in a number of settings compare women who attend for prepregnancy care with non-attenders[6], with historical controls[11], and with 'late bookers'[12]. These studies report a consistently lower incidence of congenital abnormalities in those who attended the prepregnancy clinics compared with that in the various control groups. The biases are self-evident. Those who failed to attend the Edinburgh clinic[6] were younger, less likely to be married, and more likely to smoke than those who did. Gregory *et al.*[13] argue that those who attend such clinics are highly motivated women who are likely to have better diabetic control and a better pregnancy outcome. These authors report an apparently low rate of congenital malformation in women in Nottingham[13], Paris[14] and Bristol[15] where no formal prepregnancy clinics exist. However, it may be that women in these cities are receiving the same kind of information and advice about controlling blood glucose and planning pregnancy from those who care for their diabetes.

In the absence of any controlled trials it seems reasonable to offer all women with diabetes in the reproductive age group easy access to personnel who can supply them with information on the implications of pregnancy in their individual case and to negotiate with them a personally acceptable level of blood glucose control that will reduce the risk of congenital malformation without causing them to default from care if conception fails to occur within a few months of embarking on a schedule of tight control. Whether such care takes place in a designated prepregnancy clinic or as part of the overall care of young women with diabetes is not important.

EPILEPSY

Like women with diabetes, women with epilepsy are a defined group at specific risk of complications in pregnancy. The maternal risks are the morbidity and mortality of increased seizure frequency during pregnancy, whereas the main fetal risk is of malformation. An increase in seizure frequency is most likely in women with a severe seizure disorder[16]. Bioavailability of phenytoin is more likely to be affected than that of other medications because of the alterations in protein binding, hepatic and renal clearance associated with pregnancy. Women with epilepsy intending to conceive might benefit from a review of medication and seizure control. In rare cases, where the woman has been seizure-free for two years or more, a trial of reducing or stopping anticonvulsant therapy prior to conception may be possible. The majority of women with epilepsy, however, face the prospect of embarking on a pregnancy while taking one or more medications. This is a potential source of serious anxiety for women exposed to a barrage of advice from professional and lay sources concerning the inadvisability of taking any medication in pregnancy. It is common for women with epilepsy to discontinue or abandon antiepileptic drug medication in early pregnancy because of concern about fetal abnormality. For this reason, prepregnancy care for women with epilepsy is desirable. Women and their partners are in need of accurate information concerning the risks of fetal abnormality. The prepregnancy period may be an appropriate time for such women and their partners to begin to learn about the benefits and risks of screening for fetal abnormalities.

The overall frequency of congenital abnormality in babies born to women with epilepsy is estimated at three times the background rate, i.e. 6%[16]. The risk of malformation rises with the number of drugs, with three or more drugs in combination being associated with a 10% risk of malformation[17]. Individual drugs are associated with specific abnormalities, e.g. sodium valproate and neural tube defects[18]. Therefore, in addition to the provision of information, the potential exists for a prepregnancy intervention in the form of reducing or altering the drugs in use. In practical terms, the potential to intervene may be limited, as the women on combinations of multiple medications are likely to have the most severe and most difficult to control epilepsy. Evidence that periconceptional folic acid supplementation reduces the risk of both occurrent[19] and recurrent[20] neural tube defects makes the case for the incorporation of folate supplementation into the prepregnancy care of the woman with epilepsy. However as women with epilepsy were excluded from the study[20], there is no evidence from randomized trials to support this recommendation. In view of the altered folate metabolism associated with anticonvulsants the higher 4 mg dose of folic acid is probably more appropriate in this group. To date there is no evidence to indicate the magnitude of any reduction in risk of teratogenesis that might be achieved in women on anticonvulsants or whether any benefits extend to malformations other than neural tube defects.

OTHER CHRONIC DISEASES

All women with medical conditions need information about the effects of pregnancy on the underlying condition, the effect of the condition on the outcome of the pregnancy and the potential teratogenicity of any medication. A prepregnancy consultation provides an opportunity to review the risks and benefits of discontinuing or altering medication prior to pregnancy. This is of particular importance when the drug is a major teratogen such as lithium[21] or retinoid therapy for acne[22] or when a woman is taking a new medication of which teratogenicity is unknown. Designated prepregnancy clinics are not necessary to fulfil this function. Women with diagnosed medical disorders are likely to be in regular contact with either hospital-based specialists or general practitioners whereas those on long-term medications will have prescriptions renewed on a regular basis providing the opportunity for the question of pregnancy to be raised. Prepregnancy care should become an integral part of any medical consultation for any woman in the reproductive age-group who has not been sterilized.

PREVIOUS ADVERSE PREGNANCY OUTCOME

In Ireland in 1988, the perinatal mortality rate in women with a history of one previous perinatal death was 16.6 per 1000 compared with a rate of 10.1 for women with no previous perinatal death. This figure rose to 38.5 per 1000 for those with two and 83.3 per 1000 for those with three previous perinatal deaths[23]. Given the risk of recurrence, couples who have had a previous perinatal death, fetal abnormality or extremely low birthweight baby are obvious candidates for prepregnancy care. The role of a miscarriage clinic is discussed in Chapter 12. In some obstetric units, couples who have suffered either miscarriages or perinatal deaths are seen in a pregnancy loss clinic. Counseling following a perinatal death is now widely available and although the circumstances of the death and the prognosis for future pregnancies is normally discussed on this occasion, a further consultation should be offered before any subsequent pregnancy. Information given immediately following the perinatal death may be forgotten due to distress[24], or overlaid by misinformation from other sources. New investigations or interventions may come to light in the interval between pregnancies.

Provided the obstetrician has access to all available information concerning the perinatal death it should be possible to indicate whether the death was due to a recurrent or non-recurrent cause and to give some indication of the prognosis and the potential of currently available obstetric interventions to prevent a recurrence. In some cases, highly effective intervention is available to prevent a recurrence, for example, periconceptional folate for women who have previously given birth to a baby with a neural tube defect[25]. In other cases the prepregnancy consultation provides an opportunity for relaying information about the predictive value of antenatal tests for fetal abnormality. Counseling in the case of some fetal anomalies will require referral to a geneticist.

Women who have adverse but non-lethal obstetric outcomes may not receive the same standard of care as those who have perinatal deaths. Parents of very low-birthweight babies may fail to receive potentially valuable prepregnancy care. Liaison between obstetricians and pediatricians running follow-up clinics for survivors of neonatal intensive care may help to ensure that these parents have access to the advice of a perinatologist prior to conceiving again. All categories of low-birthweight are associated with a substantial recurrence risk. Although few effective interventions exist to prevent a recurrence of either prematurity[26] or intrauterine growth retardation, assessment in the non-pregnant state may help with the diagnosis of essential hypertension, antiphospholipid syndrome or cervical incompetence.

Women with puerperal psychiatric disease are another group who merit prepregnancy assessment, ideally by a psychiatrist with access to records relating to the previous event.

A rigorous attempt should be made to differentiate between puerperal psychosis and postnatal depression or 'unhappiness'[27] as the severity, recurrence risk and effectiveness of preventive interventions vary enormously.

A minority of women find events at the time of delivery, usually of their first baby, so traumatic that they are terrified of becoming pregnant again. Some experience 'flash-backs' characteristic of post-traumatic stress disorder. Prepregnancy care may be useful in some of these cases providing obstetricians with the opportunity to review and explain events surrounding the previous delivery and agree plans for the management of a future pregnancy[28]. In some cases referral to a psychiatrist may be necessary. General practitioners, midwives, psychiatrists and family planning clinics are all potential referral sources for such women.

PREPREGNANCY CARE FOR LOW-RISK WOMEN

RUBELLA SUSCEPTIBILITY

The effectiveness of offering prepregnancy care to women without specific medical or obstetric risk factors has not been evaluated. However, some of its components are of proven value. Screening for rubella susceptibility fulfils the criteria laid down for an effective screening program[29,30] if carried out before, rather than during pregnancy when effective intervention in the form of rubella immunization is possible. The incidence of rubella susceptibility will vary with the interval from childhood immunization, and the country of origin of the woman[31,32]. The author has in the past seen rubella immunization withheld from women because they were unable to guarantee contraception for three months following immunization. The risk of congenital rubella syndrome due to conception following immunization is thought to be negligible[33].

TOXOPLASMOSIS SCREENING

Babies born to women who acquire a primary *Toxoplasma* infection during pregnancy are at risk of congenital abnormality and because of this, women in some countries, notably France, are screened in pregnancy[34]. A recent working party set up by the Royal College of Obstetricians and Gynaecologists[35] examined the case for an antenatal screening program using the criteria for an effective screening program already mentioned[29,30]. The working party did not recommend the introduction of a prenatal screening program because of the low incidence of the disease in the UK, potentially giving rise to a high incidence of false-positive test results, and because of the fact that treatment has not been evaluated[36]. The question of prepregnancy screening for *Toxoplasma* susceptibility was not addressed. Unlike prepregnancy rubella screening, no immunization is available, so the only intervention that could be offered to susceptible individuals would be advice about avoiding sources of infection. As 80% of women in Britain are susceptible, an alternative option would be to advise all women planning pregnancy to avoid handling cats' litter and eating undercooked lamb. The main risks of such a policy would be the generation of excessive anxiety.

PERICONCEPTIONAL FOLATE

Two randomized controlled trials[20,37] indicate that folic acid 4 mg/day for three months before and three months after conception reduces the risk of recurrent neural tube defects in the infant of women who have had a previously affected pregnancy. The odds ratio for recurrence is 0.27 (95% confidence interval (CI) 0.11–0.64)[25]. The relative efficacy and safety of the 4 mg dose versus the 0.34 mg dose used in an observational study[38] has not been established. At present, the 4 mg dose should be prescribed to all women at high risk whenever there is any possibility of conception. There is now evidence from a randomized trial, that occurrent as well as recurrent neural tube defects can be prevented[19], in this case by supplementation with periconceptional multivitamins including 0.8 mg folic acid. In this trial, there was a significant reduction in the prevalence of neural tube defects in the study group (odds ratio 0.13; 95% CI 0.03–0.65). The prevalence in those in the control group was close to that expected from population surveillance data. The prevalence of all congenital malformations was significantly lower in the study group (odds ratio 0.51; 95% CI 0.35–0.76) but there were no differences in other specific malformations such as cleft lip and/or cleft palate[39]. Even before this trial was published prepregnancy low-dose folate was being urged for all women[40]. No consensus has been reached concerning the best strategy for supplying a regular dose of folic acid to women in the reproductive age group. Options include fortification of foods, dietary advice and the widespread promotion of over-the-counter preparations. Potential hazards of dietary fortification strategies include the theoretical risk of precipitating subacute combined degeneration of the cord in people with pernicious anemia]41]. Promoting periconceptional medication with over-the-counter vitamin preparations might, in theory, lead to an increase in intake of potentially teratogenic vitamin A[42]. Randomized trials of all these options are indicated. Pending such trials this author would favor advising women to take 0.8 mg of folic acid daily.

OTHER VITAMINS AND TRACE ELEMENTS

At present there is no evidence to support the use of any vitamins or trace elements other than folic acid prior to pregnancy[43,44]. Excessive intake of vitamin A, either in multivitamin preparations or through eating liver may be harmful[42]. Once again, strategies for disseminating this information need to be tested scientifically.

DIETARY INTERVENTIONS

Observational data indicate that women with a high body mass index have an increased risk of delivering a macrosomic baby and of undergoing operative delivery[45], whereas a low body mass index is associated with an increased risk of low-birthweight and perinatal death[46]. There is no evidence from randomized trials to indicate whether weight reduction in overweight women and weight increase in underweight women prior to conception improves obstetric outcome. The evidence derived from randomized trials of dietary interventions in the form of energy or protein restriction in overweight women and supplementation in nutritionally deprived women has been reviewed by Kramer[47–50]. These trials refer to dietary interventions during pregnancy; no trials of the effect on pregnancy outcomes of prepregnancy dietary interventions have been carried out.

Two trials of dietary restriction in women who were obese or gaining excessive weight during pregnancy[51,52] provide no evidence of a reduction in pre-eclampsia or pregnancy-induced hypertension. The effect on birthweight was small. The caesarean section rate was not reported.

Evidence from randomized trials suggests that balanced protein supplementation alone (i.e. without energy supplementation) is unlikely to be of benefit to pregnant women or their infants and may even impair fetal growth[48]. High protein supplementation of pregnant women is even less likely to be beneficial and may increase the risk of neonatal death[49]. The available evidence provides no justification for prescribing high-protein nutritional supplements to pregnant women. Not only do such supplements appear to lack beneficial effects, the evidence suggests that they may even be harmful. Balanced protein/energy supplementation results in modest increases in maternal weight gain and fetal growth. These increases do not appear larger in undernourished women, nor do they seem to confer long-term benefits to the child in terms of growth or neurocognitive development. The available evidence is inadequate to reach conclusions concerning effects on preterm birth, fetal and infant survival, or maternal health.

In the real world, undernourished women are more likely to be advised to eat more than to be given dietary supplements. The randomized trials of dietary advice in pregnancy were reviewed by Kramer[53]. Nutritional advice to pregnant women to increase their energy and protein intakes seems capable of achieving those goals to a modest degree, but any benefits to the health of the mother or her baby remain to be demonstrated and are unlikely to be of major importance.

In the absence of randomized trials of dietary intervention before pregnancy any extrapolation of evidence from the trials of dietary interventions in pregnancy backwards to the prepregnancy period is speculative. It is unlikely, given its unwanted effects in pregnancy, that high protein supplements in the prepregnancy period would confer any advantage. It may be that normalizing weight prior to conception will have important benefits on pregnancy outcome or it may be that these effects will be as modest as those achieved by nutritional interventions during pregnancy.

SMOKING

The increase in smoking among young women and the lower success rate among women attempting to stop smoking compared with men, make it the most common women's health problem[54]. There is robust observational evidence to suggest that smoking during pregnancy is associated with a mean birthweight deficit of 175–200 g[55] and an increase in the stillbirth rate due to intrauterine growth retardation and placental complications[56]. In the past, women who smoked in pregnancy were stridently advised to stop, a strategy that has fallen into disrepute as 'victim-blaming'[55] and on more scientific grounds, because randomized trials of advice to stop smoking showed only a small effect on smoking cessation rates (odds ratio for continued smoking 0.42; 95% CI 0.24–0.74[57]). Self-help behavioral strategies have been shown to be more effective (odds ratio for continued smoking 0.35; 95% CI 0.29–0.44[58]). Overall, interventions aimed at stopping smoking in pregnancy, if they are effective, will lead to a small increase in mean birthweight. However, no effect on the incidence of low birthweight, preterm birth or perinatal mortality has yet been demonstrated with confidence[59]. This may be because the interventions are relatively ineffective, because the pregnancy outcome in smokers relates to the smoker rather than her smoking[60,61], or because smoking needs to cease prior to pregnancy in order to abolish its ill-effects. Efforts to help women to stop smoking prior to pregnancy would seem to be a reasonable component of prepregnancy care. Based on the evidence already cited, this should consist of strategies other than just advice or counseling. Non-pregnant women are also able to benefit from nicotine transdermal patches that have been proven to help women stop smoking[62,63], although once again, the overall smoking cessation rates are low.

The medical, social and economic arguments in favor of women stopping smoking are strong, irrespective of their plans for pregnancy. Therefore, any contact between smokers and health care professionals should include the offer of effective assistance with smoking cessation. This approach may ultimately be a more effective method of reducing smoking in women than measures which reinforce the concept that giving up smoking is a sacrifice that women must make for their babies.

ALCOHOL

In the United States, all alcoholic beverages are labeled with a warning that consumption of alcohol during pregnancy may damage the unborn child. Many women abstain from alcohol completely while pregnant and some women do so during the second half of every menstrual cycle, while trying to conceive. Concern about the adverse effects of alcohol in pregnancy derive from reports of fetal anomalies and intrauterine growth retardation in heavy drinkers[64,65], an increased risk of second trimester miscarriage in women reporting drinking more than one alcoholic drink per day during pregnancy[66] and an increase in intrauterine growth retardation in those drinking more than 10 units of alcohol per week[67]. Despite the fact that there was no evidence to support advice to abstain from alcohol completely, this became a standard recommendation on both sides of the Atlantic[68,69] on the basis that a safe level of drinking had not been established[68]. However, a large population-based study of prospectively recorded alcohol intake and pregnancy outcome in Australia showed no adverse association below an intake of two standard drinks per day[70]. Compared with total abstinence, occasional social drinking was associated with a possible benefit in terms of birthweight. The consistency between this study and the other smaller studies quoted above make it unnecessary to prohibit alcohol completely. Advice to avoid binge drinking and to keep weekly intake below 10 units seems valid for all women, whether planning pregnancy or not. There is good evidence from randomized trials that alcohol intake can be assessed using questionnaires and that brief intervention in the form of information on excessive drinking can reduce alcohol consumption by 24% (95% CI 18–31)[71].

POTENTIAL ADVERSE EFFECTS OF PREPREGNANCY CARE

Due to the absence of formal studies, our assessment of the potential adverse effects of prepregnancy care is speculative and anecdotal. Excessive emphasis on prepregnancy care may create a public perception that adverse obstetric outcomes can be prevented, and that unplanned pregnancies are doomed. The author has been consulted by a conscientious schoolteacher considering termination of pregnancy because she had not abstained from alcohol during the first two weeks of an unplanned pregnancy. Women who fail to take folic acid or who continue to smoke may suffer from guilt and anxiety which may adversely affect the pregnancy. Women who have not had prepregnancy care may be placed by caregivers in the same 'second-class' category currently occupied by women who have uncertain dates, who book late or who continue to smoke. Self-help measures such as stopping smoking, moderating alcohol intake and normalizing weight may be seen only as temporary measures to be undertaken for pregnancy rather than incorporated into normal life style.

PREPREGNANCY CARE – WHO, WHERE, HOW?

There is no good evidence to support the view that formal prepregnancy care for all women should become the norm. Women in the reproductive age-group who have chronic medical conditions should be regularly invited by their general practitioners or specialist clinic staff to discuss plans for pregnancy. Both contraception and prepregnancy care should become a routine part of treatment. Every effort should be made by general practitioners, obstetricians, midwives and family planning clinics to identify women whose previous obstetric experience puts them at real or perceived risk of obstetric, genetic or psychological problems in a subsequent pregnancy. Prepregnancy referral can then be arranged to the most appropriate service for their needs.

For women in general, folic acid supplementation and ascertainment of rubella status are the only prepregnancy interventions of proven efficacy. National strategies should be tested by randomized trials to make both these interventions available on a widespread basis to women in the reproductive age-group in such a way that women whose pregnancies are unplanned have the same degree of protection as those who are planning to conceive. All women should be offered assistance to stop smoking at every contact with the health services. This should not be specifically linked with prepregnancy care. Measures to identify women whose alcohol intake is excessive and interventions to reduce it should also be incorporated into routine health care as should assistance for women whose body mass index is either above the 95th or below the 5th centile. These interventions should be offered by general practitioners on an opportunistic basis when women attend for family planning, cervical screening or for any other reason. All of these self-help, preventive medicine measures should be free to all women, regardless of their plans for pregnancy.

REFERENCES

1. Chamberlain, G. (1980) The prepregnancy clinic. *Br. Med. J.*, **281**, 29–30.
2. Foresight (no date) The association for preconceptual care. Guidelines for future parents. Surrey: Foresight pp. 5–42.
3. House of Commons (1980) Second report from the Social Services Committee. Session 1979–1980. *Perinatal and Neonatal Mortality*, vol. 1, p. 127.
4. Foresight Newsletter (1986) p.1.
5. Cox, M., Whittle, M., Byrne, A. *et al.* (1992) Prepregnancy counselling: experience from 1075 cases.
6. Steel, J.S., Johnstone, F.D., Hepburn, D.A. and Smith, A.F. (1990) Can prepregnancy care of diabetic women reduce the risk of abnormal babies. *Br. Med. J.*, **301**, 1070–4.
7. Hunter, D.S. (1987) Diabetes in pregnancy, in *Effective Care in Pregnancy and Childbirth* (eds I. Chalmers, M. Enkin and M.J.N.C. Keirse), Oxford University Press, Oxford, pp. 578–93.
8. Reid, M. and Garcia, J. (1987) Women's views of care during pregnancy and childbirth, in *Effective Care in Pregnancy and Childbirth* (eds I. Chalmers, M. Enkin and M.J.N.C. Keirse), Oxford University Press, Oxford, pp. 131–42.
9. Leslie, R.D.G., John, P.N., Pyke, D.A. and White,

J.M. (1978) Haemoglobin A1 in diabetic pregnancy. *Lancet*, **ii**, 958–9.

10. Miller, E., Hare, J.W., Cloherty, J.P. *et al.* (1981) Elevated maternal haemoglobin A1c in early pregnancy and major congenital anomalies in infants of diabetic mothers. *N. Engl. J. Med.*, **304**, 1351–4.

11. Damm, P. and Molstead-Pedersen, L. (1989) Significant decrease in congenital malformations in newborn infants of an unselected population of diabetic women. *Am. J. Obstet. Gynecol.*, **161**, 1163–7.

12. Kitzmiller, J.L., Gavin, L.A., Gin, G.D. *et al.* (1991) Preconception care of diabetic pregnancies: glycemic control prevents congenital anomalies. *JAMA*, **265**, 731–6.

13. Gregory, R., Scott, A.R., Mohajer, M. and Tattersall, R.B. (1992) Diabetic pregnancy 1977–1990; have we reached a plateau? *J.R. Coll. Phys. Lond.*, **26**, 162–6.

14. Tchobroutsky, C., Vray, M.M. and Altman, J.J. (1991) Risk/benefit ratio of changing late obstetrical strategies in the management of insulin-dependent diabetic pregnancies: a comparison between 1971–77 and 1978–85 periods in 389 pregnancies. *Diabete. Metab.*, **17**, 287–94.

15. Cullimore, J., Roland, J. and Turner, G. (1990) The management of diabetic pregnancy in a regional centre: a five year review. *J. Obstet. Gynaecol.*, **10**, 171–5.

16. Brodie, M.J. (1990) Management of epilepsy during pregnancy and lactation. *Lancet*, **336**, 426–7.

17. Nakane, Y., Okuma, T., Takahashi, R. *et al.* (1980) Multi-institutional study on the teratogenicity and fetal toxicity of antiepileptic drugs: a report of a collaborative study in Japan. *Epilepsia*, **21**, 663–80.

18. Editorial (1988) Valproate, spina bifida and birth defects. *Lancet*, **ii**, 1404–5.

19. Czeizel, A.E. and Dudas, I. (1992) Prevention of the first occurrence of neural tube defects by peri-conceptional vitamin supplementation. *N. Engl. J. Med.*, **327**, 1832–5.

20. MRC Vitamin Study Research Group (1991) Prevention of neural tube defects: results of the Medical Research Council Vitamin Study. *Lancet*, **338**, 131–7.

21. Weinstein, M.R. (1976) The international register of lithium babies. *Drug Information J.*, **2**, 94–100.

22. Chalmers, R. (1992) Retinoid therapy – a real hazard for the developing embryo. *Br. J. Obstet. Gynaecol.*, **99**, 276–8.

23. Magee, H. (1988) *Perinatal Statistics 1988*. The Stationery Office, Dublin, p. 27.

24. Forrest, G. (1987) Care of the bereaved after perinatal death, in *Effective Care in Pregnancy and Childbirth*, (eds I. Chalmers, M. Enkin and M.J.N.C. Keirse), Oxford University Press, Oxford, pp. 1423–32.

25. Lumley, J. (1994) Periconceptional folic acid vs placebo, in *Pregnancy and Childbirth Module* (eds M.W. Enkin, M.J.N.C. Keirse, M.J. Renfrew and J.P. Neilson), *Cochrane Database of Systematic Reviews:* Review No. 06488, 24 September 1993. Published through 'Cochrane Updates on Disk', Update Software, 1994, Oxford, Disk Issue 1.

26. Keirse, M.J.N.C., Grant, A. and King, J.F. (1987) Preterm labour, in *Effective Care in Pregnancy and Childbirth* (eds I. Chalmers, M. Enkin and M.J.N.C. Keirse), Oxford University Press, Oxford, pp. 694–745.

27. Romito, P. (1987) Unhappiness after childbirth, in *Effective Care in Pregnancy and Childbirth* (eds I. Chalmers, M. Enkin and M.J.N.C. Keirse), Oxford University Press, Oxford, pp. 1433–46.

28. Chamberlain, G. (1993) What is the correct caesarean section rate? *Br. J. Obstet. Gynaecol.*, **100**, 403–4.

29. Wilson, J.M.G. and Jungner, G. (1968) Principles and practice of screening for disease. *Public Health Paper, No. 34.* World Health Organisation, Geneva.

30. Cadman, D., Chambers, L.W., Feldman, W. and Sackett, D.L. (1984) Assessing the effectiveness of community screening programs. *JAMA*, **252**, 1580–5.

31. O'Shea, S., Best, J.M., Banatvala, J.E. *et al.* (1984) Persistence of rubella antibody 8–18 years after vaccination. *Br. Med. J.*, **288**, 1043.

32. Lawman, S., Morton, K. and Best, J.M. (1994) Reasons for rubella susceptibility among pregnant women in West Lambeth. *J.R. Soc. Med.*, **87**, 263.

33. Banatvala, J.E. (1985) Rubella – continuing problems. *Br. J. Obstet. Gynaecol.*, **85**, 8–11.

34. Desmonts, G., Daffos, F., Forrestier, F. *et al.* (1985) Prenatal diagnosis of congenital toxoplasmosis. *Lancet*, **i**, 500–4.

35. Peckham, C.S., Hall, S., Patel, N. *et al.* (1992) *Prenatal Screening for Toxoplasmosis in the UK: Report of a Multi-disciplinary Working Group*, Royal College of Obstetricians and Gynaecologists, Department of Health, London.

36. Peckham, C. and Logan, S. (1993) Screening for toxoplasmosis in pregnancy. *Arch. Dis. Child*, **68**, 3–5.

37. Laurence, K.M., James N., Miller, M.H. *et al.* (1981) Double blind randomised controlled trial of folate treatment before conception to prevent recurrence of neural tube defects. *Br. Med. J.*, **282**, 1509–11.

38. Smithells, R.W., Shephard, S., Schhorah, C.J. *et al.* (1980) Possible prevention of neural tube defects by peri-conceptional vitamin supplementation. *Lancet*, **i**, 339–40.

39. Lumley, J. (1994) Periconceptional multivitamins (incl folate 0.8 mg) vs placebo, in *Pregnancy and Childbirth Module* (eds M.W. Enkin, M.J.N.C. Keirse, M.J. Renfrew and J.P. Neilson), *Cochrane Database of Systematic Reviews*: Review No. 06490, 27 September 1993. Published through 'Cochrane Updates on Disk', Update Software, 1994, Oxford, Disk Issue 2.

40. Report from an Expert Advisory Group (1992) Folic acid and the prevention of neural tube defects. Department of Health, London.

41. Wald, N.J. and Bower, C. (1994) Folic acid, pernicious anaemia and prevention of neural tube defects. *Lancet*, **343**, 307.

42. Acheson, D. and Poole, A.B. (1990) *Vitamin A and Pregnancy*. Department of Health Circular PL/CMO(90)11, London.

43. Hytten, F.E. (1985) Do pregnant women need Zinc supplements? *Br. J. Obstet. Gynaecol.*, **92**, 873–4.

44. Mahomed, K. and Hytten, F. (1987) Iron and folate supplementation in pregnancy, in *Effective Care in Pregnancy and Childbirth* (eds I. Chalmers, M. Enkin and M.J.N.C. Keirse), Oxford University Press, Oxford, pp. 301–17.

45. Byrne, B. and Turner, M. (1994) The influence of maternal body mass index on the course of labour in nulliparas. *Int. J. Obstet. Gynecol.*, **46**(Suppl. 2), 150.

46. Cattanach, S., Morrison, J., Anderson, M.J. *et al.* (1993) Pregnancy hazards associated with low maternal body mass indices. *Aust. N.Z. Obstet. Gynaecol.*, **33**, 45–7.

47. Kramer, M.S. (1994) Energy/protein restriction in pregnant women with high weight-for-height or weight gain, in *Pregnancy and Childbirth Module* (eds M.W. Enkin, M.J.N.C. Keirse, M.J. Renfrew and J.P. Neilson), Cochrane Database of Systematic Reviews: Review no. 07139, 5 August 1993. Published through 'Cochrane Updates on Disk', Update Software, 1994, Oxford, Disk Issue 1.

48. Kramer, M.S. (1994) Isocaloric balanced protein supplementation in pregnancy, in *Pregnancy and Childbirth Module* (eds M.W. Enkin, M.J.N.C. Keirse, M.J. Renfrew and J.P. Neilson), Cochrane Database of Systematic Reviews: Review no. 07140, 5 August 1993. Published through 'Cochrane Updates on Disk', Update Software, 1994, Oxford, Disk Issue 1.

49. Kramer, M.S. (1994) High protein supplementation in pregnancy, in *Pregnancy and Childbirth Module* (eds M.W. Enkin, M.J.N.C. Keirse, M.J. Renfrew and J.P. Neilson), Cochrane Database of Systematic Reviews: Review no. 07142, 5 August 1993. Published through 'Cochrane Updates on Disk', Update Software, 1994, Oxford, Disk Issue 1.

50. Kramer, M.S. Balanced protein/energy supplementation in pregnancy, in *Pregnancy and Childbirth Module* (eds M.W. Enkin, M.J.N.C. Keirse, M.J. Renfrew and J.P. Neilson), Cochrane Database of Systematic Reviews: Review no. 07141, 17 September 1993. Published through 'Cochrane Updates on Disk', Update Software, 1994, Oxford, Disk Issue 1.

51. Campbell, D.M. and MacGillivray, I. (1975) The effect of a low calorie diet or a thiazide diuretic on the incidence of pre-eclampsia and on birthweight. *Br. J. Obstet. Gynaecol.*, **82**, 572–7.

52. Campbell, D.M. (1983) Dietary restriction in obesity and its effects on neonatal outcome, in *Nutrition in Pregnancy* (eds D.M. Campbell and M.D.G. Gillmer), Proceedings of 10th Study Group of the RCOG, RCOG, London, pp. 243–50.

53 Kramer, M.S. (1994) Nutritional advice in pregnancy, in *Pregnancy and Childbirth Module* (eds M.W. Enkin, M.J.N.C. Keirse, M.J. Renfrew and J.P. Neilson), Cochrane Database of Systematic Reviews: Review no. 07138, 5 August 1993. Published through 'Cochrane Updates on Disk', Update Software, 1994, Oxford, Disk Issue 1.

54. Fiore, M.C., Novotny, T.E., Pierce, J.P. *et al.* (1989) Trends in cigarette smoking in the United States. The changing influence of gender and race. *JAMA*, **261**, 70–4.

55. Lumley, J. (1989) Advice for pregnancy, in *Effective Care in Pregnancy and Childbirth* (eds I. Chalmers, M. Enkin and M.J.N.C. Keirse), Oxford University Press, Oxford, pp. 237–54.

56. Raymond, E.G., Cnattingus, S. and Kiely, J.L. (1994) Effects of maternal age, parity and smoking on the risk of stillbirth. *Br. J. Obstet. Gynaecol.*, **101**, 301–6.

57. Lumley, J. (1994) Advice as a strategy for reducing smoking in pregnancy, in *Pregnancy and*

Childbirth Module (eds M.W. Enkin, M.J.N.C. Keirse, M.J. Renfrew and J.P. Neilson), 'Cochrane Database of Systematic Reviews': Review no. 03394, 2 October 1993. Published through 'Cochrane Updates on Disk', Update Software, 1994, Oxford, Disk Issue 1.

58. Lumley, J. (1994) Behavioural strategies for reducing smoking in pregnancy, in *Pregnancy and Childbirth Module* (eds M.W. Enkin, M.J.N.C. Keirse, M.J. Renfrew and J.P. Neilson), Cochrane Database of Systematic Reviews: Review no. 03397, 27 September 1993. Published through 'Cochrane Updates on Disk', Update Software, 1994, Oxford, Disk Issue 1.

59. Lumley, J. (1994) Strategies for reducing smoking in pregnancy, in *Pregnancy and Childbirth Module* (eds M.W. Enkin, M.J.N.C. Keirse, M.J. Renfrew and J.P. Neilson), Cochrane Database of Systematic Reviews: Review no. 03312, 2 October 1993. Published through 'Cochrane Updates on Disk', Update Software, 1994, Oxford, Disk Issue 1.

60. Yerushalmy, J. (1971) The relationship of patients' cigarette smoking to outcome of pregnancy-implications as to the problems of inferring causation from observed associations. *Am. J. Epidemiol.*, **93**, 443–56.

61. Yerushalmy, J. (1972) Infants with low birthweight born before their mothers started to smoke cigarettes. *Am. J. Obstet. Gynecol.*, **112**, 277–84.

62. Imperial Cancer Research Fund General Practice Research Group (1993) Effectiveness of a nicotine patch in helping people stop smoking: results of a randomised trial in general practice. *Br. Med. J.*, **306**, 1304–8.

63. Russell, M.A., Stapleton, J.A., Feyerabend, C. *et al.* (1993) Targeting heavy smokers in general practice: randomised controlled trial of transdermal nicotine patches. *Br. Med. J.*, **306**, 1308–12.

64. Jones, K.L., Smith, D.W., Ullelaland, C.N. and Streissguth, S.P. (1973) Patterns of malformation in offspring of chronic alcoholic mothers. *Lancet*, **ii**, 1267–71.

65. Jones, K.L., Smith, D.W., Stressguth, S.P. and Myrianthopoulos, N.C. (1974) Outcome in offspring of chronic alcoholic women. *Lancet*, **i**, 1076–8.

66. Evans, D.R., Newcombe, R.G. and Campbell, H. (1979) Maternal smoking habits and congenital malformations. *Br. Med. J.*, **2**, 171–3.

67. Wright, J.L., Waterson, E.J., Barrison, I.J. *et al.* (1983) Alcohol consumption, pregnancy and low birthweight. *Lancet*, **i**, 663–5.

68. Little, R.E., Streissgith, A.P. and Guzinski, G.M. (1980) Prevention of fetal alcohol syndrome: a model program. *Alcohol. Clin. Exp. Res.*, **4**, 185–9.

69. Edwards, G. (1983) Alcohol and advice to the pregnant woman. *Br. Med. J.*, **286**, 247–8.

70. Lumley, J., Correy, J., Newman, N. and Curran, J. (1985) Cigarette smoking, alcohol consumption and fetal outcome in Tasmania, 1981–2. *Aust. N.Z. J. Obstet. Gynaecol.*, **25**, 33–40.

71. *Effective Health Care Bulletin* (1993) **7**.

J.A. Coulter

INTRODUCTION

The purpose of screening patients in early pregnancy is to identify those women who have risk factors present for possible adverse pregnancy outcomes as well as to try to detect asymptomatic conditions already prevalent. Thus, it is very much a prophylactic exercise. There are many investigations which are considered standard in early antenatal care and their inclusion is not controversial such as hemoglobin estimation, blood type, rhesus status and the presence of antibodies. Disorders which are not that prevalent in the community but which can have profound effects on the fetus are also screened for, such as rubella and syphilis. In recent years there has been increasing concern about the rising incidence of hepatitis B and C as well as human immunodeficiency virus (HIV) in the general community. There is currently much debate as to whether these viral diseases should be included in screening protocols in early pregnancy and, if so, whether they should be on a voluntary or mandatory basis. Many units have already begun screening patients deemed to be at high risk. However, there is evidence that screening based on risk factor reporting alone will miss a significant number of HIV and hepatitis B-positive women and may, therefore, induce a false sense of security[1].

Until recently, the pregnancy test has been associated with a qualitative positive or negative result based on the appearance of human chorionic gonadotrophin (hCG) in the urine. However, more knowledge about the rate of rise of serum hCG levels and the levels of progesterone has led to quantitative tests which have predictive value in determining the presence of an extrauterine pregnancy. There are also many studies ongoing to determine the value of using hCG in conjunction with other hormones such as serum progesterone as a predictor of pregnancy outcome.

The use of ultrasonography, both abdominally but more especially using a transvaginal probe, has markedly improved the knowledge and management of early pregnancy. As well as confirming an intrauterine pregnancy, assessment of gestational age is becoming more important when considering the advent of maternal antenatal screening programs based on accurate dating. As there is a trend towards first trimester diagnostic procedures, such as amniocentesis and chorionic villous biopsy, early ultrasonography becomes more clinically important.

Many of the screening tests used in the first half of pregnancy are inexpensive and widely accepted. However, others are associated with controversy because of widespread psychological and socioeconomic implications and are still being evaluated[2].

Clinical Management of Early Pregnancy. Edited by Walter Prendiville and James R. Scott.
Published in 1999 by Arnold, ISBN 0 340 74100 7

THE PREGNANCY TEST

The diagnosis of pregnancy has many psychological, emotional, physical and economic consequences for a woman and her partner. It is important that a rapid sensitive and specific test be available to confirm the presence or absence of a pregnancy. Most women resort to 'home' pregnancy tests but often express concern about their accuracy and differences. Indeed, inaccurate results may be due to poorly understood instructions or just poor technique. A recent study noted that the test performance was not affected by age, education or activity[3].

The fact that hCG is present in the urine in the first week after conception makes it an excellent marker for early pregnancy. Pregnancy test kits are now available that can detect hCG concentrations as low as 25 mIU/l in urine and can be used accurately before the woman has missed her period. These kits employ monoclonal or polyclonal antibodies sensitive to a particular membrane site on the hCG molecule in an enzyme-linked immunoassay. If hCG is present in the urine it will be bound by antibody-coated particles. These may be colored and, as the complexes move along the strip, they are in turn bound by immobilized antibody on the test line giving the positive result denoted by the particular color change. Some kits have the colored particles on the immobilized antibody. The enzyme-linked immunoassay method has superseded the use of the hemagglutination–inhibition technique as the latter required high levels of hCG for a positive result[4].

Most of the commercially available kits claim close to 100% sensitivity and specificity, if used correctly. A study by Hicks *et al.*[5] found that volunteers achieved an inaccurate result approximately 10% of the time compared to laboratory testing of the same samples. There are many reasons given for false negatives and positives but user error is the most common. Furthermore, many participants questioned during studies like these claim that they read the instructions carefully but some wording may not be clearly understood.

False positive results can occur if there has been a recent birth or miscarriage. Elevated luteinizing hormone (LH) levels can lead to a false positive result as can the use of certain medications including chlordiazepoxide, promethazine and methadone[6]. The modern pregnancy tests are less susceptible to this interference as they use monoclonal antibody immunoassays. False negative results usually result because of procedural error. The test may have been performed too soon after conception. If the urine is shaken or not allowed to return to room temperature after refrigeration the test may also be falsely negative. Carbamazepine use has been known to cause a false negative result.

Laboratory-based urine pregnancy testing also employs enzyme-linked immunoassay techniques for a straightforward positive or negative result. However, serum β-hCG levels can be quantified and, when used serially, may help to predict normal from abnormal pregnancies. For example, hCG levels double every 48 h[7]. If serial sampling reveals a rise of less than 66%, the pregnancy is likely to be ectopic if ultrasonography has been unhelpful[8].

Serum hCG levels may also be used in conjunction with other hormones, such as progesterone, to produce a pregnancy test with predictive value of outcome as well as the simple task of confirming pregnancy.

HEMATOLOGICAL INVESTIGATIONS

HEMOGLOBIN AND BLOOD GROUP

When a woman is seen at the antenatal clinic for her booking visit, there are certain investigations which are now 'routine' screening tests. There is no dispute as to the value of a booking hemoglobin. By the time many women have booked the intravascular blood volume and cardiac output have already increased by up to 50%. Because of this and the increased requirement for iron during the pregnancy, some women become anaemic in the ensuing months. It is important to have a baseline hemoglobin estimation. This will need to be repeated, if indicated, during the pregnancy. If patients have predisposing risk-factors for antepartum or postpartum hemorrhage, for example, it is obviously of paramount importance to keep their hemo-globin level adequate during pregnancy. If a patient requires emergency transfusion of blood products during pregnancy it is helpful to have prior knowledge of her blood group available in the case records.

RHESUS AND ANTIBODY DETERMINATION

Rhesus isoimmunization and hemolytic disease of the newborn have become uncom-mon problems in clinical practice in recent years. The perinatal mortality rate due to this disorder has also fallen dramatically[9]. This is mostly due to the introduction of anti-D in the late 1960s but also due to improvements in antenatal diagnosis and management, such as cordocentesis and intravascular transfusion. The finding of irregular antibodies has also decreased.

Although the administration of anti-D to rhesus-negative women at times of potential sensitization has had a huge impact on the dis-order, women still continue to develop anti-bodies. Approximately 1% of rhesus-negative women become sensitized during pregnancy. Silent sensitization is thought to account for up to 50% of cases[10], with therapeutic failures and failure to give anti-D making up most of the remainder. Because of the decline in anti-D-related problems, other blood group types are assuming a greater significance in clinical prac-tice such as anti-c and anti-kell antibodies which can be associated with hemolytic disease of the newborn.

The objectives of screening women in early pregnancy for rhesus group and irregular

antibodies have been recently reviewed in Britain[11]. The objectives are as follows:

1. To identify those pregnancies at risk of fetal and neonatal hemolytic disease;
2. To identify those rhesus-negative women who may require anti-D prophylaxis in the course of their pregnancy;
3. To facilitate the provision of appropriate blood for the mother in an emergency.

Thus, serological testing should be per-formed at the first visit, not only to ascertain the rhesus group, but also to detect any irregu-lar antibodies. It has been recommended that the antibody levels, in all patients, be checked again later in the pregnancy, usually between 28 and 36 weeks to look for a rising titer. In almost every maternity unit, rhesus-negative women are included in such a protocol. As to whether these women should be checked more frequently is still a matter for debate. Women who have had a previously affected baby form a special group and should be referred to a specialist center early in the preg-nancy.

URINARY INVESTIGATION

Screening of the urine is not routinely per-formed in all centers in early pregnancy. The basis for screening is to detect asymptomatic bacteriuria which can lead to upper or lower urinary tract infection during pregnancy.

Many anatomical and physiological changes combine to render the urinary tract more sus-ceptible to infection, especially in the second and third trimesters. Compression of the ureters at the pelvic brim due to the enlarging uterus and ovarian veins lead to mild hydroureter and hydronephrosis, this being more pronounced on the right side. The effect of progesterone is to decrease smooth muscle tone and peristalsis in the ureter and bladder. The pregnant woman tends to incompletely empty her bladder as pregnancy progresses. Increasing proteinuria and glycosuria as well as the changes mentioned above are known to facilitate the growth and delay the excretion of bacteria from the urinary tract.

Asymptomatic bacteriuria is defined as the presence of >100 000 colony-forming units per milliliter of urine in two consecutive midstream samples, in the absence of clinical infection. It is common in pregnancy, being present in approximately 6% of women (range 2–11%)[12]. Significant morbidity associated with asymptomatic bacteriuria has been described in pregnant women[13]. Between 30 and 40% of these women will develop pyelonephritis later in pregnancy if the asymptomatic bacteriuria is not adequately treated. There are many studies associating asymptomatic bacteriuria with preterm labor and intrauterine growth restriction but, also, there are many which fail to confirm the association[14]. There is no doubt that women developing clinical pyelonephritis are at increased risk of complications such as preterm labor, intrauterine growth retardation and, thus, perinatal mortality.

Based on our current knowledge, it seems appropriate to screen for asymptomatic bacteriuria in pregnancy. The most appropriate time would appear to be at the end of the first trimester or beginning of the second trimester. Culture of the urine is the most efficient screen. Patients should be treated according to sensitivities of the organisms whether there is pyuria or not. After treatment a repeat culture should be performed to ensure cure. Those patients requiring treatment should be screened again later in pregnancy as the infection is more likely to recur. The optimal frequency of screening is, as yet, undetermined.

CONGENITAL INFECTIONS

HUMAN IMMUNODEFICIENCY VIRUS

As the prevalence of HIV infection increases, health care providers in maternity units will encounter more and more pregnant seropositive women. Indeed, in the United States, the greatest increase in HIV infection has been among heterosexual women[15]. Anonymous surveys have measured seropositivity rates in areas of the UK between 1990 and 1992; in London the rate is 2.1 per 1000 and that outside London is 0.13 per 1000[16]. However, it is difficult to estimate the prevalence of infection in other communities in the absence of universal screening. Nevertheless, although the number of women who would be affected by a positive HIV result during screening in pregnancy is small, there are demonstrable benefits for both the woman and her baby.

When the results of the ACTG 076 trial were published in 1994, it became clear that the vertical transmission rate of HIV to the fetus would fall from 25% to 8% if prophylactic zidovudine therapy was given to the pregnant woman diagnosed as HIV positive[17]. Transmission to the fetus is dependent on maternal viral load. There is evidence to show that early aggressive treatment with nucleoside analogs and protease inhibitors substantially reduces viral load[18] and could further decrease transmission rates to the fetus. To date, however, many of these therapies have not been evaluated in pregnancy.

Based on these findings, it seems logical that screening of pregnant women in early pregnancy would have substantial benefits for both mother and, especially, the fetus. There is considerable debate as to the type of screening model that should be employed. This controversy is more related to the social and political rather than the medical implications of screening. Universal screening proponents claim that the healthcare benefits to the mother as well as the potential savings of caring for the increased number of infected babies outweigh the medical and sociopolitical costs. Opponents of mass screening suggest that there is considerable potential for (a) prejudice and discrimination against HIV-positive patients and (b) familial disharmony, loss of maternal employment and jeopardy of the mother/baby relationship.

Screening protocols based on patient-reported risk factors have been shown to exclude many seropositive women[19]. However, in many obstetric units it is the screening method of choice. This is probably due to a reluctance to establish a protocol and to leave the decision to screen to the discretion of the obstetrician.

Routine voluntary testing is a widely acceptable method of screening to both maternity health care providers and patients alike[20]. The concept is dependent on patient education and counseling and places the decision firmly with the pregnant woman and her partner. The hope is that if the woman understands vertical transmission of HIV and the risk to her baby then she will be more likely to accept screening. Routine voluntary screening of pregnant women is currently recommended by the American College of Obstetricians and Gynecologists[21] and the American Academy of Pediatrics[22].

Mandatory antenatal HIV screening has its advocates[23], but, overall, it has serious difficulties. It is likely that if mandatory screening was introduced universally, the number of women attending for antenatal care would drop significantly. Furthermore, screening centers would have a legal and moral obligation to counsel, treat, follow-up and provide social services for those pregnant women diagnosed as HIV positive. Many women would reject this lack of autonomy to decide for themselves and their babies that which may be in their best long-term interests.

Counseling of the woman before and after a screening HIV test is of paramount importance. It often falls to junior personnel in busy antenatal clinics, where neither the time nor the facilities are available, to comprehensively educate the woman to make an informed choice regarding screening. The ideal time is at the initial antenatal visit. To discuss the result the woman must be seen in person. If the result is negative, further education regarding future sexual practices and/or the use of drugs is possible. If the result is positive, the question of prophylactic medication as well as their responsibilities to family, friends and partner has to be discussed. The option of terminating the pregnancy also warrants consideration.

As well as the obvious benefits to the fetus of screening for HIV in early pregnancy, the opportunity to educate women as part of an antenatal screening program may help change public attitudes about sexual behavior and use of drugs, even when the test result is negative. However, health care providers must be ever vigilant of the negative social implications of a positive test result for a pregnant woman when considering an HIV screening program.

HEPATITIS B

The incidence of hepatitis B viral infection (HBV) has been rising in most countries worldwide despite a slight leveling out in industrialized countries due to a change in sexual practices, especially in homosexuals. Heterosexual spread of the virus continues to rise[24]. Although over 90% of adults who contract HBV infection recover and 10% go on to develop chronic sequelae of the disease, the opposite is true for neonates infected during pregnancy and childbirth. Thus, the benefit to the fetus of maternal screening can be overwhelming given that neonatal prophylaxis and immunization is effective in over 90% of cases[25]. Even though the prevalence of hepatitis B is known to be higher in Southeast Asians, Africans, intravenous drug users and those with multiple sexual partners, risk assessment (not unlike HIV) will fail to identify about half the carriers of the HBV surface antigen. Universal screening is currently recommended in the USA[26] but some argue that the current prevalence of neonatal disease in the UK (only two cases in children under one year in England and Wales in 1991) does not warrant such a program.

Nevertheless, if the benefit is mostly to the fetus, whose mortality risk would otherwise be high in the long term, then it would be relatively inexpensive to screen women at their first antenatal visit. With all of the controversy surrounding the screening for HIV, it would seem prudent to screen for HBV and receive a higher return on investment.

RUBELLA

First and early second trimester maternal infection with rubella is associated with a high risk of fetal transmission and congenital abnormality. Since the introduction of a vaccine in the USA in 1969, the incidence of rubella has dropped enormously. Now, over 99% of women booking for antenatal care are seropositive and the incidence of congenitally affected babies has dropped accordingly. During 1990 there were only seven cases reported in the UK and ten in the USA. However, there were only three cases reported in the USA in the previous 2 years[27]. There is concern that the incidence is rising due to the emergence of groups who are not availing themselves of immunization. Screening for asymptomatic infection in seronegative women is not considered worthwhile as the risk of congenital disease is very low and it appears to be confined to those with a rash. The main purpose of screening for rubella antibody in early pregnancy is to identify those women who are seronegative and, thus, will require immunization postnatally.

SYPHILIS

In Western Europe up to one in 2000 pregnancies are complicated by active syphilis. Congenital syphilis is rare but serious and largely preventable. In the USA the incidence of both the active and congenital forms has increased steadily since the mid 1980s[28]. Infection of the fetus can occur at any gestation, usually in the early stages of the disease (primary, secondary or early latent), and can lead to miscarriage, stillbirth, preterm labor, intrauterine growth restriction or congenital syphilis. The disease is treatable in pregnancy with penicillin and can lead to maternal cure in 98% of cases. Treatment will usually prevent congenital disease[29]. However, fetal damage already caused may be irreversible.

It is considered advisable and cost-effective to screen for syphilis in early pregnancy[30]. Screening tests are based on treponemal and non-treponemal antibody identification. Nontreponemal serology such as VDRL (Venereal Disease Research Laboratory) and RPR (Rapid Plasma Reagin) have sensitivities and specificities of approximately 60 and 75% and 84 and 99%, respectively. There are many causes of false positives. Thus, if the initial test is positive, a treponemal test such as TPHA (*Treponema pallidum* hemaglutination assay) is used to confirm the result.

Because primary infection late in the pregnancy may not be detected by current screening programs, it would be advisable to re-test high-risk women in the third trimester.

TOXOPLASMOSIS

Infection with *Toxoplasma gondii* is very often asymptomatic except in the immunocompromised adult or the fetus. Epidemiological evidence suggests that up to 50% of the world's population has been infected at some time, with serological evidence of infection in up to 90% in certain populations. Infection of the placenta is thought to lead to congenital infection of up to 50% of newborns. The rate of fetal infection rises with each trimester: 17% in the first compared to 63% in the third. Of the infected infants, the majority are asymptomatic at birth (75%) but about 15% are severely affected. There is some evidence that up to 40% of even the asymptomatic children may have some long-term learning difficulties or develop eye lesions.

Primary toxoplasmosis is usually acquired from ingesting uncooked meat containing cysts or exposure to cat feces containing oocysts. Prenatally, and in early pregnancy, women should be educated about the need to avoid inadequately cooked meats, gardening without gloves, handling cats' litter and to wash vegetables before use.

Certain countries already have screening programs in place, such as France and Austria, where seropositivity rates are high. Seroconversion and confirmation of infection allow decisions regarding treatment or termination of pregnancy to be made. The reported incidence of primary infection in pregnancy is about 2 per 1000 in the UK{31]. Based on a quoted infection rate in the fetus of up to 50% and the fact that about 15% are severely affected at birth, it is difficult to reconcile the fact that only approximately six cases of congenital infection are reported in the UK each year[32]. It now appears likely that fetal transmission rates have been overestimated as well as the clinical significance of fetal infection. A working party set up by the Royal College of Obstetricians and Gynaecologists[33] concluded that, at present, screening for toxoplasmosis should not be introduced in the UK.

ULTRASONOGRAPHY

The use of ultrasonography in early pregnancy is considered more comprehensively in Chapter 5. However, there are certain features that the basic ultrasonographic examination should demonstrate. The confirmation of an intrauterine pregnancy coupled with basic measurements of gestational age would be the commonest reported findings. However, evaluation of fetal number with possible chorionicity and amnionicity, localization of the placenta and examination of the adnexal structures are also practical and worthwhile. Transvaginal ultrasonography is becoming increasingly popular in clinical practice as experience with the technique grows. The improved resolution due to the higher frequency used and the closer proximity to the relevant organs has afforded ultrasonographers a greater diagnostic ability in early pregnancy.

The use of crown–rump length to estimate gestational age is most accurate when over 1.0 cm. If less than this, then gestational sac size is often quoted. Early pregnancy dating scans have tended to become the norm in clinical practice in recent years. They are important in establishing accurate dates in patients presenting for antenatal diagnostic tests, e.g. biochemical screening for fetal trisomy. Obstetric diagnostic interventions are now being performed in the late first trimester and early second trimester. Amniocentesis and chorionic villous biopsy are performed under ultrasound control. The measurement of fetal nuchal translucency between 9 and 11 weeks' gestation is becoming popular as one of the methods of screening for trisomy 21[34]. As the medical risks of termination of pregnancy are considerably higher as gestational age increases, earlier diagnostic screening tests like these that have become available quite recently offer considerable advantages to both patient and obstetrician.

BIOCHEMICAL SCREENING FOR TRISOMY 21

Down's syndrome is the commonest cause of severe mental retardation in school children. It occurs as a result of trisomy of chromosome 21, most often due to non-dysjunction before conception (95% of cases). The incidence of trisomy 21 (T21) is approximately 1.3 per 1000 births but there is a recognized association between risk of T21 and advancing maternal age. The risk of giving birth to a Down's syndrome baby is around 1/1000 at 30 years, 1/350 at 35 years and 1/100 at 40 years. Since the mid 1980s, when the association of low maternal alpha fetoprotein (AFP) levels with fetal trisomies was recognized[35], there has been considerable interest in the development of antenatal diagnostic screening programs in an effort to allow mothers to decide whether to continue the pregnancy or not.

More recent studies have identified the association of other fetoplacental markers with trisomic fetuses. As the Down's syndrome pregnancy is perceived as being less mature than normal, the fetal production of AFP and estriol are considered to be lower than expected and the placental production of hCG higher than expected. Risk of T21 based on maternal age alone was initially the basis of screening but, more recently, the biochemical parameters have become incorporated into a computerized screening test. Maternal age, serum hCG, estriol and serum AFP are incorporated in the 'triple test'. This is designed to determine a woman's risk of carrying a T21 fetus. It is carried out at approximately 16 weeks' gestation and the result is expressed as a probability ratio. Some authors dispute the relevant contribution of estriol to the screening test and claim that a 'dual test' is just as accurate as the 'triple test'[36]. Earlier screening programs used maternal age combined with AFP levels and improved the antenatal diagnosis to about 40%. More recently, the 'triple test' has been shown to identify about 60% of cases antenatally. The complex computerization is required as the different parameters at different gestational ages and maternal weight must be taken into account. The idea of expressing each parameter as a multiple of the median (MoM) has contributed to the ascribing of probability in the computer program.

Based on the probability result the decision to proceed with a more definitive diagnostic test is made. There has been much research into the 'optimal' cut-off level. Most centers have adopted 1:250 as the most cost-effective cut-off level[37]. Thereafter, the woman is offered a diagnostic karyotyping test – amniocentesis. As mentioned previously, the availability of ultrasonographic diagnosis of increased nuchal-fold thickness has meant that an earlier screening tool with a reported detection rate of 80% is now in clinical practice. Lower than expected levels of maternal AFP and hCG together are found in association with other chromosomal abnormalities such as trisomy 18 and triploidies.

The measurement of maternal serum AFP has another important screening implication – the detection of neural tube defects (NTD). As over 90% of babies with a NTD are born to couples without a previous family history, antenatal screening between 16 and 18 weeks has become cost-effective. Based on an initial calculation of ≥ 2.0 MoM (the cut-off varies in different centers), a repeat test is usually performed in conjunction with ultrasonography and a decision about amniocentesis made. A normal scan can eliminate over 95% of the maternal serum AFP-associated risk. However, approximately 10% of spinal defects are covered by skin and do not leak AFP and up to 15% of open neural tube defects may not be identified.

AMNIOCENTESIS

Amniocentesis is the procedure whereby fluid is withdrawn from the amniotic sac, for the culture of fetal cells or measurement of AFP levels. In early pregnancy the most common indication for amniocentesis is for fetal karyotyping, usually for genetic reasons. These indications include:

1. Maternal age;
2. Following a 'triple test';
3. A previous history of chromosomal anomaly;
4. A scan suggestive of structural abnormality;
5. Balanced translocation in either parent.

In later pregnancy, other indications include investigation of rhesus disease and assessment of fetal lung maturity (lecithin/sphingomyelin ratio). Amniocentesis is most commonly performed under direct ultrasound guidance. Thus, the operator can visualize the pool of liquor suitable for sampling, reducing the risk of fetal and placental injury. Up to relatively recently, amniocentesis was performed between 15 and 17 weeks' gestation. There are theoretical advantages to this timing. First, the maternal biochemical screening tests are usually advised at 16 weeks. Second, there is more liquor present at this later gestation, with better visualization of the needle, fetus, placenta and cord. Amniocentesis at approximately 16 weeks does, however, have a major drawback: fetal cell culture must be achieved before karyotyping can be performed. This can take up to 3 weeks in some centers. If termination of pregnancy is the decision, then the procedure has to be performed late in the second trimester.

Because of this, there has been a great deal of interest in performing amniocentesis at an earlier gestation. Adding to this innovation have been improvements in the technique of cell culture and karyotyping, so that in most centers results are available in 10 days. There are theoretical reservations to this 'early' amniocentesis. Is it as safe to the pregnancy and does it give as good a yield as the later amniocentesis?

The procedure-related fetal loss rate following amniocentesis at 15–17 weeks is quoted at approximately 1%, overall. Many studies have been performed to date comparing early (10–12 weeks) amniocentesis to mid-trimester (15–17 weeks). Most would seem to indicate that there is no significant difference in fetal loss and diagnostic yield rates[38,39]. However, there is conflicting evidence from the USA that early amniocentesis (11–14 weeks) significantly increases the fetal loss rate over mid-trimester amniocentesis (16–19 weeks) – 2.2% versus 0.2%[40]. Currently, there are many prospective randomized, controlled trials in progress that should help to answer this question.

CHORIONIC VILLOUS SAMPLING

Biopsy of the placenta provides trophoblastic tissue to the clinician for investigation. It can be performed transcervically at between 9 and 11 weeks' gestation and transabdominally throughout pregnancy. The technique involves introducing a narrow cannula into the placental site, preferably below the insertion of the cord and away from the placental edge. Suction is applied and the cannula is moved to and fro in order to shear off some trophoblastic tissue. The indications for chorionic villous sampling (CVS) are generally those for amniocentesis, i.e. karyotyping. However, the availability of actively growing placental tissue has

other advantages. Karyotyping may be performed by direct preparation with a result in 48 h. Cell culture can also be performed to back-up the analysis of minor chromosomal abnormalities as the number of mitoses in direct preparation is less, leading to less accurate results. Inherited inborn errors of metabolism can be detected by direct assay of the cultured chorionic villi. Also, conditions associated with abnormal genes can be detected by gene probing of the DNA of chorionic villi (an advantage over amniocentesis). However, AFP levels cannot be assessed by CVS. Mosaicism of the placenta may occur in up to 2% of cases. This can give rise to misleading diagnoses of trisomies – usually 2, 16 and 20. These trisomies, which are considered lethal to the fetus, do not seem to affect the placenta. Therefore, care must be taken in the interpretation of results.

Despite the advantages of CVS, the safety of the procedure has been questioned. At 9–11 weeks' gestation approximately 2% of pregnancies will miscarry once a viable fetus has been seen by ultrasonography. Chorionic villous biopsy is thought to increase this risk by up to another 2%. This compares to a 1% fetal loss rate with amniocentesis. However, there is recent evidence that CVS in experienced hands is not associated with higher risk than early amniocentesis[41].

CONCLUSION

In most countries screening investigations in early pregnancy are well accepted by patients and maternity health care workers. Even though the detection rate of asymptomatic disease in the mother is often quite low, the implications for the fetus can be overwhelming. The costs of such 'routine' antenatal tests may seem prohibitive but compare favorably to the potential costs to Health Authorities of caring for children affected by disorders that can be detected, and sometimes managed, antenatally. The majority of early pregnancy screening tests have been commonplace for quite some time. However, included more recently are a number of investigations that involve ethical considerations, e.g. HIV and hepatitis B. A positive result has long-term medical, social and psychological implications not just for the fetus but also for the mother.

As obstetric and pediatric expertise continues to improve, antenatal detection of fetal and maternal disorders has become an important part of antenatal care and prophylactic and therapeutic measures are increasingly becoming available in clinical practice.

REFERENCES

1. Wiznia, A.A., Crane, M., Lambert, G. *et al.* (1996) Zidovudine use to reduce perinatal HIV type I transmission in an urban medical center. *JAMA*, **275**, 1504–8.

2. Amstey, M.D. (1991) Politics of HIV testing. *Contemp Ob/Gyn*, **5**, 11.

3. Daviaud, J., Fournet, D., Ballongue, C. *et al.* (1993) Reliability and feasability of pregnancy home-use tests: laboratory validation and diagnostic evaluation by 638 volunteers. *Clin. Chem.*, **39**, 53–9.

4. Caoila, S. (1992) The pharmacist and the home-use pregnancy tests. *Am. Pharm.*, **32**, 57–60.

5. Hicks, J. and Iosefsohn, M. (1989) Reliability of home pregnancy-test kits in the hands of laypersons. *N. Engl. J. Med.*, **320**, 320–1.

6. Linhard, A. (1993) Evaluation of home pregnancy tests. *Ugeskr. Laeger.*, **155**, 1550–3.

7. Hamori, M., Stuckensen, J.A., Rumpf, D. *et al.* (1989) Early pregnancy wastage following late implantation of embryos after IVF-ET. *Hum. Reprod.*, **4**, 714–17.

8. Kadar, N., De Vore, G., Romero, R. *et al.* (1981) Discriminatory hCG zone: its use in the sonographic evaluation for ectopic pregnancy. *Obstet. Gynecol.*, **58**, 156–61.

9. CESDI (1995) *Confidential Enquiry into Stillbirths and Deaths in Infancy*. Department of Health, London.

10. Murphy, K.W. and Whitfield, C.R. (1994) Rhesus disease in this decade. *Contemp. Rev. Obstet. Gynaecol.*, **6**, 61–7.

11. British Committee for Standards in Haematology (1996) Guidelines for blood grouping and red cell antibody testing during pregnancy. *Transfusion Med.*, **6**, 71–4.

12. Sweet, R.L. (1977) Bacteruria and pyelonephritis during pregnancy. *Semin. Perinatol.*, **1**, 25–40.

13. Patterson, T.F. and Andriole, V.T. (1987) Bacteruria in pregnancy. *Infect. Dis. Clin. North. Am.*, **1**, 807–22.

14. Canadian Task Force on Periodic Health Care Examination (1994) Screening for asymptomatic bacteruria in pregnancy, in *The Canadian Guide to Clinical Preventative Health Care*, Canada Communication Group, Ottawa, pp. 100–7.

15. Centers for Disease Control (1996) Update: mortality attributable to HIV infection among persons aged 25–44 years – US, 1994. *MMWR*, **45**, 121–4.

16. Public Health Laboratory Service (1993) Unlinked anonymous monitoring of HIV prevalence in England and Wales, 1990–1992. *Commun. Dis. Rep.*, **3**, R1–11.

17. Connor, E.M., Sperling, R.S., Gelbar, R. *et al.* (1994) Reduction of maternal infant transmission of human immunodeficiency virus with zidovudine treatment. *N. Engl. J. Med.*, **331**, 1173–80.

18. Gulick, R.M., Mellors, J., Havlir, D. *et al.* (1996) Potent and sustained antiretroviral activity of indinavir (IDV), zidovudine (ZDV), and lamividine (3TC). *XIth International Conference on AIDS*, Vancouver, Canada, July 1996. Abstract Th.B 931.

19. Barbacci, M., Repke, J.T. and Chaisson, R.E. (1991) Routine prenatal screening for HIV infection. *Lancet*, **i**, 709–11.

20. Lindsay, M.K., Adefris, W., Paterson, H.B. *et al.* (1991) Determinants of acceptance of routine voluntary human immunodeficiency virus testing in an inner city prenatal population. *Obstet. Gynecol.*, **78**, 678–80.

21. The Committee on Obstetric Practice (1994) Zidovudine for the prevention of vertical transmission of human immunodeficiency virus. *ACOG Committee Opinion*, no. 148, December.

22. American Academy of Pediatrics Provisional Committee on Pediatric AIDS (1995) Prenatal human immunodeficiency virus testing. *Pediatrics*, **95**, 303.

23. Krasinski, K., Borkowsky, W., Beleenroth, D. *et al.* (1988) Failure of voluntary testing for HIV to identify infected parturient women in a high risk population. *N. Engl. J. Med.*, **318**, 185.

24. Alter, M.J., Coleman, P.J., Alexander, W.J. *et al.* (1989) Importance of heterosexual activity in the transmission of hepatitis B and non-A, non B hepatitis. *JAMA*, **262**, 1201–5.

25. Beasley, R.P., Hwang, L.Y., Lee, G.C. *et al.* (1983) Prevention of perinatally transmitted hepatitis B infections with hepatitis B immune globulin and hepatitis B vaccine. *Lancet*, **ii**, 1099–102.

26. Centers for Disease Control and Prevention (1995) US Public Health Service recommendation for human immunodeficiency virus counseling and voluntary testing for pregnant women. *MMWR*, **44**(RR-7), 1–12.

27. Centers for Disease Control (1991) Increase in rubella and congenital rubella syndrome – United States, 1988–1990. *MMWR*, **40**, 93–9.

28. Centers for Disease Control (1988) Syphilis and congenital syphilis – United States, 1985–1988. *MMWR*, **37**, 486–9.

29. Thompson, S.E. (1976) Treatment of syphilis in pregnancy. *J. Am. Venereal Dis. Assoc.*, **3**, 159–66.

30. Garland, S.M. and Kelly, V.N. (1989) Is antenatal screening for syphilis worthwhile? *Med. J. Aust.*, **151**, 368–72.

31. Ades, A.E. (1992) Methods for estimating the incidence of primary infection in pregnancy: a reappraisal of toxoplasmosis and cytomegalovirus data. *Epidemiol. Infect.*, **108**, 367–75.

32. Hall, S.M. (1990) Congenital toxoplasmosis. *Br. Med. J.*, **305**, 291–7.

33. Royal College of Obstetricians and Gynaecologists (1992) Prenatal screening for toxoplasmosis in the UK. Report of a multidisciplinary working group. RCOG, London.

34. Pandya, P.P., Goldberg, H., Nicolaides, K.H. *et al.* (1995) The implementation of first-trimester scanning at 10–13 weeks' gestation and the measurement of fetal nuchal translucency thickness in two maternity units. *Ultrasound Obstet. Gynecol.*, **5**, 20–5.

35. Merkatz, J.R., Nitowsky, H.M., Macri, J.N. *et al.* (1984) An association between low maternal serum alpha-fetoprotein and fetal chromosomal abnormalities. *Am. J. Obstet. Gynecol.*, **14**, 886–94.

36. Spencer, K., Coombes, E.J., Mallard, A.S. *et al.* (1992) Free beta human choriogonadotrophinin in Down's syndrome screening: a multicentre study of its role compared with other biochemical markers. *Ann. Clin. Biochem.*, **29**, 506–18.

37. Sheldon, T.A. and Simpson, J. (1991) Appraisal of a new scheme for prenatal screening for Down's syndrome. *Br. Med. J.*, **302**, 1133–6.

38. Johnson, J.M., Wilson, R.D., Winsor, E.J. *et al.* (1996) The early amniocentesis study: a randomised clinical trial of early amniocentesis versus midtrimester amniocentesis. *Fetal Diagn. Ther.*, **11**, 85–93.

39. Diaz Vega, M., De La Cueva, P., Leal, C. *et al.* (1996) Early amniocentesis at 10–12 weeks' gestation. *Prenat. Diagn.*, **16**, 307–12.

40. Brumfield, C.G., Lin, S., Conner, W. *et al.* (1996) Pregnancy outcome following genetic amniocentesis at 11–14 vs 16–19 weeks' gestation. *Obstet. Gynecol.*, **88**, 114–18.

41. Nikolaides, K.H., Brizot, M.L., Patel, F. *et al.* (1996) Comparison of chorionic villous sampling and early amniocentesis for karyotyping in 1,492 singleton pregnancies. *Fetal Diagn.. Ther.*, **11**, 9–15.

ISSUES RELATED TO MEDICATION: PRE-CONCEPTIONAL AND FIRST TRIMESTER

J.C. Jennings and L.P. Martinez

The use of prescription and over-the-counter medications during pregnancy is common. It is estimated that between 45 and 100% of women use at least one or more drugs during a pregnancy. Potential exposures include medications prescribed by a healthcare provider, non-prescription drug products, herbal remedies, nutritional supplements, substances of abuse, and commonly ingested beverages containing caffeine or alcohol. Few pregnancies progress to term without the use of at least one medication. The mean number of medications used in the US is approximately six. If vitamins and minerals are excluded, the average number of drugs used during a pregnancy decreases to about three to four with analgesics being the most commonly reported exposure. Other commonly used categories of drugs include cough/cold products, antacids, antihistamines/antinauseants, barbiturate sedatives, and antibiotics[1]. The proportion of women reporting use of either prescription or over-the-counter medications has been shown to be highest in the first trimester with a trend toward less use in the second and third trimesters[2]. Therefore, it is not uncommon for health care professionals to be asked to answer questions related to these issues. However, answering these questions can often pose difficulty due to limited availability of data. This chapter is designed to review the basic components of evaluating risks related to medication exposures during pregnancy.

Suggestions for evaluating risks and discussing issues related to medication exposures are addressed including obtaining medication histories, reviewing literature, summarizing evidence and counseling patients.

MEDICATION USE DURING PREGNANCY

When one considers medication use during pregnancy, often the initial concern is teratogenicity. A teratogen is defined as an agent external to the fetus's genome that induces structural malformations, growth deficiency and/or functional alterations during antenatal development[3]. It is usually difficult to prove causation and to identify an agent as a teratogen. The list of drugs known to be teratogens is relatively short (Table 3.1).

Drug exposure during pregnancy may produce the following teratogenic effects: structural abnormalities; pregnancy loss/fetal death; intrauterine growth retardation/low birthweight/small for gestational age; functional abnormalities. Other potential concerning effects include prematurity, premature rupture of membranes, and transient pharmacologic effects[3]. It is well known that there is a 3–4% risk with any pregnancy of having a child with a clinically significant structural defect (Holmes, personal communication). This background risk should be noted and included as an essential component of all patient education. This percentage includes all malformations due

Clinical Management of Early Pregnancy. Edited by Walter Prendiville and James R. Scott.
Published in 1999 by Arnold, ISBN 0 340 74100 7

Table 3.1 Known drug teratogens

Drug	Potential defect	Critical period	% Affected
Angiotensin converting enzyme inhibitors	Renal dysgenesis Oligohydramnios Skull ossification defects	Second to third trimester	Not established
Alcohol, chronic	Craniofacial dysmorphology CNS abnormalities Heart defects	<12 weeks	10–15
	Low birthweight Developmental delay	>24 weeks	
Aminopterin	Spontaneous abortion	<14 weeks	Not established
	Craniofacial dysmorphology Limb defects Craniosynostosis Neural tube defects	First trimester	
	Low birthweight	>20 weeks	
Androgens/ Norprogesterones	Masculinization of external female genitalia	>10 weeks	0.3
Carbamazepine	Spina bifida	<pc 30 days*	1
Carbimazole/ methimazole	Hypothyroidism Goiter		Not established
Cigarette smoking	Miscarriage	<20 weeks	Not established
	Low birthweight	>20 weeks	
Cocaine	Prune belly sequence Genitourinary abnormalities	Association questionable	Not established
	Abruptio placenta	Second to third trimester	
	Intracranial hemorrhage Premature labor/delivery	Third trimester	
Diethylstilbestrol	Uterine abnormalities Vaginal adenosis Vaginal adenocarcinoma Cervical ridges Male infertility	<12 weeks	
Etretinate	*See* isotretinoin		
Isotretinoin	Fetal death Hydrocephalus CNS defects Microtia/anotia Small or missing thymus Conotruncal heart defects Micrognathia	>15 pc days*	45–50
Lithium	Ebstein anomaly	<8 weeks	<1

Table 3.1 continued

Drug	Potential defect	Critical period	% Affected
Methotrexate	Craniosynostosis Underossified skull Craniofacial dysmorphology Limb defects	6–9 pc weeks	Not established
Penicillamine	Cutis laxa		Not established
Phenytoin	Craniofacial dysmorphology Hypoplastic phalanges/nails	First trimester	10–30
	Vitamin K deficiency with resultant hemorrhage	Second to third trimester	
Solvents, abuse (entire pregnancy)	SGA Developmental delay		Not established
Streptomycin	Hearing loss	Third trimester	Not established
Tetracycline	Stained teeth and bone	≥20 weeks	Not established
Thalidomide	Limb reduction defects Limb hypoplasia Ear anomalies	38–50 post-last menstrual period days	15–25
Thiouracil	Spontaneous abortion	First trimester	Not established
	Stillbirth	>20 weeks	
	Goiter		
Trimethadione	Developmental delay V-shaped eyebrows Low set ears Irregular teeth	First trimester	Not established
Valproic acid	Spina bifida	<30 pc days[*]	<1
	Craniofacial dysmorphology Preaxial defects	First trimester	
Warfarin	Nasal hypoplasia Stippled epiphyses	6–9 weeks	Not established
	CNS defects secondary to cerebral hemorrhage	>12 weeks	

[*]pc, post conceptual.
CNS, central nervous system; SGA, small for gestational age.

to any cause. Malformations may be genetic in origin or result from exposures to drugs, chemicals, maternal infections or maternal disease states. Thus, clearly drug use during pregnancy can be associated with increased risks to the fetus. A common misconception is that the majority of birth defects are caused by drug exposures. This frequently causes feelings of extreme guilt for mothers of infants born with defects since they assume that this is the result of something that they took during their pregnancy. However, drug exposures make up 5% or less of the causes of clinically significant congenital structural defects in humans (Table 3.2).

The outcome of a pregnancy following fetal

Table 3.2 Causes of clinically significant birth defects in humans

Etiology	Risk (%)
Mendelian disorders: single gene	20
Cystic fibrosis	
Achondroplasia	
Craniofacial syndromes	
Chromosomal disorders	10
Trisomies 13, 18, 21	
Turner syndrome	
Environmental causes	5
Infections	<1
Rubella	
Toxoplasmosis	
Cytomegalovirus	
Varicella	
Maternal states	2
Insulin-dependent diabetes mellitus	
Phenylketonuria	
Hyperthermia	
Radiation	<1
Drugs and chemicals	2
Unknown causes	65

Adapted from Maria Louisa Martinez-Frias and Lewis Holmes personal communications.

Table 3.3 Factors involved in determining teratogenicity

Dose and route of administration
Timing of exposure
Duration of exposure
Concurrent exposure to other agents
Species susceptibility
Maternal metabolism
Placental transport
Placental metabolism
Fetal metabolism
Clinical consistency

exposure to a drug or multiple drugs is difficult to predict and is influenced by many variables. The factors used in determining whether an agent causes malformations in humans are considered in Table 3.3. When evaluating the medical literature regarding the teratogenicity of a particular agent, these items should be considered.

DOSE

The dose influences the quantity of drug that is available to cross the placenta and the final drug concentration to which the fetus is exposed. This concentration is variable based on maternal serum concentrations. Each specific drug has its threshold dose above which fetal effects can occur and below which no effects are seen. The existence of a threshold dose for teratogenicity has been demonstrated repeatedly in animal models and more recently in humans. For example, administration of methotrexate once a week in doses for the management of rheumatoid arthritis or psoriasis has not been associated with fetal harm in humans. However, higher doses of methotrexate used for chemotherapy or to induce abortion have been shown to induce malformations[4].

Unfortunately, identifying the doses of a drug that were actually consumed in a studied population is difficult. Many published studies report the names of medications but are unable to include accurate doses due to their methods of obtaining data by retrospective review and patient report. The result is that studies often provide little, if any, information about doses taken by the study participants. It is also important to note that dose equivalence between species can only be determined based on pharmacokinetic studies and dose–response curves in humans and the species being studied. Therefore, animal data reported as milligram/kilogram doses are rough approximations of dose equivalence in humans[5].

ROUTE OF ADMINISTRATION

The means by which the pregnant woman is using the drug can have a significant impact on the amount of drug available in the maternal circulation to which the fetus could be exposed. Common routes of administration include oral, intravenous, subcutaneous, inhaled, intranasal, topical and transdermal. The product bioavailability can vary significantly depending on the drug and the route by which it is administered. If drugs of abuse are being injected, the risk to the fetus of possible maternal infections such as human immunodeficiency virus, hepatitis, and syphilis should be discussed.

Route of administration of a drug is not typically identified in published studies. This is particularly true for studies of antenatal substance abuse.

TIMING OF EXPOSURE

The timing of fetal exposure to a drug is possibly the most important factor in determining teratogenic risk. All teratogens exert specific influences on selected embryonic or fetal tissues or organ systems. However, malformations of a specific structure can usually only be produced during the critical period when the structure is undergoing tissue differentiation. Tissues or organ systems develop at limited times during gestation producing very narrow windows of time when defects can be induced. For instance, thalidomide, a sedative once used for hyperemesis gravidarum, primarily affects limb bud development[6]. Therefore, maternal use of thalidomide after the limbs have formed does not result in limb reductions.

Teratogenic effects are more often observed as syndromes or a variety of defects that correspond to fetal tissue or organ system development at the time of drug exposure. Since the major events of organogenesis occur in the first eight weeks of fetal development, it is during this period that the embryo is most vulnerable to teratogens that affect structural development. Although the first 14 days after conception is a period of low teratogenicity as embryonic cells have not yet started to differentiate; most drugs exert their main effects on structural development during the first trimester. First trimester exposures may result in more severe malformations since this is the critical period of tissue differentiation and organ system development. Drug exposures during the second and third trimesters may cause less severe physiologic deficits. However, caution should be exercised when administering certain drugs even late in pregnancy since they may place the health of the fetus at risk[7]. Those drugs that exert their main teratogenic effect on functional development, i.e. tobacco, alcohol, amphetamines, lithium, angiotensin converting enzyme inhibitors, are of more concern late in pregnancy.

To establish an association between a drug and a particular congenital defect, it is important to know that the drug was used at a time when that defect could have been induced. Unfortunately, studies purporting to show an association often do not determine the timing of the exposure in any more detail than to delineate the trimester of use. This can be a significant problem. In many situations, knowing only that an exposure occurred at some time during the first trimester can be of little help in determining if the exposure and outcome are linked. For example, if the outcome being investigated is a neural tube defect, the timing of the exposure is crucial since neural tube defects can only be induced during the first 28 days after conception[7].

DURATION OF EXPOSURE

Since functional as well as structural development of the fetus can be affected by some drugs, the duration of an exposure can have a significant impact. Smoking more than ten cigarettes each day can affect the growth of the fetus if the smoking continues beyond the twentieth week of gestation[8]. Alcohol can affect functional brain development and thus daily consumption of alcohol that continues beyond 24 weeks in the pregnancy is associated with developmental and learning disorders[9].

The total amount of time that a fetus is exposed to a drug and its metabolites can be more significant than the drug's rate of placental transfer. The concentration of drug to which the fetus is exposed has the potential to be higher depending on the length of therapy and maternal serum concentrations. Therefore, chronic medication use may present a higher risk of teratogenicity than single dose therapy[10].

CONCURRENT EXPOSURE TO OTHER AGENTS

It is vital to know whether a reported association between a drug and a particular pregnancy outcome is related to the drug itself or to some other collateral exposure. Multiple drug exposures during pregnancy as well as maternal states add confounding factors making it difficult to detect a sole causative agent. There is also concern of additive effects (Table 3.4). The severity of a maternal state may influence pregnancy outcome and also may be noted by the number of drugs required to control the condition. For example, it is difficult to sort out whether certain malformations such as oral clefts and minor ventral septal heart defects are associated with anticonvulsant medications, the seizure disorder for which the prescription is used, or some familial/genetic predisposition[11].

Table 3.4 Maternal states known to increase teratogenic risk

Cytomegalovirus
Diabetes mellitus
Herpes
Hypertension
Hyperthermia
Hypo/hyperthyroidism
Lymphocytic chorionic meningitis
Parvovirus
Phenylketonuria
Rubella
Seizure disorder
Syphilis
Systemic lupus erythematosus
Toxoplasmosis
Varicella
Venezuelan equine encephalitis

Early studies of caffeine implicated the consumption of more than six cups of coffee a day during pregnancy with low birthweight babies[12]. However, it was soon discovered that pregnant women who were ingesting large quantities of coffee were also smoking more than 20 cigarettes (one pack) per day. When the non-smokers who drank more than six cups of coffee daily were analyzed, no effect on birthweight was observed[13,14]. This demonstrates the importance of identifying potential confounding factors.

SPECIES SUSCEPTIBILITY

Studies of pregnancy outcomes in animals are not predictive of human outcomes since teratogenic agents tend to demonstrate species specific effects. Genetic variability among species produces differences in drug absorption, distribution and metabolism. It is problematic to extrapolate animal data to humans since pharmacokinetic profiles vary depending on the drug and the species. Other differences are seen due to the animals' ability to carry multiple fetuses and variations in placental development and function. This can account for the variations in teratogenic effects observed between animal models and humans[5]. Animal models are useful in detecting the mechanism(s) by which known teratogens exert their influence, but are not beneficial in determining which drugs may be teratogenic in humans[3].

OTHER FACTORS

The dose of the drug that truly reaches the fetus is influenced by maternal absorption, distribution and metabolism, placental transfer and the ability of the fetus to metabolize or eliminate the drug and its metabolites. Substances most commonly cross the placenta by simple diffusion. Factors that influence transfer of drugs across the placenta include lipid solubility (lipophilic drugs diffuse more readily), molecular size (drugs with MW <

1000 cross easily), plasma protein binding (only free unbound drugs can cross) and pH and degree of ionization (unionized drugs cross more easily)[10]. Most medications cross the placenta to some extent based on these factors. For many years it was assumed that the placenta acted as a barrier, preventing exogenous agents access to the developing embryo and fetus. With the rubella and thalidomide tragedies, it became apparent that this was not so. Then came the era when the placenta was seen as a sieve that allowed everything to reach the fetus. It is now known that the placenta also metabolizes many drugs and other exogenous agents which decreases placental transport. This understanding of the placenta as more than a barrier or sieve is leading to ground-breaking work in teratology[15]. The drug concentrations to which the fetus is exposed have the potential to be higher depending on the length of therapy and maternal serum concentrations. These two elements determine if the threshold for teratogenic potential is reached. Thus, placental transfer of a medication does not solely imply teratogenicity. The ability of the fetus to metabolize or eliminate a drug or its metabolites is not fully developed until days to weeks after birth. Therefore, fetal accumulation of the drug may lengthen the actual exposure time beyond just the days on which the mother ingests an agent. Although it has not yet been demonstrated in humans, fetal ability to metabolize drugs may be a reason for the variability of teratogenic insult observed from one antenatally exposed individual to another.

CLINICAL CONSISTENCY

Most of the identified human teratogens show patterns of abnormalities presenting as syndromes rather than isolated or non-specific single defects. These patterns that are statistically rare events have been the hallmark by which teratogens have been 'discovered'. Two examples can illustrate this point.

First, isotretinoin, a vitamin A congener used to treat severe cystic acne, was marketed in the United States beginning in 1982. Within three years of its release, a report of three cases appeared in the medical literature[16]. The infants exposed antenatally who were described in these reports all had malformations that were rare even when isolated, i.e. anotia, microtia, conotruncal heart defects, but in combination were extremely rare. It was possible based on just three reports to begin to suspect that isotretinoin was a human teratogen. This suspicion has since been established.

Second, during the 1960s through the late 1970s the antinausea product Bendectin®, (doxylamine, dicyclomine, pyridoxine combination), was used by approximately one-third of all pregnant women. Case reports of malformations among children exposed to Bendectin® *in utero* became very common in the literature. Yet, the cases reported demonstrated no pattern of defects and epidemiologic analyses found the rate of malformations in the exposed groups to be no higher than the expected rate of 4% (the background risk for malformations referred to earlier[17]. This clearly demonstrated the lack of teratogenicity of the product.

Therefore, the degree of certainty of cause depends on the rarity of the exposure and the distinctiveness of the outcome. A pattern of multiple defects, i.e. a syndrome, adds weight to the theory of cause because as the effect becomes more specific or unique coincidence becomes less likely[18].

Because these factors can vary from species to species and from woman to woman, teratogenicity is difficult to predict based on data from animal studies or case reports alone. Only a few drugs are considered definitely hazardous (Table 3.1), although most medications have an unknown teratogenic potential in humans. Therefore, commonly used drug references are frequently not helpful in guiding the choice of therapy during pregnancy. Statements such as 'safety for use in pregnancy has not been established' complicate therapeutic decisions. The obvious conclusion is that all medications should be used with caution during pregnancy and given only at minimum effective doses and for the shortest duration necessary when there is a legitimate need and a specific indication for the drug. Yet, it is not reasonable to expect that this can always be achieved in practice. In clinical practice it is useful to place medications into three categories based on studies, case reports, chemical properties of the drug, and the woman's therapeutic need: drugs with known adverse effects, drugs with suspected adverse effects and drugs without known adverse effects at customary doses.

OBTAINING A MEDICATION HISTORY

The first step toward assessing teratogenic risk is taking a detailed medication history. When performing a medication history one should consider all of the factors that may influence teratogenic risk. The history should consist of the date of the last menstrual period, gestational age at the time of the exposure, all drug exposures including prescription and nonprescription products, dosage and route of administration, length of the exposure, any maternal states that may alter drug clearance or pose teratogenic risk and the indication for the medication use.

The date of the last menstrual period is used to estimate the gestational age at the time of the drug exposure. This and the length of the exposure are used to determine if the use was during a critical period. All aspects of the drug use including names of prescription and nonprescription medications, potential occupational exposures, substance of abuse, dosages, routes of administration, and start and stop dates should be documented. Also, any maternal states that may alter drug clearance, i.e. renal or hepatic disease, or pose a teratogenic risk should be noted. The indication for the drug use and its importance to the patient should be ascertained to decide if it is essential. It is important to note the indication for use of any medication since some infections

and disease states can adversely affect the developing fetus (Table 3.4). In addition, agents used to treat disease states that pose a risk to the mother or fetus if left untreated should be viewed differently from those used for non-essential reasons.

One study demonstrated that typical methods of drug history documentation by physicians caring for pregnant patients identified only 30% of actual drug exposures to the fetus. These authors concluded that the antenatal medical record is a poor source of information regarding actual drug exposures in the preconceptional period and during early pregnancy and that the usual methods of collecting medication histories are unacceptable[19].

REVIEWING LITERATURE AND SUMMARIZING EVIDENCE

Review of the available literature begins with identifying reference materials and information services that can be utilized. Sources of information on the potential effects of drug use during pregnancy incorporate the use of books, journals, computer references, product labeling, and teratogen information services.

Reference books and computer databases can be used as initial steps to acquire references, but it is important to look at the primary sources and evaluate the data before making a final conclusive statement regarding the agent's use during pregnancy. Journals supply data as case reports, studies and review articles. Careful interpretation of data is required when utilizing studies or case reports to identify human teratogens. One should closely evaluate the quality of the data to avoid making decisions or recommendations based on poor data. Data may be considered poor if they are published in an obscure journal, or poorly peer reviewed, if the outcome is nonspecific, if there is poor documentation of data, or if the results have never been duplicated. There is the potential for several types of bias in this type of literature. A bias toward publication of reports showing associations between congenital anomalies and drugs, as opposed to those finding no associations; recall bias for drug names, dose and timing of exposure especially with retrospective patient interviews; and the tendency for a mother who gives birth to a child with a structural defect to attribute the defect to an exposure or event during her pregnancy should all be considered[1]. Thus, it is important to examine all sources of data critically.

A problem exists with the sole use of product labeling to assess teratogenic risk. Manufacturers' product labeling utilizes the United States Food and Drug Administration (FDA) Use-in-pregnancy Ratings or 'pregnancy categories'. The FDA rating (A, B, C, D, X) system is 'based on the degree to which available information has ruled out risk to the fetus, balanced against the drug's potential benefits to the patient'[20]. The ratings combine several risk statements into a single assessment intended to provide both maternal and fetal risk information. Therefore, 'pregnancy categories' do not necessarily correlate with actual teratogenic risk. A published comparison of the FDA ratings to risk ratings developed by 'a consensus of expert opinion' showed that correlation between the two rating systems was no greater than that expected by chance. Due to this incongruity, the authors suggest that the FDA ratings should not be used to provide counseling regarding potential teratogenic effects to pregnant women who have already taken a medication. It is recommended that when assessing only teratogenic risk, counseling should be based on a more comprehensive literature evaluation and does not necessarily need to consider the therapeutic benefit of the drug[21]. An additional problem is that as more information becomes available about a particular drug, changes are not usually made in the FDA Use-in-pregnancy Ratings, i.e. hormonal agents, benzodiazepines.

Another source for teratogenic evaluations of drugs is the Teratology or Teratogen Information Service (TIS). The main function of teratogen information services is to provide information and consultation to health professionals and the public regarding concerns about drug, chemical, or environmental exposure during pregnancy. There are many such services in the United States, Canada and Europe. Most of these programs are operated by genetics or perinatal units and utilize dysmorphologists, pharmacologists, obstetricians, industrial medicine specialists, epidemiologists and others specializing in clinical teratology risk assessments. To identify the nearest TIS, the Pregnancy RiskLine in Salt Lake City, Utah may be contacted at (801) 328-2229.

When reviewing the available information for a particular drug, the focus should remain on human data. It is often difficult to gather enough data in humans to provide a clear answer. However, findings from animal studies are not necessarily applicable to humans. It is important to understand that teratogenicity in animals does not always indicate teratogenicity in humans. Therefore, one should never use animal data as an ultimate answer and should not counsel a patient that a drug is a cause of birth defects based on animal data alone.

COUNSELING PATIENTS

Patient counseling regarding drug use during pregnancy can range from basic and simple for those agents which are known to be safe to extremely complex for medications suspected of being or known to be teratogens. When counseling a patient about the risk of medication exposure during pregnancy, the basic approach should address the 3–4% background risk of congenital malformations, the risk versus benefit of the medication used including both maternal and fetal issues, and notification of the pediatrician of the medication exposure. However, the most important point of patient counseling is to avoid unnecessarily alarming the patient. Since most of the questions regarding pregnancy exposures are raised by patients after the exposure has occurred[22], the potential for heightened anxiety to be produced by speculation from animal data, FDA categories, or case reports is certainly real. If uncertainty arises when addressing the issue, the patient should be referred to other appropriate resources for information, such as a teratogen information service.

As mentioned previously, drug exposures early in pregnancy may result in a higher potential for structural teratogenicity since this is the critical period of tissue differentiation and organ system development. Because many women are not yet aware that they are pregnant for much of this critical period, preconceptional counseling becomes very important for women during their reproductive years. This counseling should not be limited to only those planning a pregnancy, but should be extended to all women since more than 50% of pregnancies in the United States are not planned[23]. Multiple common drugs and medical illnesses can adversely affect fetal outcome. The importance of discussing the possibility of pregnancy with women who require management of medical conditions has been recognized. Often, the correction or improvement of the condition before conception can improve maternal health during pregnancy and result in a more positive fetal outcome. For example, strict periconceptional control of conditions such as diabetes mellitus and phenylketonuria improves pregnancy outcome[24,25]. Many women are so concerned that their medications may pose a teratogenic risk that they stop taking drugs that may instead increase the likelihood of fetal well-being. For instance, women with systemic lupus erythematosus who discontinue their medications may put their embryo/fetus at an increased risk for congenital heart block due to the high maternal levels of circulating lupus anticoagulant that they subsequently produce[26].

Preconceptional counseling also affords the opportunity for medications to be changed from those that carry teratogenic potential to those that do not, or at least, have less potential to cause fetal harm. It is generally thought that the best medication for a particular woman planning a pregnancy is that drug which best controls her condition, since a strong predictor of pregnancy outcome is maternal health.

The preconceptional evaluation should identify behavioral, psychosocial, genetic and medical conditions that may place the woman or fetus at risk. By addressing the problems before pregnancy, this allows the opportunity to intervene and lessen or eliminate the potential risk[27].

Counseling should always be client-centered. It is important to know the patient's concerns in order to better educate and allay anxieties. Initially assess the patient's knowledge, understanding, and area of concern by asking what they have already heard about the drug. For example, if the patient has heard that oral contraceptives cause heart or limb defects, it will probably not be acceptable to say, 'birth control pills do not cause birth defects'. Addressing what she has already heard and why what you are telling her is different will provide her with much better information upon which to base decisions regarding her pregnancy. This information may influence choices for a woman such as whether to continue a pregnancy, consent to appropriate antenatal diagnostic testing, and select an obstetrician, perinatologist, family practitioner or nurse midwife for antenatal care.

REFERENCES

1. Schardein, J.L. (1993) *Chemically Induced Birth Defects*, 2nd edn, Marcel Dekker, New York.
2. Rubin, J.D., Ferencz, C., Loffredo, C. *et al.* (1993) Use of prescription and non-prescription drugs in pregnancy. *J. Clin. Epidemiol.*, **46**, 581–9.
3. Wilson, J.G. and Fraser, F.C. (1978) *Handbook of Teratology*. Plenum Press, New York.
4. Feldkamp, M. and Carey, J.C. (1993) Clinical teratology counseling and consultation case report: low dose methotrexate exposure in the early weeks of pregnancy. *Teratology*, **47**, 533–9.

5. Brent, R.L. and Beckman, D.A. (1990) Environmental teratogens. *Bull. NY Acad. Med.*, **66**, 123–63.

6. Lenz, W.D. and Knapp, K. (1962) Die Thalidomid-Embryopathie. *Dtsch. Med. Wochenschr.*, **87**, 1232–42.

7. Warkany, J. (1986) Hyperthermia, in *Teratogen Update: Environmentally Induced Birth Defect Risks* (eds J.L. Sever and R.L. Brent), Alan R. Liss, New York, pp. 181–7.

8. Werler, M.M., Pober, B.R. and Holmes, L.B. Smoking and pregnancy. *Teratology*, **32**, 473–81.

9. Coles, C. (1994) Critical periods for prenatal alcohol exposure: evidence from animal and human studies. *Alcohol Health Res. World*, **18**, 22–9.

10. Livezey, G.T. and Rayburn, W.F. (1992) Principles of perinatal pharmacology, in *Drug Therapy in Obstetrics and Gynecology*, 3rd edn (eds W.F. Rayburn and F.P. Zuspan), Mosby Year Book, St Louis, MO, pp. 3–12.

11. Kelly, T.E. (1984) Teratogenicity of anticonvulsant drugs. I. Review of the literature. *Am. J. Med. Genet.*, **19**, 413–34.

12. Furuhashi, N., Sato, S., Suzuki, M. *et al.* (1985) Effects of caffeine ingestion during pregnancy. *Gynecol. Obstet. Invest.*, **19**, 187–91.

13. Barr, H.M., Streissguth, A.P., Martin, D.C. and Herman, C.S. (1984) Infant size at 8 months of age; relationship to maternal use of alcohol, nicotine, and caffeine during pregnancy. *Pediatrics*, **74**, 336–41.

14. Mills, J.L., Holmes, L.B., Aarons, J.H. *et al.* (1993) Moderate caffeine use and the risk of spontaneous abortion and intrauterine growth retardation. *JAMA*, **269**, 593–7.

15. Koren, G., Klein, J. and Graham, K. (1994) Biological markers of intrauterine exposure to cocaine and cigarette smoking, in *Maternal–Fetal Toxicology. A Clinician's Guide*, 2nd edn (ed. G. Koren), Marcel Dekker, New York, p. 388.

16. Birth defects caused by isotretinoin – New Jersey. (1988) *MMWR*, **37**(11), 171–7.

17. Shiono, P.H. and Klebanoff, M.A. (1989) Bendectin and human congenital malformations. *Teratology*, **40**, 151–5.

18. Brent, R.L. (1986) Methods of evaluating the alleged teratogenicity of environmental agents, in *Teratogen Update: Environmentally Induced Birth Defect Risks* (eds J.L. Sever and R.L. Brent), Alan R. Liss, New York, pp. 199–201.

19. Bodendorfer, T.W., Briggs, G.G. and Gunnings, J.E. (1979) Obtaining drug exposure histories during pregnancy. *Am. J. Obstet. Gynecol.*, **135**, 490–4.

20. *Physicians' Desk Reference* (1995) Medical Economics, Inc., New Jersey.

21. Friedman, J.M., Little, B.B., Brent, R.L. *et al.* (1990) Potential human teratogenicity of frequently prescribed drugs. *Obstet. Gynecol.*, **75**, 594–9.

22. Koren, G., Bologna, M., Long, D. *et al.* (1989) Perception of teratogenic risk by pregnant women exposed to drugs and chemicals during the first trimester. *Am. J. Obstet. Gynecol.*, **160**, 1190–4.

23. Jones, E.F., Forrest, J.D., Henshaw, S.K. *et al.* (1988) Unintended pregnancy, contraceptive practice and family planning services in developed countries. *Fam. Plann. Perspect.*, **20**, 53–67.

24. Willhoite, M.B., Bennert, H.W., Palomaki, G.E. *et al.* (1993) The impact of preconception counseling on pregnancy outcomes. *Diabetes Care*, **16**, 450–5.

25. Platt, L.D., Koch, R., Azen, C. *et al.* (1992) Maternal phenylketonuria collaborative study, obstetric aspects and outcome: the first 6 years. *Am. J. Obstet. Gynecol.*, **166**, 1150–62.

26. Scott, J.S., Maddison, P.J., Taylor, P.V. *et al.* (1983) Connective tissue disease, antibodies to ribonucleoprotein, and congenital heart block. *N. Engl. J. Med.*, **309**, 209.

27. Kuller, J.A. (1994) Preconceptional counseling and intervention. *Arch. Intern. Med.*, **154**, 2273–80.

FURTHER READING

Briggs, G.G., Freeman, R.K. and Yaffe, S.J. (eds) (1994) *Drugs in Pregnancy and Lactation*, Williams and Wilkins, Baltimore.

Friedman, J.M. and Polifka, J.E. (eds) (1994) *Teratogenic Effects of Drugs: A Resource for Clinicians (TERIS)*, Johns Hopkins University Press, Baltimore.

Koren, G. (ed.) (1994) *Maternal–Fetal Toxicology: A Clinician's Guide*. Marcel Dekker, New York.

Remington, J.S. and Klein, J.O. (eds) (1990) *Infectious Disease of the Fetus and Newborn Infant*, Saunders, Philadelphia.

Institute of Medicine (1996) *Fetal Alcohol Syndrome: Diagnosis Epidemiology, Prevention and Treatment*, National Academy Press, Washington, DC.

EMBRYOLOGY AND PATHOLOGY OF SUCCESSFUL AND FAILED PREGNANCY

C.M. Craven and K. Ward

INTRODUCTION

Outstanding advances are occurring in our understanding of early human development and the pathophysiology of early pregnancy loss. In an increasing number of cases, an etiology of the pregnancy loss can be determined by the gross and microscopic examination, karotype and molecular genetic investigation. The careful documentation of normal and abnormal findings are valuable to those who care for and counsel patients with pregnancy loss. This chapter defines and discusses successful and failed pregnancy and makes recommendations for the pathologist's examination.

DEFINITIONS

Definitions direct our thoughts. In pregnancy failure, the terminology used aids in understanding of the etiology of the loss. We define that conception occurs with the fertilization of the ovum. The time after conception is the developmental age. Gestational age is the time calculated from the last menstrual period, and by convention exceeds the developmental age by 2 weeks[1,2].

The pre-embryonic period is defined as the first two weeks after fertilization. During this time, the fertilized oocyte becomes a blastomere, or morula, during its first series of divisions, in the second to fourth day after

fertilization. Next, the blastomere becomes a blastocyst as a central cavity is formed. The cells on the outer layer differentiate to become trophoblasts. An embryonic disc is formed from the inner cell mass. Folding of the disc at the end of the second week of development marks the beginning of the embryonic period. At 8 weeks after fertilization, most organ development is completed or well underway, and the conceptus is termed a fetus. It has a crown–rump length of 30 mm and a gestational age of 10 weeks. The fetal period continues until birth and is marked by growth, central nervous system development and finally pulmonary maturation[3,4].

Pregnancy begins with the implantation of the conceptus into endometrium, with the invasion of trophoblasts into maternal tissues. Clinical evidence of a pregnancy is supported by the appearance of the β-chain of human chorionic gonadotropin (β-hCG) in the maternal serum or urine. This 'positive' pregnancy test occurs by the synthesis of the gonadotropin by the syncytiotrophoblasts. The test does not prove a viable pregnancy as syncytiotrophoblasts may produce hormone without a fetus or in neoplastic trophoblastic disease. Early clinical confirmation of a pregnancy may be made by the ultrasonographic observation of heart motion or fetal motion[5,6].

Most generally, abortion is defined as the termination of pregnancy by any means before

Clinical Management of Early Pregnancy. Edited by Walter Prendiville and James R. Scott.
Published in 1999 by Arnold, ISBN 0 340 74100 7

the fetus is sufficiently developed to survive. In many countries, the definition is restricted to loss occurring before 20 weeks[7]. Spontaneous abortion occurs when the conceptus is involuntarily lost. The products of conception may be incompletely expelled and the abortion termed incomplete. The embryo may die or be resorbed and the trophoblast shell continue to be viable. This is termed an anembryonic pregnancy or 'blighted ovum'. Recurrent spontaneous abortions occur in women having three or more consecutive abortions[8].

INCIDENCE

The incidence of pregnancy failure depends on the definitions used for pregnancy and pregnancy loss, and the clinical population studied. The probability of the delivery of a live newborn to a healthy, sexually active, fertile woman per menstrual cycle has been estimated at 20–30%[9,10]. This model suggests that in 70–80% of cycles, an ovum is released, but fertilization, implantation and continued pregnancy does not occur. Failure of fertilization, in the presence of sperm, is estimated to occur 10% of the time[11]. This failure of conception contributes to infertility, but not to pregnancy failure.

After fertilization, the developing blastocyst travels from the fallopian tube into the uterine cavity. Postfertilization and preimplantation loss of the conceptus has been estimated at 12–15%[11]. Hertig *et al.*[12] undertook a histologic study of conception and implantation. They found a maximum total fertility rate to implantation of 58%. In their series, 42% of possible pregnancies were lost because of a failure of fertilization or implantation. Studies in infertile women undergoing the transfer of a conceptus after artificial insemination or *in vitro* fertilization (IVF) show an implantation rate of 7–47%, averaging about 20%[13–16].

Mesrogli and Dieterle[13] measured early pregnancy factor (EPF) to document the transfer of a viable conceptus. EPF is a protein produced by the cleaving embryo which can be detected in maternal serum 24–48 h after embryo transfer. These investigators found that 17 of 52 embryos expressing EPF implanted successfully and the remaining two thirds were lost. The studies of assisted fertilization and IVF pregnancies may not be directly applied to healthy fertile women; however, they do indicate that many fertilized ova fail to implant.

Currently, the clinical hallmark of implantation is the detection of β-hCG. This assay is used as presumptive evidence of pregnancy. Once this test became available, pregnancies and pregnancy losses were diagnosed earlier, at a time which previously they had been clinically silent[17–20]. These 'preclinical' pregnancy failure rates varied from 8 to 57% (Table 4.1). The differences in the estimates may be due to differences in methodology or definition of a positive test. It is clear, however, that many pregnancies fail early. As many of these are clinically unsuspected, the expelled tissue has not been studied to determine a possible etiology.

About 1 in 6 clinically recognized pregnancies fail. Warburton and Fraser[21], using data gathered in the 1950s and 1960s, found an overall abortion rate of 14.7%. A study by Mills *et al.*[22] reviewing fertility in women with diabetes found an early pregnancy failure rate of 16.0% in the control group and 15.5% in those with diabetes.

The incidence of pregnancy failure is not the same in all women. Reviewing families with at least one live birth, Warburton and Fraser[21] found a 32.2% risk of abortion in a woman who had three previous abortions. Poland *et al.*[23] found that women who had only reproductive failures and pregnancy losses had a 46% rate of subsequent spontaneous abortion. A prospective study confirms these trends: women without pregnancy failures had a spontaneous abortion rate of 4%, and those without successful pregnancies had an abortion rate of 24%[24]. Another significant predicting factor for abortion is maternal age: women ≥ 40 years have a spontaneous abortion rate twice that of

Table 4.1 Different rates of abortion in clinically diagnosed pregnancies and in those diagnosed by β-hCG

Study	No. of women	β-hCG for positive test	Clinical pregnancies	Clinical abortions	β-hCG pregnancies	Preclinical abortions	Total abortions
Chartier [17]	147	>4 mIU	71	14/71 (20%)	90	19/90 (21%)	33/90 (37%)
Miller [18]	197	>5 μg/l once or >2μg/l twice	102	15/102 (15%)	152	50/152 (33%)	65/152 (43%)
Edmonds [19]	82	>56 IU/l	51	6/51 (12%)	118	67/118 (57%)	73/118 (62%)
Whittaker [20]	91	>16 mU/ml	85	11/85 (13%)	92	7/92 (8%)	18/92 (20%)

women <20 years[21]. Cashner and Wilson[25] also documented an increased risk of spontaneous abortions in older women.

The appearance of β-hCG in the serum or urine is only presumptive evidence of pregnancy. Anembryonic pregnancy or neoplastic trophoblastic disease produces β-hCG in the absence of an embryo. Historically, a definitive diagnosis of a viable pregnancy has been the clinical detection of fetal heart beats or movement. Transabdominal or endovaginal ultrasound examination of cardiac activity has been used recently to prove a viable pregnancy. With transabdominal ultrasound, cardiac activity may be reliably visualized after seven or eight weeks of gestation. The identification of cardiac activity has a favorable prognosis for pregnancy: the rate of spontaneous abortions is only 2–3% in women who have a viable fetus documented by transabdominal ultrasound between 8 and 16 weeks[5,24–26].

Endovaginal ultrasonography has allowed detection of cardiac activity at an earlier gestational age of 4–5 weeks[6]. When these earlier ages were studied, the incidence of spontaneous abortions increased. Merchiers *et al.*[27] reported that 9% of embryos with heart activity had subsequent first trimester pregnancy loss. This study reported an overall abortion rate of 17%[27].

These studies document that pregnancy failure is common. For 100 pregnancies begun, about 40 are lost in the first trimester. Preclinical pregnancy loss, at or about the time of the normal menses occurs in about 25% of all pregnancies. Between 12 and 15% of pregnancies are lost thereafter in the first 8 weeks. Those pregnancies which progress further than 8 weeks' gestation with a normal fetus have a later abortion rate of 3%.

FERTILIZATION AND PREIMPLANTATION

For fertilization to occur, the oocyte must leave the ovary, be swept into the fallopian tube, and encounter serviceable sperm (Figure 4.1)[28]. Usually, fertilization occurs within 24 h after ovulation, taking place in the third of the tube adjacent to the ovary. The unfertilized ovum is surrounded by its zona pellucida and carries its first polar body. The oocyte has completed its first meiotic division and has begun the second one (Figure 4.2)[3]. The sperm penetrates the zona pellucida and fuses its plasma membranes with those of the ovum (Figure 4.3). Its nucleus and other cellular contents enter the egg's cytoplasm. Fertilization activates the ovum to complete meiosis II and to discharge its second polar body (Figure 4.4). The next step for a successful pregnancy is cleavage: the division of the fertilized egg to form the multicellular blastomere (Figure 4.5). Normally, 4 days are required to reach the 16-cell stage.

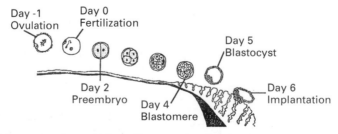

Figure 4.1. Travels of the ovum through the Fallopian tube. Fertilization occurs in the tube on day 0. The passage of the fertilized ovum to the uterine cavity is associated with its differentiation to a blastocyst. Adapted from Oppenheimer and Lefevre [28].

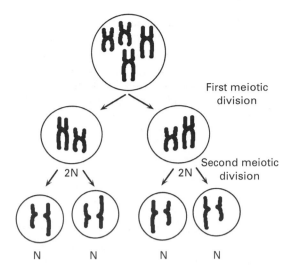

First meiotic division

2N   2N   Second meiotic division

N   N   N   N

Figure 4.2. Normal meiosis. In the testes, meiosis results in the formation of four haploid sperm. In the ovary, meiosis yields a single haploid ovum and non-functional polar bodies.

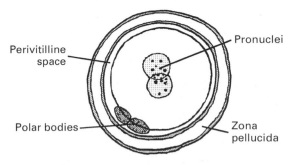

Perivitilline space

Pronuclei

Polar bodies

Zona pellucida

Figure 4.4. Normal fertilized ovum. At 12 h of age, there are two visible pronuclei derived from the ovum and sperm. These become associated with pairing of the maternal and paternal chromosomes and DNA synthesis begins. Adapted from Veeck [42].

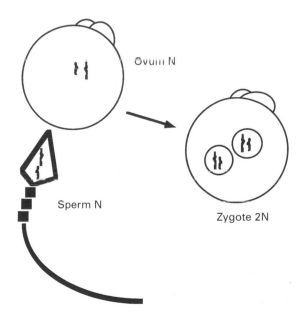

Ovum N

Sperm N

Zygote 2N

Figure 4.3. Normal fertilization. The number of chromosomes is here reduced to two for simplicity. Normally, the union of the haploid sperm and ovum creates the euploid zygote.

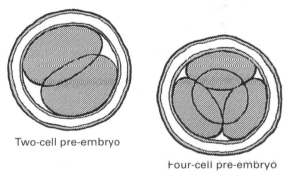

Two-cell pre-embryo

Four-cell pre-embryo

Figure 4.5. Normal blastomeres. The first two mitotic divisions of the fertilized ovum occur in the first two days of development [42].

IMPLANTATION

In the four days after fertilization, the pre-embryo travels through the tube and enters the cavity of the uterus (Figure 4.1). In preparation for implantation on day 5, the blastomere sheds the zona pellucida. The blastomere develops a central cavity, becoming a blasto-cyst. Differentiation occurs, with the surface cells transforming to trophoblasts[28]. Concur-rently, the endometrium is in preparation for implantation (Figure 4.6)[29]. Estradiol has stimulated the epithelial cells to proliferate, and has prepared the stromal cells for their response to progesterone. The epithelium is in

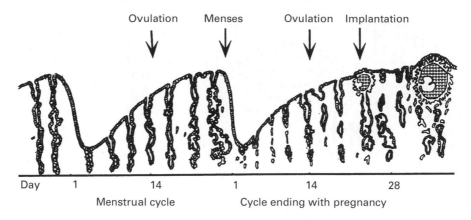

Figure 4.6. Endometrial tissue findings in a menstrual cycle and in pregnancy. The endometrium proliferates in the first 14 days of the cycle, and becomes secretory after ovulation. If implantation does not occur, the tissue is lost in the menses. With implantation, the endometrium is transformed to decidua. Adapted from Oppenheimer and Lefevre [28].

a secretory phase and there is a rich vascular network of spiral arteries and other vessels.

Adhesion and invasion of the blastocyst is mediated by cellular interaction of the trophoblasts with epithelial cells and endometrial extracellular matrix. Initially, there is apposition of the trophoblast to the endometrial epithelial cells (Figure 4.7a)[30]. The trophoblasts intrude between epithelial cells and penetrate to the basement membrane. Trophoblasts secrete enzymes to degrade the basement membrane and the extracellular matrix to promote invasion (Figure 4.7b)[31]. The endometrial epithelium at the surface closes over the implantation site (Figure 4.7c).

MATERNAL VASCULAR CONNECTION

The trophoblastic shell forms the initial cellular junction between the embryo and the endometrium. The trophoblasts are the precursor cells for the placenta and membranes.

Those trophoblasts of the implantation pole form the placenta proper, while the trophoblasts on the anti-implantation pole become the chorionic membranes[32].

In early placental development, there is proliferation of the mononuclear cytotrophoblasts in the trophoblastic shell. Multinucleated syncytiotrophoblast cells are seen on the blastocyst surface. Spaces or lacunae appear between the cytotrophoblasts in the trophoblastic shell. Some cytotrophoblasts, termed X-cells, migrate away from the shell into the decidua and erode into maternal vessels. Maternal red cells may be seen in the trophoblastic lacunae in the second postconception week[32].

Trophoblastic infiltration of the endometrium and myometrium is associated with alteration of the maternal vessels (Figure 4.8)[33]. The spiral arteries undergo a transformation with loss of the intima and media. The normal muscular and elastic tissue is replaced by fibrinoid material. The vascular

Figure 4.7. Blastocyst implantation in the uterus. (a) There is adhesion of the trophoblasts to the surface uterine epithelial cells. (b) The trophoblasts invade into the endometrial stroma. (c) The blastocyst becomes embedded in the endometrium. The surface epithelium is repaired. By the second week of development, trophoblasts have formed the trophoblastic shell, a precursor of the placenta. Adapted from Oppenheimer and Lefevre [28].

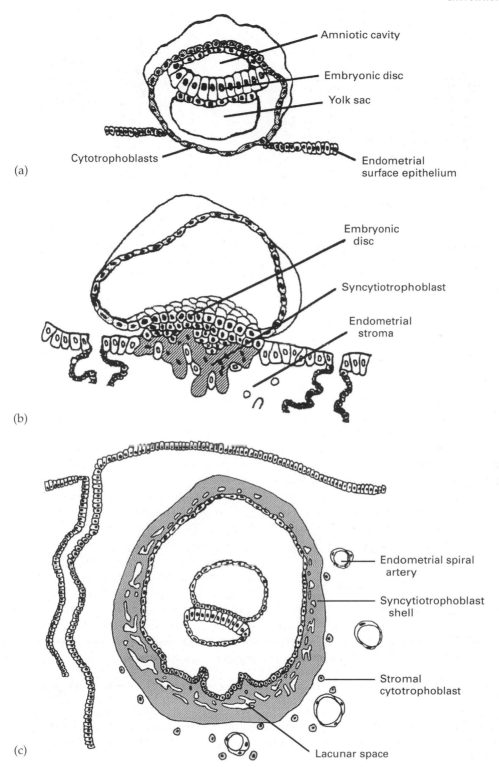

(a)

Amniotic cavity

Embryonic disc

Yolk sac

Cytotrophoblasts

Endometrial
surface epithelium

(b)

Embryonic
disc

Syncytiotrophoblast

Endometrial
stroma

(c)

Endometrial spiral
artery

Syncytiotrophoblast
shell

Stromal
cytotrophoblast

Lacunar space

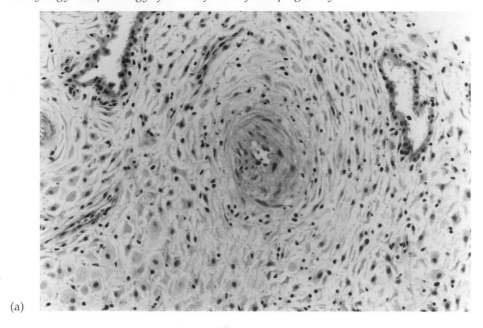

(a)

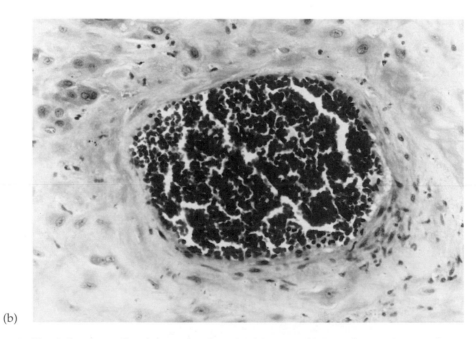

(b)

Figure 4.8. Physiologic transformation of endometrial arteries. (a) In early pregnancy, the spiral artery has a well-defined wall with concentric rings of smooth muscle cells. (b) Pregnancy transforms these small arteries to dilated vessels whose smooth muscular walls are replaced by fibrinoid material. Hematoxylin and eosin, original magnification ×40.

lumen becomes dilated and there is infiltration by cytotrophoblasts. The endothelium becomes discontinuous. In this manner, the arteries are transformed into uteroplacental vessels which directly open into the placental intervillous space. Similar vessel wall transformation is seen in the uterine veins which drain the placenta[32].

FETAL VILLOUS DEVELOPMENT

Concurrent with the invasion of the trophoblasts into the decidua and the establishment of a maternal vascular connection, cells within the trophoblastic shell are beginning to form placental villi. In the second postconception week, cords of trophoblasts grow into, and expand the lacunae[32]. Some cords of trophoblasts remain attached to the trophoblastic shell and become the anchoring villi. Budding of other cytotrophoblasts into the lacunae form the primary villi. Extraembryonic mesenchymal cells grow into these buds of trophoblasts, transforming the primary villi into secondary villi. Fetal vascular cells grow into the mesenchyme on postconception days 18–20, forming tertiary villi. Umbilical vessels connect to the embryonic vessels by growing into the chorionic plate and villi. The villous tissue proliferates by budding and branching like limbs on a tree.

With maturation of the placenta, the trophoblast layer adjacent to the intervillous space becomes progressively thinner and the villous diameter decreases. Fetal capillaries enlarge and become apposed to the trophoblastic surface (Figure 4.9). There is a decrease in the distance from the maternal blood space to the fetal blood space, from 50–100 μm in the 2nd month of gestation to 4–5 μm in the last month[32].

EMBRYONIC DEVELOPMENT

It is self-evident that a successful pregnancy requires an embryo. However, in addition to the new life provided with birth, the embryo contributes in an essential and functional manner to the maintenance of the pregnancy. Evidence for this statement is provided by the failure of anembryonic pregnancies to progress. Supportive evidence is that there are certain congenital anomalies which are never seen in continuing pregnancies and must be incompatible with early interuterine life. Surveying organ systems, most major and minor structural abnormalities are seen in the fetus and newborn. However, some anomalies are not diagnosed, or are diagnosed only under special conditions.

For example, the fetal circulatory system appears critical for maintenance of a pregnancy. Acardia is seen only in twin pregnancy with twin-to-twin blood transfusion indicating that a heart is required for fetal life. In a similar manner, a fetus may survive with a two-vessel umbilical cord but a one-vessel cord is not seen. And babies are not born with aplastic anemia. It seems that a pump, vessels and blood cells are required to provide nutritional exchange for the embryo.

Anembryonic pregnancies occur, but are seen with decreasing frequency with later gestation[34–36]. Some proportion of these may represent an embryonic defect that was incompatible with intrauterine life. This abnormal development may lead to death and resorption. With the loss of an embryo, the gestational sac is expelled. The embryo may therefore provide a trophic effect to maintain the normal function of the placental tissues.

PATHOLOGY OF PREGNANCY FAILURE

ROLE OF THE CONCEPTUS IN PREGNANCY FAILURE

Chromosome abnormalities

In 1959, Hertig *et al.*[12] reported the results of a 17-year histologic study of human fertilized ovum. They had studied the uteruses and uterine contents of fertile women at risk for

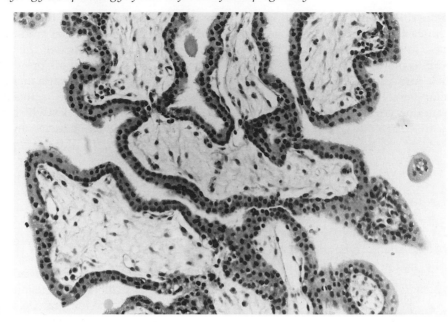

(a)

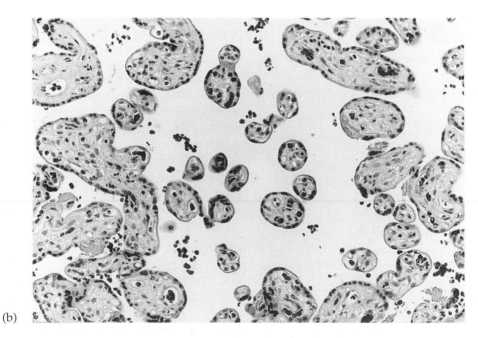

(b)

Figure 4.9. Normal placental villi. (a) Villi in the first trimester have a bilayered trophoblastic surface. The villous core is loose mesenchyme, and the fetal blood vessels are inconspicuous. (b) In the term placenta, with growth and maturation the villi are smaller. The trophoblast layer is thinned and dilated fetal capillaries lie immediately below the trophoblastic layer for nutritional exchange. Hematoxylin and eosin, original magnification ×40.

pregnancy. Morphologic abnormalities of the preimplantation blastocyst and the implanted embryo were seen frequently: half of the blastocysts and one quarter of the embryos were abnormal by light microscopy. This suggested that the morphologic defects were intrinsic to the conceptus rather than secondary to the local or endocrine environment, and were the cause of spontaneous abortion.

Mikado[37] investigated whether there were detectable abnormalities of the chromosomes to explain abortion. Tissue cultures of amnion, cord, skin, muscle and lung were set up for karyotype. Tissue from 150 spontaneous abortions were cultured and 45% were evaluable. Of these, 17 (25%) had gross chromosomal aberrations, which were more common in the younger age groups. These findings suggested that '. . . a considerable number of embryos die at early stages due to extremely abnormal morphogenesis and reduced viability, often associated with gross chromosomal aberrations.' Other workers have repeated this study with spontaneously aborted tissues and have obtained similar results (Table 4.2)[36,38–41].

Overall, about half the aborted conceptions were abnormal. Trisomies were the most frequent type of karyotypic abnormalities, with triploidy and monosomy X being the next two groups in abnormal occurrence. These findings of chromosomal abnormalities confirm Hertig's hypothesis that defects in the zygote were responsible for some abortions. The kinds of abnormalities detected indicate failures in meiosis, fertilization and early zygote division. Non-dysjunction of the gamete in meiosis may explain the numerical errors of the chromosomes: triploidy and monosomy X (Figure 4.10). Fertilization of the ovum by two sperm may yield triploidy (Figure 4.11). Tetraploidy and mosaicism may occur because of abnormalities of the early divisions of the fertilized ovum. The number of spontaneous abortions, and the number of those with karyotypic abnormalities has led Boue *et al.*[38] to suggest that one of three conceptions fails because of abnormal chromosome numbers.

There are morphologic and other findings associated with abnormal fertilization. As *in vitro* fertilization (IVF) studies have shown, normal fertilization produces an ovum with two pronuclei (Figure 4.4) whereas abnormal meiosis and fertilization is associated with abnormal pronuclear numbers (Figure 4.12a and b)[42]. *In vitro*, triploid pre-embryos cleave at an accelerated rate. Those pre-embryos which cleave more slowly than normal have a decreased potential to produce a successful pregnancy[42]. These differences from normal in the IVF pre-embryos are associated with decreased pregnancy potential. These *in vitro* observations likely duplicate those *in vivo*, as Hertig *et al.* demonstrated histologically similar abnormal fertilized ova in their hysterectomy specimens[12].

Studies consistently identify factors associated with abnormal chromosomes: parental age, gestational age of the conceptus, and the

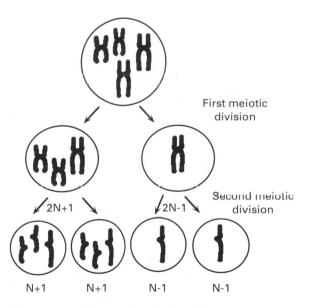

Figure 4.10. Abnormal meiosis with non-dysjunction of chromosomes. Non-dysjunction of individual chromosomes during meiosis results in gametes with aneuploidy. Trisomy results from fertilization with an N + 1 gamete. Monosomy X may result from the N − 1 gamete.

Table 4.2 Cytogenetic findings in spontaneous abortion tissues

Study	Gestational age (weeks)	Successful karyotype (%)	Abnormal karyotype (%)	Distribution of karyotypic abnormality (%)			
				Trisomy	Triploidy	Monosomy	Other
Boue [38]	<12	N.R.*	921/1498 (62)	52	20	15	13
Creasy [39]†	<24	941/1767 (53)	287/941 (31)	50	13	24	13
Hassold [40]‡	<24	1000/1120 (89)	463/1000 (46)	46	15	11	28
Kajii [36]	<30	402/565 (71)	215/402 (54)	31	7	10	52
Byrne [41]	<28	1356/3472 (39)	540/1356 (40)	49	16	16	19

* N.R. = Not reported.
† Data on singleton pregnancies.
‡ Study excluded 'blighted ovum'.

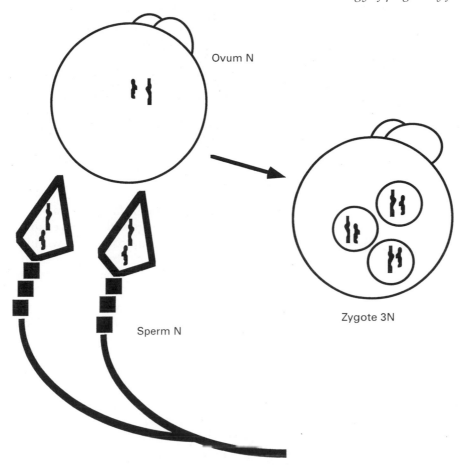

Ovum N

Zygote 3N

Sperm N

Figure 4.11. Abnormal fertilization resulting in triploidy. Fertilization by two sperm produces a zygote with 3N aneuploidy.

abortus tissue findings. Parental age, especially maternal age, is associated with chromosome abnormalities in general, and trisomies in particular. Mikado *et al.*[37] speculate that the aging of the ovum is the most important defect leading to abortion. The study by Boue *et al.*[38] found the parental age correlation for trisomies, but not triploidies, tetraploidies, monosomy X or translocation. They speculate that the association between paternal age and chromosomes is related to older men fertilizing older women rather than a problem of old men's sperm. Other studies also have documented the association of maternal age and

trisomies[36,40]. These findings may explain the increased incidence of spontaneous abortions in women over 40[43].

The gestational age of the conceptus also correlates with the frequency of abnormal chromosomes. The earlier the spontaneous abortion, the more likely the occurrence of an abnormal karyotype. Creasy *et al.*[39] found that a normal-appearing embryo had a 59% incidence of chromosome abnormality, whereas an older, normal fetus had a 2% incidence. Two studies have found a peak incidence of chromosome abnormalities at about 11 weeks' gestational age, with the proportion of abnormalities

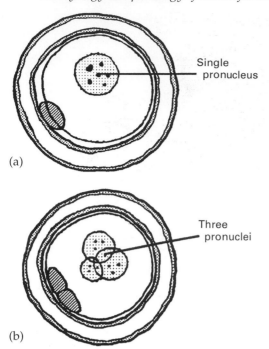

(a)

(b)

Figure 4.12. Abnormal fertilized ovum due to abnormal fertilization. (a) A single pronucleus is seen in a haploid zygote. (b) Three pronuclei in triploidy. Adapted from Veeck [42].

Table 4.3 Anatomic classification of abortions [35]

Group I: Incomplete specimen
Group II: Ruptured empty sac
Group III: Intact empty sac
Group IV: Embryo or fetus present
    A. Normal embryo or fetus
    B. Deformed embryo
    C. Embryo or fetus with anomalies
    D. Fragmented or autolyzed tissue

suggests that a set of embryonic chromosomal abnormalities is fatal *in utero*.

The findings at the gross examination of the abortion tissue correlated with the frequency of chromosome abnormalities. Most examiners have used the Anatomic Classification proposed by Fujukura *et al.*[35] (Table 4.3). There is a correlation with the gross findings, as is shown in Table 4.4. Abnormal chromosomes are more commonly found with malformations. However, no study has defined a single morphologic category with a particular chromosomal abnormality. A grossly normal fetus has a >95% chance of normal chromosomes[39,41].

Histology of the villi has a rough correlation with the chromosome findings which is best expressed in the trophoblastic molar pregnancy. Hydatidiform villous changes are diagnosed when villi are swollen and filled with fluid that lead to the formation of a central cistern[44]. Complete moles have a generalized

dropping sharply to near 0% after 20 weeks' gestation[36,39]. Some pregnancies which abort later have monosomy X or triploidies. These are karyotypes seen occasionally in newborns. Conversely, some karyotypes of the younger abortions are never seen at term. This

Table 4.4 Classification of abortion tissue and chromosomal abnormalities

Anatomic classification	Abnormal Karyotype (%)	
	Creasy [39]	Byrne [41]
Group I: Incomplete specimen	29	45
Group II: Ruptured empty sac	49	54
Group III: Intact empty sac	64	61
Group IV: Embryo or fetus present		
Embryo, normal	54	59
Embryo, abnormal	69	73
Fetus, normal	3	2
Fetus, abnormal	18	32

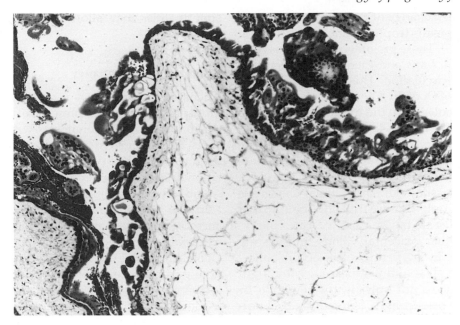

Figure 4.13. Villous morphology in a complete hydatiform mole. The enlarged villous has a hyperplastic trophoblastic cell layer. The trophoblasts are cytologically abnormal. The villous core is hydropic and lacks fetal vessels. Hematoxylin and eosin, original magnification ×20.

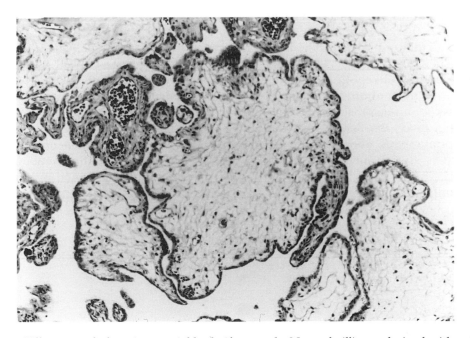

Figure 4.14. Villous morphology in a partial hydatiform mole. Normal villi are admixed with enlarged hydropic ones. The surface of the large villous is irregular with scalloping and indentations of the trophoblastic layer. Hematoxylin and eosin, original magnification ×20.

hydatidiform change of the villi with cytologically atypical trophoblastic proliferation (Figure 4.13). These pregnancies do not have an embryo or a fetus and there is no evidence in the villi of circulation. The karyotype of these tissues is 46 XX or 46 XY.

Partial moles have the hydatidiform change in some villi (Figure 4.14), and are associated with an embryo or fetus. Partial moles are common in triploidy, but 5% of triploidies are not associated with molar villous changes[44]. Further, if tissue with partial molar changes is karotyped, only 42% are triploid. About 13% of partial moles are trisomic and 19% are eukaryotic[45]. Other placental villous findings are not helpful in predicting a karyotypic abnormality[46]. The villous histology by light microscopy is not sufficiently sensitive or specific in predicting a chromosomal abnormality to replace routine cytogenetics. The application of *in situ* hybridization techniques to the abortus tissue may detect aneuploidy directly[47].

In recurrent spontaneous abortions, chromosome studies have been attempted to define whether the karyotype of an abortion predicts risk to the couple of further abnormal pregnancies[40,48,49]. Most generally, a normal karyotype is likely to be repeated as normal in the next abortion. There is an increased risk for a second abnormal chromosome finding, given the first is abnormal. In 3–5% of spontaneous abortions, structural abnormality of the chromosomes is found, which may be detected as a familial translocation[50,51]. Detection of these abnormalities may allow specific counseling and treatment.

Anembryonic pregnancy

Anembryonic pregnancy is diagnosed during ultrasonography by the presence of a collapsed or abnormal gestational sac without fetal parts[25,52]. Current technology allows the diagnosis of anembryonic pregnancy at 8 gestational weeks. Its overall incidence at ultrasound in women who abort is 11–15%[53,54].

In the presonography era, incidence of anembryonic pregnancy was estimated from material submitted for pathology review (Table 4.5). In the <10 weeks of gestation abortion specimens, intact empty chorionic sacs are found about 10% of the time[34–36]. In the tissue from later abortions, the frequency of intact empty chorionic sacs decreases to 2–5%[35,55]. Presumably, without an embryo, there is earlier uterine expulsion of the trophoblastic tissue.

On occasion, the pathologist receives the empty chorionic sac intact in anembryonic pregnancy. Nishimura and Shiota[56] determined that the sacs were smaller than would be predicted for gestational age, suggesting growth retardation of the trophoblasts. In general, the chorionic villi were found to be decreased in number and hydropic.

More frequently, the tissue submitted for pathology review is fragmented and incomplete. The villi frequently are abnormal with hydrops and great variation in size. In some cases the villi show signs of intrauterine

Table 4.5 Incidence of anembryonic pregnancies in pathology studies

Study	Number of SAB	Gestational age (weeks)	Empty sacs (%)	Ruptured sacs without embryo (%)	Total (%)
Fujikura [35]	54	5–10	5	32	37
Fantel [34]	393	<8	13	28	41
Kajii [36]	639	<9	10	36	46
Fujikura [35]	308	11–20	5	20	25
Birber [55]	1025	<20	2	18	20

SAB = Spontaneous abortions.

retention with fibrosis of the villi and syncytial knots[57]. Without embryonic heart beat, the blood vessels within the villi become abnormal. The capillaries disappear from the terminal villi, and the vessels in the intermediate and stem villi become fibrotic[58].

Embryonic maldevelopment

An aborted embryo is usually malformed. The Central Laboratory for Human Embryology at the University of Washington has found that only 15% of 2–8 week embryos appeared normal[43]. This proportion differs greatly from the finding in the aborted fetus, where more than 70% were morphologically normal. Embryos also differed in their pattern of malformation, exhibiting major malformations and generalized growth retardation. The fetus more commonly had a single anomaly. Poland *et al.*[59] made similar observations about embryonic malformations. Of the 1126 embryos studied, 77% were growth disorganized, 7% had systemic defects such as central nervous system abnormalities or musculoskeletal abnormalities and 16% were normal.

These embryonic findings are not unexpected, given the high frequency of chromosomal defects in early pregnancy loss. However, an abnormal karyotype alone is not sufficient to explain the congenital malformations. Poland's study determined that 42% of abnormal embryos had normal chromosomes. Byrne *et al.*[41] found that 27% of the abnormal embryos had normal chromosomes. Fatal embryonic malformations occur frequently. The pathologist is in the observer's role, without an explanation at present to explain the defects seen. Documentation of the malformations may allow future clinical or laboratory studies to clarify the disorder.

Trophoblastic abnormalities

Spontaneous abortions are associated with features of abnormal trophoblastic function. Hustin *et al.*[60] reviewed 184 cases of spontaneous abortion in which there was a completely intact gestational sac embedded in endometrium for examination. In these cases, the trophoblastic shell was hypocellular and discontinuous. There was an abnormal direct contact between the maternal decidua and the intervillous space. There was decreased infiltration of the decidua by the cytotrophoblastic X-cells. There was no correlation of these histologic findings with the presence of normal or abnormal chromosomes. Khong *et al.*[61] confirmed the findings of abnormal X-cell migration and a lack of maternal vessel changes in the placental bed of women with recurrent abortions.

Other markers of trophoblastic cell dysfunction are seen in failed pregnancies. Normally, trophoblasts synthesize placental products β-hCG, pregnancy specific beta-1 glycoprotein (SP-1), and pregnancy-associated plasma proteins (PAPP-A)[62,63]. Maternal serum levels of these decrease in anembryonic pregnancies and in those pregnancies which end in abortion[53,64].

Another trophoblastic cause of failed pregnancy is the hydatiform mole. The term 'hydatiform mole' derives from the Latin: hydatis = a drop of water and mole = a shapeless mass. Molar pregnancies have been separated into complete and partial moles based on clinical, genetic and pathologic findings[65,66]. Complete molar pregnancies are found in approximately 1/1500 pregnancies in the United States, and detected in 2% of spontaneous abortions[59]. Women often have first trimester bleeding, an increased uterine size and a characteristic ultrasonograph[67]. The maternal serum β-hCG levels are generally elevated above normal for gestational age. Grossly, the specimen is large and characterized by swollen, vesicular villi. The histology shows enlarged edematous villi (Figure 4.13). The villi display a central cistern, which is a prominent acellular central space. They usually are avascular. There is haphazard proliferation of cytologically abnormal trophoblasts on the surface of the villi[65].

Women with partial moles commonly present with spontaneous abortion or missed abortion[68]. Uterine size is generally small for dates and serum β-hCG is in the low or normal range. The tissue volume is small and some normal placental tissue is present. A fetus may be present and congenital abnormalities are often detected. Histologically, there is a mix of normal and abnormal villi. The central cisterns are less conspicuous than in complete moles. Trophoblast hyperplasia is less marked and there may be scalloping of the villi (Figure 4.14)[65.].

Complete and partial moles are the result of abnormal fertilization of the conceptus. Most complete moles are euploid and 46,XX. The genotype results from the fertilization of an empty ovum by a single sperm, with duplication of the paternal haploid DNA (Figure 4.15). Some 3–13% of complete moles are 46,XY; these moles are formed by the fertilization of an empty ovum by two sperm. Tetraploidy is also common in true moles. Most partial moles are triploid with a maternal component, as discussed previously. Recently, the study of molar pregnancies has been aided by flow cytometry which can rapidly measure DNA content in individual cells[69].

MATERNAL CAUSES OF PREGNANCY FAILURE

Vascular abnormalities

In normal pregnancy, the maternal spiral arteries are transformed from vessels with well-defined endothelium, elastic membranes and smooth muscle layers to uteroplacental arteries. These dilated vessels have lost their organized smooth muscle layers and elastic membranes. Their intravascular lumen is lined discontinuously by endothelium, and walls are lined by fibrinoid material and trophoblasts[70,71].

A failure of this transformation has been seen in the placental bed in women who have had pregnancy-induced hypertension or delivered small-for-gestational age infants[72]. Two studies have reported similar findings in abortion tissue. Hustin *et al.*[60] reviewed 184 cases of spontaneous abortions, and found that the maternal vessels did not show normal physiologic transformation. This finding was associated with a decrease in trophoblast infiltration. There was no correlation of the lack of vessel transformation with normal or abnormal fetal chromosomes. Khong *et al.*[61] reviewed the placental bed tissue of women with recurrent abortions. They found a failure of maternal vascular transformation in all five of their second trimester abortions, and in two of seven first trimester losses. Another study of maternal vessels in abortus specimens found abnormalities of the arteries in 14% of the specimens examined[73].

The establishment of uterine placental vascular connection is critical for normal pregnancy, and its failure may cause abortion. The mechanism of the transformation of spiral arteries is unknown. Some investigators

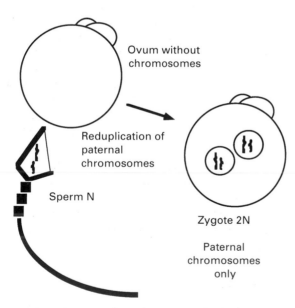

Figure 4.15. Abnormal fertilization in complete hydatiform mole. A single sperm fertilizes an empty ovum, with duplication of the paternal haploid DNA. The result is an euploid zygote with paternal chromosomes.

believe it is under the direct influence of the migrating interstitial trophoblast[71], whereas others have demonstrated that physiologic transformation is independent of the depth of trophoblast penetration[74]. The lack of association between abnormal embryonic chromosomes and vascular abnormalities suggests that trophoblasts are not the sole determinant of the vascular change[60]. Rather, a cellular interaction between the maternal endothelial cells and the invading trophoblasts occurs. One example of this is demonstrated by an induced expression of surface cellular adhesion molecules by both cell types in early placentation[75].

Autoimmune disease

The maternal immune system normally recognizes self and non-self. A foreign antigen typically provokes an immune response with the generation of antibodies or cytotoxic lymphocytes. Self-antigens are tolerated without an immune response. In normal pregnancies, the fetal antigens do not provoke an untoward immune response from the mother[76]. Autoimmune diseases such as systemic lupus erythematosus, polymyositis dermatosis, scleroderma and mixed connective tissue diseases are associated with abortion and late pregnancy loss[77]. The presence of autoantibodies such as antiphospholipid antibodies or anticardiolipin antibodies has been associated with failed pregnancies[78–84]. Some women with recurrent fetal loss and anticardiolipin antibodies also produce antibodies directed against the trophoblast[85]. The etiology of pregnancy loss in the presence of autoantibodies is unclear as there is not a direct correlation between autoantibody titer and reproductive failure.

When examined, the tissues from these abortions show signs of ischemia[86]. Fetal loss is confirmed, but there is typically no malformation or chromosome abnormality. The placentas showed signs of hypoxia: infarction, villous fibrosis, increased syncytial knots and perivillous fibrin. In some cases, the maternal decidual vessels failed to show normal physiologic changes and demonstrated spiral artery vasculopathy, so called 'acute atherosis'. These findings suggest that pregnancy loss is a consequence of placental vascular disorders rather than an immune attack on the conceptus[86–88].

Alloimmune disease

Another mechanism for pregnancy loss may be due to genetic dissimilarity between the mother and the fetus. To investigate a possible immune mechanism for abortion, surveys of women with recurrent pregnancy failure have been made. Studies indicate that most women with successful pregnancies have lymphocytotoxic antibodies, as detected in a mixed lymphocyte culture. Women with reproductive failure lack these antibodies[89]. A model has been proposed on the assumption that paternal antigens are expressed by fetal cells[89]. Normally, a maternal immune mechanism is formed to prevent immune recognition and rejection of the fetus. Pregnancy failure may occur when these antibodies are not formed. Maternal immunization with paternal cells may stimulate production of immune protection and allow for a pregnancy success. Clinical trials have been designed and executed, some with a favorable response[89–94]. This subject is critically evaluated in Chapter 10. There have been no reports on histology on the tissue from the abortions of women with this mechanism of pregnancy loss, or from the cases of lymphocyte treated women who have had failed pregnancies[89–94].

Infectious disease

Maternal infections have been associated with abortions. The incidence of this association varies by study, and no investigation has conclusively proven that infections induce recurrent pregnancy loss. Harger *et al.*[95]

found *Ureaplasma urealyticum* in cervical cultures of 48% of women with two or more consecutive pregnancy losses. Quinn *et al.*[96,97] detected *U. urealyticum* and *Mycoplasma hominis* in couples with abortions, and treatment improved pregnancy outcome in those with infections. Quinn's group also found that chlamydial antibody occurred in women with recurrent spontaneous abortions: 57.6% compared to 33.7% in normal pregnant woman. In the second trimester, an association has been demonstrated between the colonization with group B streptococci and spontaneous abortion[98].

For the pathologist, the finding of an inflammatory infiltrate in the tissue sections raises concern about infection. Lymphocytes are normally present in decidua, and neutrophils may be present in the decidual tissue as it is expelled. However, neutrophils in the chorion or amnion are always a sign of infection[99]. The organisms associated with recurrent abortion, *U. urealyticum*, *M. hominis*, and group B streptococci induce similar histologic findings of acute inflammation in abortion specimens (Figure 4.16)[100,101]. For streptococci and other common bacteria and fungi, routine tissue Gram stains are effective in demonstrating the organisms. The tissue diagnosis of a *Mycoplasma* infection has been impaired by the lack of a specific histologic stain[99]. Molecular biologic analysis of the abortus tissue with *in situ* hybridization of probes to the infectious genome may allow diagnosis of a specific infection[102].

Chronic infection has also been seen in abortions. In a tissue specimen, chronic villitis is diagnosed by the finding of a lymphoplasmacytic infiltrate in the villi. Syphilis and other spirochetic infections have been diagnosed in some abortion specimens which demonstrate chronic infection[103,104]. Cytomegalovirus is infrequently seen in abortion specimens[105] and may be specifically diagnosed by immunologic stains or detection of viral genome[106,107].

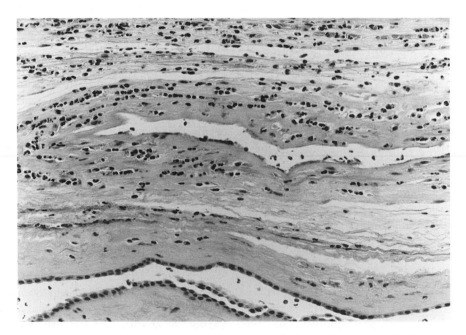

Figure 4.16. Acute amnionitis. The amniotic membranes are thickened by layers of infiltration polymorphonuclear leukocytes. Hematoxylin and eosin, original magnification ×40.

Endocrine diseases

Maternal endocrine abnormalities have been associated with pregnancy failure[108]. Uncontrolled diabetes mellitus has increased rates of spontaneous abortions[22,109] and fetal anomalies are seen in 6–9% of the specimens examined. These include congenital heart disease, spinal bifida, caudal regression syndrome, renal anomalies and the VATER association[110]. No significant differences in the rates of abortion were seen in diabetic women with good metabolic control compared to non-diabetic women[22].

Thyroid disease has rarely been associated with pregnancy failure. Hypothyroidism is not associated with habitual abortions in women and in thyrotoxicosis, abortion is only seen infrequently[111,112]. In one series, women with thyroid autoantibodies had an abortion rate of 17% compared to a control rate of 8.4%[113]. This increased rate of miscarriage in this population may be related to an underlying autoimmune disease rather than a primary endocrine disease.

Luteal phase defect is another endocrine abnormality associated with recurrent spontaneous abortion. This condition is characterized by inadequate progesterone production by the corpus luteum[114]. The lack of progesterone leads to a failure of maturation of the endometrium for implantation. Endometrial biopsy has been used to evaluate luteal phase defect. The diagnosis is made by demonstrating a discrepancy between the ovulatory and histologic dating of two days or more. The technique has an accuracy rating of only 23–35%[108]. Although there have been difficulties with diagnosis of the defect and its treatment, the condition has been diagnosed and successfully treated by the administration of progesterone[115–119].

Structural abnormalities of the uterus

Both congenital and acquired structural abnormalities of the uterus are found in many women with a history of repeated spontaneous abortions[120,121]. Uterine abnormalities or cervical incompetence are seen in 18% of women with recurrent abortion[112]. Most were Mullerian fusion anomalies. Other structural abnormalities present were retroversion, fibroids or synechiae. When studied by hysterosalpingogram and hysteroscopy, uterine abnormalities were detected in 27% of women with recurrent pregnancy losses[95]. In general, the tissue specimens obtained in these cases are freshly aborted, without signs of retention or trophoblastic disease[122].

EXAMINATION OF PRODUCTS OF CONCEPTION

The pathologist's goal in the examination of tissue from a failed pregnancy is to document the pregnancy and to demonstrate a possible cause for the abortion. The information provided by the pathologist is of value for reproductive counseling of couples with recurrent abortion. For the health care providers, even the 'negative' pathology findings are valuable. The usefulness of the tissue report for reproductive counseling is dependent on the thoroughness of the pathologist's examination of the abortion tissue.

There are excellent texts and monographs about the handling of the abortion tissue and the following discussion is not intended to replace those, but rather to indicate how a specimen may be handled to increase the information derived from its examination[7,122,123].

SPECIMEN ACQUISITION

For the pathologist to interpret the gross and microscopic findings, an adequate maternal clinical history is essential. Information about the pregnancy and the past obstetric and medical history is required for the consultation (Table 4.6). In most cases, the re-examination of previous pathology materials and reports will enrich the current interpretation.

Table 4.6 Pregnancy history for the pathologist

Maternal age
Obstetric history
Details of previous abortions
Details of current pregnancy:
    Last menstrual period
    Bleeding, illness, drugs, other
Ultrasonography findings
Specimen acquisition
    Spontaneous
    Elective, technique
Other medical or surgical history

The examination of products of conception for reproductive counseling should be handled without fixative, as for a frozen section. Everything expelled spontaneously or obtained from surgery should be submitted. A woman with repeated abortion may be warned to obtain and bring in any expelled tissue in a clean container for examination. The specimen should be kept moist with a small amount of sterile saline, and transported cold to the pathology laboratory[1].

GROSS EXAMINATION

The tissue should be maintained in a sterile manner, to allow submission of tissue for cytogenetics. The gross tissue is delicate and will tear or fragment with handling. To prevent this and allow the tissue to expand, the specimen may be floated in a sterile Petri dish in sterile saline. Magnification of the specimen with a hand lens or dissection microscope demonstrates fine features. The gross tissue findings are ephemeral, and photographs are required.

If a single intact specimen is obtained, it is usually a decidual cast. This should be opened from the narrow end to release the chorionic sac. The size of the sac should be measured, and compared to a standard table[56]. The diameter of the sac normally correlates with gestational age, but with the death of the embryo there is a decreased rate of sac growth.

The surface of the normal sac is evenly covered by villi. Abnormal villi have swollen, clubbed or cystic tips. In some specimens, the villi may be hypoplastic and sparsely distributed.

Within the sac, there may be an embryo, cord, amniotic sac or yolk sac. The presence or absence of these embryonic structures should be documented with photographs. An embryo should be classified as having normal or abnormal external findings with the referral to embryonic development tables[4]. We use the Anatomic Classification by Fujikura and associates (Table 4.3)[35]. Several other anatomic classifications are also available[35,39,41,59]. However, there has not been an association of a particular morphology with a specific chromosome abnormality, and no classification scheme appears generally superior to another. Examination of the internal organs may be possible in some cases, and the heart tube is often preserved when other structures are autolyzed[59].

Most commonly, an incomplete and fragmented specimen is received. The sac, if present, is ruptured or collapsed. The specimen's contents should be described and photographed. An occasional specimen consists only of decidua, and the evidence of conception is made by the microscopic examination.

Tissues may be submitted for chromosomes when the history suggests recurrent spontaneous abortion, a previously morphologically abnormal pregnancy, or an earlier abnormal karyotype of an abortus[123]. Specimens with abnormal embryonic or fetal findings should be submitted as well. Clinical consultation may indicate those additional cases which require karyotype: *in vitro* fertilization, chromosome abnormalities in the parents, previous amniocentesis or chorionic villus sampling for chromosomes, and so on. Tissue from the embryo, amniotic membranes, or villi may be submitted for culture[7,123]. Villous tissue with hydropic change, or abortion tissue in the appropriate clinical setting may be submitted for flow cytometry for a rapid analysis of triploidy[124].

HISTOLOGIC EVALUATION

There was an initial enthusiasm for the ability of the villous histology to predict the chromosome findings of the abortus[125], but subsequent observers have been unable to make a correlation[44,46,126]. At present, cytogenetic studies remain the best method for detecting chromosomal abnormalities. *In situ* hybridization techniques are being developed which may allow the detection of anueploidy directly in the abortus tissue[47]. The findings of villous edema, fibrosis or fetal hypovascularity should be noted, as they have a bearing on the length of time of embryonic death and retention[58]. In addition, the tissue should be examined histologically for inflammation, infection or infarction.

The final pathology report should estimate the gestational age, presence or absence of an embryo or fetus and whether it is morphologically normal or not. The time of embryonic death may be estimated. Villous histology should be described. Special studies for karyotype, DNA content or infection should be reported.

CONCLUSION

The role of the pathologist in the evaluation of a failed pregnancy is to thoroughly examine the abortion tissue, to assist in the selection of special studies and to correlate anatomic findings with the clinical setting. The documentation of either normal and abnormal gross and histologic findings are invaluable to those who care for women with recurrent abortion. On the basis of such information, families make critically important decisions. Examination of abortus tissue should be made with the same care and diligence that the pathologist searches for cancer and other diseases.

REFERENCES

1. Kalousek, D.K., Baldwin, V.J., Dimmick, J.E. *et al.* (1992) Embryofetal–perinatal autopsy and placental examination, in *Development Pathology of the Embryo and Fetus* (eds J.E. Dimmick and D.K. Kalousek), J.B. Lippincott, Philadelphia, pp. 799–824.
2. Kalousek, D.K., Lau, A.E. and Baldwin, V.J. (1992) Development of the embryo, fetus and placenta, in *Developmental Pathology of the Embryo and Fetus* (eds J.E. Dimmick and D.K. Kalousek), J.B. Lippincott, Philadelphia, pp. 1–25.
3. Kaplan, S. and Bolender, D. (1992) Embryology, in *Fetal and Neonatal Physiology* (eds R.A. Polin and W.W. Fox), W.B. Saunders, Philadelphia, pp. 19–36.
4. England, M.A. (1994) The human, in *Embryos, Color Atlas of Development* (ed. J.B.L. Bard), Mosby-Year Book Europe Limited, London, pp. 207–20.
5. Simpson, J.L., Mills, J.L., Holmes, L.B. *et al.* (1987) Low fetal loss rates after ultrasound – proved viability in early pregnancy. *JAMA*, **258**, 2555–7.
6. Rempen, A. (1990) Diagnosis of viability in early pregnancy with vaginal ultrasound. *J. Ultrasound Med.*, **9**, 711–16.
7. Benirschke, K. and Kaufmann, P. (1990) Abortion, placentas of trisomies and immulogical considerations of recurrent reproductive failure, in *Pathology of the Human Placenta*, 2nd edn (eds K. Benirschke and P. Kaufmann), Springer-Verlag, New York, pp. 754–81.
8. Mishell, D.R. (1993) Recurrent abortion. *J. Reprod. Med.*, **38**, 250–9.
9. Cooke, I.D., Suliaman, R.A., Lenton, E.A. and Parsons, R.J. (1981) Fertility and infertility statistics. *Clin. Obstet. Gynecol.*, **8**, 531–48.
10. Cunningham, F.G., MacDonald, P.C., Leveno, K.J. *et al.* (1991) *Williams Obstetrics*, 19th edn. Appleton & Lange, Norwalk, pp. 661–90.
11. Little, A.B. (1988) There's many a slip 'twixt implantation and the crib. *N. Engl. J. Med.*, **319**, 241–2.
12. Hertig, A.T., Rock, J., Adams, E.C. and Menkin, M.C. (1959) Thirty-four fertilized human ova, good, bad and indifferent from 210 women of known fertility. *Pediatrics*, **23**, 202–11.
13. Mesrogli, M. and Dieterle, S. (1993) Embryonic losses after in vitro fertilization and embryo transfer. *Acta Obstet. Gynecol. Scand.*, **72**, 36–38.
14. Tan, S., Doyle, P., Maconochie, N. *et al.* (1994) Pregnancy and birth rates of five infants after in vitro fertilization in women with and without previous in vitro fertilization

pregnancies: a study of eight thousand cycles at one center. *Am. J. Obstet. Gynecol.*, **170**, 34–40.

15. Buster, J.E., Bustillo, M., Rodi, I.A. *et al.* (1985) Biologic and morphologic development of donated human ova recovered by nonsurgical uterine lavage. *Am. J. Obstet. Gynecol.*, **153**, 211–17.

16. Formigli, L., Formigli, G. and Roccio, C. (1987) Donation of fertilized uterine ova to infertile women. *Fertil. Steril.*, **47**, 162–5.

17. Chartier, M., Roger, M., Barrat, J. and Michelon, B. (1979) Measurement of plasma human chorionic gonadotropin (hCG) and beta-hCG activities in the late luteal phase. *Fertil. Steril.*, **31**, 134–7.

18. Miller, J.F., Williamson, E. and Glue, J. (1980) Fetal loss after implantation. *Lancet*, **ii**, 554–6.

19. Edmonds, D.K., Lindsay, K.S., Miller, J.F. *et al.* (1982) Early embryonic mortality in women. *Fertil. Steril.*, **38**, 447–53.

20. Whittaker, P.G., Taylor, A. and Lind, T. Unsuspected pregnancy loss in healthy women. *Lancet*, **i**, 1126–7.

21. Warburton, D. and Fraser, F.C. (1964) Spontaneous abortion risk in man: data from a reproductive histories collected in a medical genetics unit. *Hum. Genet.*, **16**, 1–25.

22. Mills, J.L., Simpson, J.L., Driscoll, S.G. *et al.* (1988) Incidence of spontaneous abortions among normal women and insulin-dependent diabetic women whose pregnancies were identified within 21 days of conception. *N. Engl. J. Med.*, **319**, 1617–23.

23. Poland, B.J., Miller, J.R., Jones, D.C. and Trimble, B.K. (1977) Reproductive counseling in patients who have had a spontaneous abortion. *Am. J. Obstet. Gynecol.*, **127**, 685–91.

24. Regan, L., Braude, P.R. and Trembath, P.L. (1989) Influence of past reproductive performance on risk spontaneous abortion. *Br. Med. J.*, **299**, 541–5.

25. Cashner, K.A., Christopher, C.R. and Dysert, G.A. (1987) Spontaneous fetal loss after demonstration of a live fetus in the first trimester. *Obstet. Gynecol.*, **70**, 827–35.

26. Christiaens, G.C.M.L. (1984) Spontaneous abortion in proven intact pregnancies. *Lancet*, **ii**, 571–2.

27. Merchiers, E.H., Dhont, M., De Sutter, P.A. *et al.* (1991) Predictive value of early embryonic cardiac activity for pregnancy outcome. *Am. J. Obstet. Gynecol.*, **165**, 11–14.

28. Oppenheimer, S.B. and Lefevre, G. (1989) *Introduction to Embryonic Development*, 3rd edn, Allyn and Bacon, New York, pp. 83–114.

29. Hunt, J.S. and Roby, K.F. (1994) Implantation factors. *Clin. Obstet. Gynecol.*, **37**, 635–45.

30. Coutifaris, C., Babalola, G.O., Abisogun, A.O. *et al.* (1991) *In vitro* systems for the study of human trophoblast implantation. *Ann. NY Acad. Sci.*, **262**, 191–201.

31. Fisher, S.J. and Damsky, C.H. (1993) Human cytotrophoblast invasion. *Semin. Cell. Biol.*, **4**, 183–8.

32. Benirschke, K. and Kaufmann, P. (1990) Early development of the human placenta, in *Pathology of the Human Placenta*, 2nd edn (ed. K.K.P. Benirschke), Springer-Verlag, New York, pp. 13–21.

33. Brosens, I., Robertson, W.B. and Dixon, H.G. (1967) The physiological response of the vessels of the placental bed to normal pregnancy. *J. Path. Bact.*, **93**, 569–79.

34. Fantel, A.G. and Shepard, T.H. (1987) Morphological analysis of spontaneous abortuses, in *Spontaneous and Recurrent Abortion* (eds M.K. Bennett and D.K. Edmonds), Blackwell Scientific, Boston, pp. 8–28.

35. Fujikura, T., Froehlich, L.A. and Driscoll, S.G. (1966) A simplified anatomic classification of abortions. *Am. J. Obstet. Gynecol.*, **95**, 902–5.

36. Kajii, T., Niikawa, N., Takahara, H. *et al.* (1980) Anatomic and chromosomal anomalies in 639 spontaneous abortions. *Hum. Genet.*, **55**, 87–98.

37. Mikado, K. (1970) Anatomic and chromosomal anomalies in spontaneous abortions. *Am. J. Obstet. Gynecol.*, **106**, 243–54.

38. Boue, J., Boue, A. and Lazar, P. (1975) Retrospective and prospective epidemiological studies of 1500 karotyped spontaneous human abortions. *Teratology*, **12**, 11–26.

39. Creasy, M.R., Crolla, J.A. and Alberman, E.D. (1976) A cytogenetic study of human spontaneous abortions using banding techniques. *Hum. Genet.*, **31**, 177–96.

40. Hassold, T., Chen, N., Funkhouser, J. *et al.* (1980) A cytogenetic study of 1000 spontaneous abortions. *Ann. Hum. Genet.*, **44**, 151–64.

41. Byrne, J., Warburton, D.J.K., Blanc, W. and Stein, Z. (1985) Morphology of early fetal deaths and their chromosomal characteristics. *Teratology*, **32**, 297–315.

42. Veeck, L.L. (1991) *Atlas of the Human Oocyte and Early Conceptus*, vol. 2, Williams and Wilkins, Baltimore, p. 445.

43. Fantel, A.G., Shepard, T.H., Vadheim-Roth, C. *et al.* (1980) Embryonic and fetal phenotypes: prevalence and other associated factors in a large study of spontaneous abortion, in *Human Embryonic and Fetal Death* (eds I.H. Porter and E.B. Hook), Academic Press, New York, pp. 71–87.

44. Jacobs, P.A., Szulman, A.E., Funkhouser, J. *et al.* (1982) Human triploidy: relationship between parental origin of the additional haploid complement and development of partial hydatidiform mole. *Ann. Hum. Genet.*, **46**, 223–31.

45. Rehder, H., Coerdt, W., Eggers, R. *et al.* (1989) Is there a correlation between morphological and cytogenetic findings in placental tissue from early missed abortions? *Hum. Genet.*, **82**, 377–85.

46. Fox, H. (1993) Histologic classification of tissue from spontaneous abortions: a valueless exercise? *Histopathology*, **22**, 599–600.

47. Elias, S. and Simpson, J.L. (1993) Prenatal diagnosis using fetal cells in maternal blood, in *Essentials of Prenatal Diagnosis* (eds S. Elias and J.L. Simpson), Churchill Livingstone, New York, pp. 381–92.

48. Speroff, L., Glass, R.H. and Kase, N.G. (1994) Recurrent early pregnancy losses, in *Clinical Gynecologic Endocrinology and Infertility*, 5th edn (eds L. Speroff, R.H. Glass and N.G. Kase), Williams & Wilkins, Baltimore, pp. 841–51.

49. Warburton, D., Kline, J., Stein, Z. *et al.* (1987) Does the karotype of a spontaneous abortion predict the karotype of a subsequent abortion? Evidence from 273 women with two karyotyped spontaneous abortions. *Am. J. Hum. Genet.*, **41**, 465–83.

50. Parisi, V.M. and Creasy, R.K. (1988) Repetitive reproductive loss, in *Medical Counseling Before Pregnancy* (eds D.R. Hollingsworth and R. Resnik), Churchill Livingstone, New York, pp. 25–7.

51. Byrne, J.L.B. and Ward, K. (1994) Genetic factors in recurrent abortion. *Clin. Obstet. Gynecol.*, **37**, 693–704.

52. Filly, R.A. (1994) Ultrasound evaluation during the first trimester, in *Ultrasonography in Obstetrics and Gynecology* (ed. P.W. Caller), W.B. Saunders, Philadelphia, pp. 63–85.

53. Stabile, I. (1992) Anembryonic pregnancy, in *The Embryo* (eds M. Chapman, G. Grudzinskas and T. Chard), Springer-Verlag, London, pp. 35–43.

54. Howe, R.S., Isaacson, K.J., Albert, J.L. and Coutifaris, C.B. (1991) Embryonic heart rate in human pregnancy. *J. Ultrasound Med.*, **10**, 367–71.

55. Birber, F.R. and Driscoll, S.G. Evaluation of the spontaneous abortion and of the malformed fetus, in *Diseases of the Fetus and Newborn* (eds G.B. Reed, A.E. Claireaux and A.D. Bain), C.V. Mosby, St Louis, pp. 59–74.

56. Nishimura, H. and Shiota, K. (1984) Early embryonic death, pathology and associated factors, in *Spontaneous Abortion* (ed. E.S.E. Hafez), MTP Press, New York, pp. 115–31.

57. Jouppila, P. and Herva, R. (1980) Study of blighted ovum by ultrasonic and histopathologic methods. *Obstet. Gynecol.*, **55**, 574–8.

58. Szulman, A.E. (1991) Examination of the early conceptus. *Arch. Pathol. Lab. Med.*, **115**, 696–700.

59. Poland, B.J., Miller, J.R., Harris, M. and Livingston, J. (1981) Spontaneous abortion, a study of 1961 women and their conceptuses. *Acta Obstet. Gynecol. Scand. Suppl.*, **102**, 5–32.

60. Hustin, J., Jauniaux, E. and Schaaps, J.P. (1990) Histologic study of the maternal–embryonic interface in spontaneous abortion. *Placenta*, **11**, 477–86.

61. Khong, T.Y., Liddell, H.S. and Robertson, W.B. (1987) Defective haemochorial placentation as a cause of miscarriage: a preliminary study. *Br. J. Obstet. Gynaecol.*, **94**, 649–55.

62. Wasmoen, T.L. (1992) Placental proteins, in *Fetal and Neonatal Physiology* (eds R.A. Polin and W.W. Fox), W.B. Saunders, Philadelphia, pp. 87–95.

63. Silver, R.M., Heyborne, K.D. and Leslie, K.K. (1993) Pregnancy specific beta-1 glycoprotein (SP-1) in maternal serum and amniotic fluid. *Placenta*, **14**, 583–9.

64. Johnson, M.R., Riddle, A.F., Grudzinskas, J.G. *et al.* (1993) Role of trophoblast dysfunction in the aetiology of miscarriage. *Br. J. Obstet. Gynaecol.*, **100**, 353–9.

65. Mazur, M.T. and Kurman, R.J. (1994) Gestational trophoblastic disease and related lesions, in *Blaustein's Pathology of the Female Genital Tract* (ed. R.J. Kurman), Springer-Verlag, New York, pp. 1049–73.

66. Lewis, J.L. (1993) Diagnosis and management of gestational trophoblastic disease. *Cancer*, **71**, 1639–47.

67. O'Quinn, A.G. and Bernard, D.E. (1994) Gestational trophoblastic diseases, in *Current Obstetric and Gynecologic Diagnosis and Treatment* (eds A.H. DeCherney and M.L. Pernoll), Appleton & Lange, Norwalk, pp. 967–76.

68. Szulman, A.E. and Surti, U. (1982) The clinico-pathologic profile of the partial hydatidiform mole. *Obstet. Gynecol.*, **59**, 597–602.

69. Lage, J.M. and Popek, E.J. (1993) The role of DNA flow cytometry in evaluation of partial and complete hydatidiform moles and hydropic abortions. *Semin. Diagn. Pathol.*, **10**, 267–74.

70. Brosens, I. (1964) A study of spiral arteries of the decidua basalis in normotensive and hypertensive pregnancies. *J. Obstet. Gynecol. Br. Commw.*, **71**, 222–30.

71. Pijnenborg, R., Bland, J.M., Robertson, W.B. and Brosens, I. (1983) Uteroplacental arterial changes related to early migration in early human pregnancy. *Placenta*, **4**, 397–414.

72. Khong, T.Y., De Wolf, F., Robertson, W.B. and Brosens, I. (1986) Inadequate maternal vascular response to placentation in pregnancies complicated by pre-eclampsia and by small-for-gestational age infants. *Br. J. Obstet. Gynaecol.*, **93**, 1049–59.

73. Nadji, P. and Sommers, S.C. (1973) Lesions of toxemia in first trimester pregnancies. *Am. J. Clin. Pathol.*, **59**, 344–9.

74. Gerretsen, G., Huisjes, H.J., Hardonk, M.J. and Elema, J.D. (1983) Trophoblast alterations in the placental bed in relation to physiologic changes in spiral arteries. *Br. J. Obstet. Gynaecol.*, **90**, 34–9.

75. Burrows, T.D., King, A. and Loke, Y.W. (1994) Expression of adhesion molecules by endovascular trophoblasts and endothelial cells: implications for vascular invasion during implantation. *Placenta*, **15**, 21–33.

76. Gill, T.J. (1994) Reproductive immunology and immunogenetics, in *Physiology of Reproduction*, 2nd edn (eds E. Knobil and J.D. Neill), Raven Press, New York, pp. 783–812.

77. Gleicher, N., Pratt, D. and Dudkiewicz, A. (1993) What do we really know about autoantibody abnormalities and reproductive failure: a critical review. *Autoimmunity*, **16**, 115–40.

78. Branch, D.B., Scott, J.R., Kochenour, N.K. and Hershgold, E. (1985) Obstetric complications associated with the lupus anticoagulant. *N. Engl. J. Med.*, **313**, 1322–6.

79. Cowchock, S., Smith, J.B. and Gocial, B. (1986) Antibodies to phospholioids and nuclear antigens in patients with repeated abortions. *Am. J. Obstet. Gynecol.*, **155**, 1002–10.

80. Lockshin, M.D., Druzin, M.L., Goei, S. *et al.* (1985) Antibody to cardiolipin as a predictor of fetal distress or death in pregnant patients with systemic lupus erythematosus. *N. Engl. J. Med.*, **313**, 152–6.

81. Lubbe, W.F., Pattison, N. and Liggins, G.C. (1985) Antiphospholipic antibodies and pregnancies. *N. Engl. J. Med.*, **313**, 1350–3.

82. MacLean, M.A., Cumming, G.P., McCall, F. *et al.* (1994) The prevalence of lupus anticoagulant and anticardiolipin antibodies in women with a history of first trimester miscarriages. *Br. J. Obstet. Gynaecol.*, **101**, 103–6.

83. Out, H.J., Bruinse, H.W., Christiaens, G.C.M.L. *et al.* (1991) Prevalence of antiphospholipid antibodies in patients with fetal loss. *Ann. Rheum. Dis.*, **50**, 553–7.

84. Parazzini, F., Acaia, B., Faden, D. *et al.* (1991) Antiphospholipid antibodies and recurrent abortion. *Obstet. Gynecol.*, **77**, 854–8.

85. McCrae, K.R., DeMichele, A.M., Pandhi, P. *et al.* (1993) Detection of antitrophoblastic antibodies in the sera of patients with anticardiolipin antibodies and fetal loss. *Blood*, **82**, 2730–41.

86. Branch, D.W. (1994) Thoughts on the mechanism of pregnancy loss associated with the antiphospholipid syndrome. *Lupus*, **3**, 275–80.

87. McFaul, P.B., Patel, N. and Mills, J. (1993) An audit of the obstetric outcome of 148 consecutive pregnancies from assisted conception: implications for neonatal services. *Br. J. Obstet. Gynaecol.*, **100**, 820–5.

88. Silver, R.M. and Branch, D.W. (1994) Recurrent miscarriage: autoimmune considerations. *Clin. Obstet. Gynecol.*, **37**, 745–60.

89. Scott, J.R., Rote, N.S. and Branch, D.W. (1987) Immunologic aspects of recurrent abortion and fetal death. *Obstet. Gynecol.*, **70**, 645–56.

90. Cauchi, M.N., Lim, D., Young, D.E. *et al.* (1991) Treatment of recurrent aborters by immunization with paternal cells – controlled trial. *Am. J. Reprod. Immunol.*, **25**, 16–17.

91. Ho, H.N., Gill, T.J., Hsieh, H.J. *et al.* (1991) Immunotherapy for recurrent spontaneous abortion in a Chinese population. *Am. J. Reprod. Immunol.*, **25**, 10–15.

92. Mowbray, J.F., Gibbings, C., Liddell, H. *et al.* (1985) Controlled trial of treatment of recurrent spontaneous abortion by immunization with paternal cells. *Lancet*, **i**, 941–3.

93. Smith, J.B. and Cowchock, F. (1988) Immunologic studies in recurrent spontaneous abortion. *J. Reprod. Immunol.*, **14**, 99–113.

94. Unander, A.M. and Linholm. A. (1986)

Transfusion of leukocyte rich erythrocyte concentrates: successful treatment in selected cases of habitual abortions. *Am. J. Obstet. Gynecol.*, **154**, 516–20.

95. Harger, J.H., Archer, D.F., Marchese, S.G. *et al.* (1983) Etiology of recurrent pregnancy losses and outcome of subsequent pregnancies. *Obstet. Gynecol.*, **62**, 574–81.

96. Quinn, P.A., Shewchuk, A.B., Shuber, J. *et al.* (1983) Serologic evidence of *Ureaplasma urealyticum* infection in women with spontaneous pregnancy loss. *Am. J. Obstet. Gynecol.*, **145**, 245.

97. Quinn, P.A., Shewchuk, A.B., Shuber, J. *et al.* (1983) Efficacy of antibiotic therapy in preventing spontaneous pregnancy loss among couples colonized with genital mycoplasma. *Am. J. Obstet. Gynecol.*, **145**, 239–44.

98. Daugaard, H.O., Thomden, A.C., Henriques, U. and Ostergaard, A. (1988) Group B streptococci in the lower urogenital tract and late abortions. *Am. J. Obstet. Gynecol.*, **158**, 28–31.

99. Benirschke, K. and Kaufmann, P. (1995) Infectious diseases, in *Pathology of the Human Placenta*, 3rd edn (eds K. Benirschke and P. Kaufmann), Springer-Verlag, New York, 537–623.

100. Romano, N., Romano, F. and Carollo, F. (1971) T-strain of mycoplasma in bronchopneumonic lungs of an aborted fetus. *N. Engl. J. Med.*, **285**, 950–2.

101. Knudsin, R.B., Driscoll, S.G. and Ming, P. (1967) Strain of mycoplasma associated with human reproductive failure. *Science*, **157**, 1573–4.

102. Mies, C. (1994) Molecular biological analysis of paraffin-embedded tissues. *Hum. Pathol.*, **25**, 555–60.

103. Abramowsky, C., Beyer-Patterson, P. and Cortinas, E. (1991) Nonsyphilitic spirochetosis in second trimester fetuses. *Pediatr. Pathol.*, **11**, 827–38.

104. Young, S.A. and Crocker, D.W. (1994) Occult congenital syphilis in macerated stillborn fetuses. *Arch. Pathol. Lab . Med.*, **118**, 44–7.

105. Altshuker, G. and McAdams, A.J. (1971) Cytomegalic inclusion disease in a nineteen-week fetus. *Am. J. Obstet. Gynecol.*, **111**, 295–8.

106. Chehab, F.F., Xiao, X., Kan, Y.W. and Yen, T.S.B. (1989) Detection of cytomegalovirus infection in paraffin-embedded tissue specimens with the polymerase chain reaction. *Mod. Pathol.*, **2**, 75–8.

107. Muhlemann, K., Miller, R.K., Metlay, L. and Menegus, M.A. (1992) Cytomegalovirus infection of the human placenta, an immunocytochemical study. *Hum. Pathol.*, **23**, 1234–7.

108. Coulam, C.B. and Stern, J.J. (1994) Endocrine factors associated with recurrent spontaneous abortions. *Clin. Obstet. Gynecol.*, **37**, 730–44.

109. Miodovnik, M., Skillman, C., Holroyde, J.C. *et al.* (1985) Elevated maternal glycohemoglobin in early pregnancy and spontaneous abortion among insulin dependent women. *Am. J. Obstet. Gynecol.*, **153**, 439–42.

110. Perrin, E.V.D.K.B. and Gilbert-Barness, E. (1989) Congenital anomalies and dysmorphology, in *Diseases of the Fetus and Newborn* (eds G.B. Reed, A.E. Claireaux and A.D. Bain), C.V. Mosby, St Louis, pp. 75–88.

111. Montoro, M., Collea, J.V., Frasier, S.D. and Mestman, J.H. (1981) Successful outcome of pregnancy in women with hypothyroidism. *Ann. Intern. Med.*, **94**, 31–4.

112. Stray-Pedersen, B. and Stray-Pedersen, S. (1984) Etiologic factors and subsequent reproductive performance in 195 couples with a prior history of habitual abortion. *Am. J. Obstet. Gynecol.*, **148**, 140–6.

113. Stagnaro-Green, A., Roman, S.H., Cobin, R.H. *et al.* (1990) Detection of at-risk pregnancy by means of highly sensitive assays for thyroid autoantibodies. *JAMA*, **264**, 1422–5.

114. Horta, J.L.H., Fernandez, J.G., de Leon, B.S. and Cortes-Gallegos, V.C. (1977) Direct evidence of luteal insufficiency in women with habitual abortion. *Obstet. Gynecol.*, **49**, 705–8.

115. Daya, S., Ward, S. and Burrows, E. (1988) Progesterone profiles in luteal phase defect cycles and outcome of progesterone treatment in patients with recurrent spontaneous abortion. *Am. J. Obstet. Gynecol.*, **158**, 225–32.

116. Daya, S. (1989) Efficacy of progesterone support for pregnancy in women with recurrent miscarriage. A meta-analysis of controlled trials. *Br. J. Obstet. Gynaecol.*, **96**, 275–80.

117. Check, J.H., Chase, J.W., Wu, C. *et al.* (1987) The efficacy of progesterone in achieving successful pregnancy: propholactic use during luteal phase in anovulatory women. *Int. J. Fertil.*, **32**, 135–8.

118. Check, J.H. and Adelson, H.G. (1987) The efficacy of progesterone in achieving successful pregnancy: in women with pure luteal phase defects. *Int. J. Fertil.*, **32**, 139–41.

119. Goldstein, P., Berrier, J., Rosen, S. *et al.* (1989) A meta-analysis of randomized control trials of

progestational agents in pregnancy. *Br. J. Obstet. Gynaecol.*, **96**, 265–74.

120. Mann, E.C. (1959) Habitual abortion: a report in two parts of 160 patients. *Am. J. Obstet. Gynecol.*, **77**, 706–18.

121. Wall, R.L. and Hertig, A.T. (1948) Habitual abortion: a pathologic analysis of 100 cases. *Am. J. Obstet. Gynecol.*, **56**, 1127–33.

122. Knowles, S. (1993) Spontaneous abortion and the pathology of early pregnancy, in *Fetal and Neonatal Pathology*, 2nd edn (ed. J.W. Keeling), Springer-Verlag, New York, pp. 95–110.

123. Kalousek, D.K. and Neave, C. (1991) Pathology of the abortion, the embryo and the previable fetus, in *Textbook of Fetal and Perinatal Pathology* (eds J.S. Wigglesworth and D.B. Singer), Blackwell Scientific, Boston, pp. 123–60.

124. De Vita, R., Calugi, A., Eleuteri, P. and Vizzone, A. (1993) Flow cytometric and cytogenetic analyses in human spontaneous abortions. *Hum. Genet.*, **91**, 409–15.

125. Ornoy, A., Salamon-Arnon, J., Ben-Zur, Z. and Kohn, G. (1981) Placental findings in spontaneous abortions and stillbirths. *Teratology*, **24**, 243–52.

126. Minguillon, C., Eiben, B., Bahr-Porsch, S. *et al.* (1989) Predictive value of chorionic villus histology for identifying chromosomally normal and abnormal spontaneous abortion. *Hum. Genet.*, **82**, 373–6.

5

PAIN AND BLEEDING IN EARLY PREGNANCY

B.T. Stuart

INTRODUCTION

Vaginal bleeding complicates 20% of diagnosed pregnancies[1] and figures from the Coombe Women's Hospital, Dublin, indicate that of those patients referred to hospital with vaginal bleeding in early pregnancy, only one third will have a viable pregnancy confirmed by having fetal heart activity demonstrated by ultrasonography (Table 5.1). Documented fetal heart activity is also a good prognostic sign, as even in the presence of vaginal bleeding, the subsequent miscarriage rate is only 12%[2]. Ultrasonographic imaging of the uterus and adnexae in cases of early pregnancy bleeding will, in most instances, enable a diagnosis to be made and appropriate treatment to be arranged. A transvaginal scan (TVS) can visualize the gestational sac as early as 4 weeks after the last menstrual period, the yolk sac by 5 weeks and a fetal node by 6 weeks after the last menstrual period[3]. With transabdominal ultrasonography the fetus can usually be seen by the 7th week after the last menstrual period and fetal heart activity detected soon after that[4].

Vaginal bleeding and abdominal pain are two of the most common complications of early pregnancy. Both are serious complaints that merit detailed investigation to determine the causation and prognosis for the pregnancy. In both instances an ultrasound examination plays a primary role in this investigation[5].

ABDOMINAL PAIN DUE TO PREGNANCY-RELATED CAUSES

Abdominal pain in early pregnancy may be due to both pregnancy related and other causes. The commonest obstetrical causes include miscarriage (especially in the second trimester) and ectopic pregnancy whereas fibroids, ovarian cysts and tumors are also recognized causes of abdominal pain in early pregnancy. Causes not directly obstetric in nature but often associated with pregnancy include appendicitis, renal and ureteric calculi, urinary retention, inflammatory bowel disease, colonic cancer and rupture of the splenic artery.

ECTOPIC PREGNANCY

Ectopic pregnancy is the commonest life-threatening cause of lower abdominal pain in

Table 5.1 Percentage of 2935 consecutive patients, clinically diagnosed as having an ongoing pregnancy, in whom fetal heart activity was and was not detected by ultrasound

	%
Fetal heart activity detected	37.2
Fetal heart activity not detected	62.8

Clinical Management of Early Pregnancy. Edited by Walter Prendiville and James R. Scott.
Published in 1999 by Arnold, ISBN 0 340 74100 7

early pregnancy. The incidence of ectopic pregnancy increased threefold in the US between 1970 and 1983[6] to a rate of 14 per 1000 reported pregnancies. Ectopic pregnancy is dealt with more fully in Chapter 7 and comment here is limited to some observations concerning the diagnosis of ectopic pregnancy.

RISK FACTORS FOR ECTOPIC PREGNANCY

There are certain well-defined groups at increased risk of ectopic pregnancy. Factors known to be associated with an increased susceptibility to ectopic pregnancy include a previous ectopic pregnancy[7], history of pelvic inflammatory disease[8], the progesterone only contraceptive pill, intrauterine contraceptive devices[9], infertility, tubal surgery[10] and *in vitro* fertilization[11]. The diagnosis of ectopic pregnancy remains problematic for the spectrum of clinical presentation is wide, symptoms vary and physical signs are often unconvincing. The diagnosis of ectopic pregnancy depends on a high degree of clinical awareness, the 'ectopic mindedness' suggested by Zlatnik. However, the combination of rapid hormonal assay (progesterone and human chorionic gonadotrophin (hCG)) and transvaginal ultrasonography has transformed the investigation of suspected ectopic pregnancy from a physical and surgical approach, often involving early recourse to laparoscopy, to a non-invasive bedside protocol. This is particularly true for the unruptured ectopic. This subject is dealt with more fully in Chapter 6.

DIAGNOSIS OF ECTOPIC PREGNANCY

Any woman of child-bearing age with lower abdominal pain should be suspected of having an ectopic pregnancy. Most textbooks of obstetrics and gynecology contain flow charts relating to the diagnosis of ectopic pregnancy[12]. The availability of emergency maternal β-hCG assay greatly simplifies the management of cases of suspected ectopic pregnancy for a negative test excludes pregnancy. Urinary ELISA pregnancy tests are also very reliable and a negative test effectively excludes a diagnosis of pregnancy[13]. Ultrasound imaging of the pelvis is commonly used in cases of suspected ectopic pregnancy. Before 6 weeks transvaginal scanning (TVS) is to be preferred to transabdominal scanning as the higher resolution available leads to an increase in diagnostic rates[14]. The presence of intrauterine fetal echoes with fetal heart activity makes the diagnosis of ectopic pregnancy unlikely (quoted as 1:30 000) but the finding of an intrauterine echo-free space is not helpful in excluding an ectopic pregnancy as this may represent a pseudogestation sac or endometrial cyst and may co-exist with ectopic pregnancy[15,16]. The size of the intrauterine sac is also not helpful as the pseudogestation sac of ectopic pregnancy can be quite large (Figure 5.1) although it will contain neither fetal echoes nor fetal heart activity. The demonstration of an embryo in the adnexae makes the diagnosis of ectopic pregnancy certain and will be found in some 20% of cases of ectopic pregnancy if TVS is used[17].

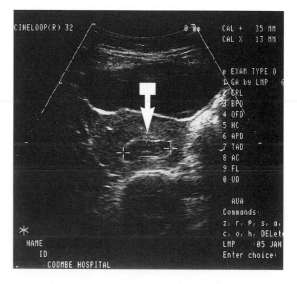

Figure 5.1. Large pseudogestation sac in a case of ectopic pregnancy.

DIAGNOSIS OF ECTOPIC PREGNANCY BEFORE TUBAL RUPTURE

Conservative treatment of ectopic pregnancy offers the best hope for the patient's future fertility and strenuous efforts are now being made toward making a diagnosis of ectopic pregnancy before tubal rupture. Early diagnosis provides the possibility of conserving the tube at laparotomy, removing the ectopic pregnancy laparoscopically[18], or treating it medically with methotrexate[19]. The relative inability of even the latest high resolution transvaginal probes to improve the early diagnosis of ectopic pregnancy has led several groups to explore other avenues of diagnosis. Many of these methods are based on the serial measurement of β-hCG either in isolation, or in association with ultrasonographic findings. Trophoblast tissue associated with ectopic pregnancy secretes less hCG than that associated with intrauterine pregnancy[20] and the rate of increase and 'doubling time' in serum β-hCG concentration can be used to differentiate between patients with intrauterine and extrauterine pregnancies[21]. In the study quoted, an increase of more than 285 IU/l per day was highly diagnostic of intrauterine pregnancy (positive predictive value 95.4%) whereas a value less than this figure suggested ectopic pregnancy (positive predictive value 94.7%).

Low levels of maternal serum progesterone are also found in cases of ectopic pregnancy and abnormal intrauterine pregnancy and a cut-off point of 15 ng/ml has been used to distinguish between normal and abnormal gestations[22]. A number of authors have described simple algorithms for the early and non-invasive management of ectopic pregnancy[23].

In a further effort to improve the early diagnosis of ectopic pregnancy with ultrasound both pulsed Doppler and colour flow methods have been used. Ectopic pregnancy is associated with increased blood flow to the affected tube and an associated reduction in tubal vascular resistance that can be detected with transvaginal pulsed Doppler[24].

VAGINAL BLEEDING IN EARLY INTRAUTERINE PREGNANCY

In the presence of an intrauterine gestation the differential diagnosis of vaginal bleeding in early pregnancy depends on the presence or absence of fetal heart pulsations. Whereas echo free areas can be visualized within the uterus with TVS as early as 4.5 weeks[25] these areas are not diagnostic of intrauterine pregnancy as both the pseudogestation sac of ectopic pregnancy and an endometrial cyst can give a very similar appearance. The presence of fetal heart activity in an intrauterine gestation sac is both diagnostic of intrauterine pregnancy and a good prognostic sign. In the absence of vaginal bleeding the subsequent miscarriage rate after the identification of fetal heart activity is 2% in singleton pregnancies and 21% in twin pregnancies[26]. Even in the presence of vaginal bleeding the demonstration of fetal heart activity is associated with a successful outcome in the majority of cases with only 12% of such pregnancies resulting in pregnancy failure[2]. Using TVS, fetal heart activity can usually be demonstrated by 41–43 days menstrual age[27] when the mean gestation sac diameter is approximately 14 mm.

ABSENT FETAL HEART ACTIVITY

The absence of fetal heart activity in a gestation sac larger than 15 mm is usually indicative of early pregnancy failure although the precise gestation at which the fetal heart will be detected may vary depending on the availability of TVS, the quality of the scanning equipment and the experience and expertise of the sonologist. If there is doubt as to whether the fetal heart is present or absent it is prudent to arrange a repeat ultrasound examination in 7–10 days as this examination should dispel all doubts.

GESTATION SAC SIZE

The gestation sac begins to grow at approximately 29 days menstrual age and increases at a rate of a millimeter a day so that it is possible to calculate gestational age from the mean sac diameter using Rossavik's simple formula[28]:

Gestational age (days)
$$= \text{Gestational sac diameter (mm)} + 29$$

Thus, it is a simple matter to calculate expected gestational sac size for any gestation prior to 10 weeks. A small sac size for gestational age is associated with increased risk of early pregnancy failure[29] though obviously it is imperative to ensure that this does not represent wrong dates. A repeat ultrasound examination will confirm poorer than expected growth in sac size between examinations.

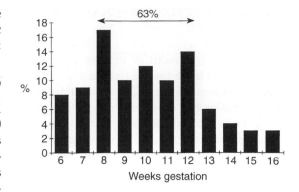

Figure 5.2. Percentage of patients presenting with bleeding in early pregnancy at each week of gestation.

BLEEDING IN EARLY PREGNANCY

Although today's obstetrician need only refer to one of the older textbooks to learn of the diagnostic and therapeutic dilemmas faced by our predecessors in the management of vaginal bleeding in early pregnancy the basic principle remains the same in that 'loss of blood, no matter how slight, in the early months of pregnancy, should always be regarded with suspicion'[30]. Two thirds of cases of early pregnancy bleeding referred to hospital, present between the 8th and 12th weeks of pregnancy and the percentage of patients referred to the author's hospital with early pregnancy bleeding during each week of gestation from the 6th to the 16th week inclusive are shown in Figure 5.2.

Bimanual or digital pelvic examination unaided by biochemical or ultrasound assessment of such cases often results in the inappropriately optimistic clinical diagnosis of 'threatened abortion'. Even in patients who present with vaginal spotting not associated with pain, the rate of pregnancy loss is 58% whereas if the bleeding was painful this figure rose to 80%, even in cases where the cervix was closed at the time of vaginal examination[31]. In a series of almost 3000 patients with early pregnancy bleeding, scanned at the Coombe Women's Hospital between January 1989 and December 1994 and in whom a diagnosis of 'threatened abortion' was made following clinical examination based on the finding of an enlarged pregnant uterus and a closed cervix, only 37% had an ongoing pregnancy, defined by the presence of fetal heart activity in an intrauterine gestation, at ultrasound examination the same day (Table 5.1). This figure is similar to those published two decades ago from the author's hospital which showed that of patients admitted to hospital with early pregnancy bleeding only 32.5% of pregnancies continued[32].

Transabdominal ultrasonographic findings in 2935 consecutive cases of early pregnancy bleeding who had been diagnosed as having a 'threatened abortion' on the basis of history and clinical examination are shown in Table 5.2. The diagnosis of threatened abortion is confirmed by ultrasonography if fetal heart activity is present in an intrauterine gestation; incomplete abortion refers to the presence of retained products of conception; anembryonic pregnancy to the finding of a gestation sac of >20 mm size without an embryo; missed abortion to the presence of an embryo with no cardiac activity; complete abortion to a uterus with no residual tissue in a patient with a positive urinary pregnancy test and molar pregnancy to cases demonstrating the

Table 5.2 Ultrasonographic diagnosis in 2935 consecutive cases of early pregnancy bleeding scanned at the Coombe Women's Hospital

	%
Threatened abortion	37.2
Incomplete abortion	27.1
Anembryonic pregnancy	19.9
Missed abortion	7.5
Complete abortion	7.4
Molar pregnancy	0.9

characteristic 'snow storm' effect *in utero*. Although some authors prefer the term 'early pregnancy failure' or 'early fetal death'[33] the above description has the merit of defining not only the etiology of the miscarriage but also the need for further treatment such as evacuation of retained products of conception. The author also recognizes that many now prefer to use the term 'miscarriage' rather than 'abortion' although older books use these terms to define pregnancy loss in the second and first trimesters respectively[30].

THREATENED ABORTION

This diagnosis is frequently made in clinical practice either as a result of taking a history of slight vaginal spotting or consequent upon the finding of a closed cervix at subsequent vaginal examination. A definitive diagnosis of threatened abortion should, however, only be made following ultrasonographic examination which shows the presence of fetal heart activity in an intrauterine pregnancy. If present, this is usually seen quite readily during the examination and is easier to document on videotape than with M-mode which, in the author's opinion is a more cumbersome way of documenting fetal heart activity in early pregnancy than the A-mode scans found on earlier generations of ultrasound machines.

A normal fetal heart rate for the gestation is a good prognostic indicator but the finding of a fetal bradycardia at the time of scan is associated with increased subsequent fetal loss.

Tables of normal fetal heart rates in early pregnancy (6 weeks to 11 weeks) with lower limit cut-off values have been published[34]. There is no evidence that bed rest is beneficial in the treatment of threatened abortion[35]. Early fetal death subsequently occurs in 12% of patients with ultrasound-confirmed threatened abortion[2]. There is little treatment to offer the patient with threatened abortion. During the 1940s and 1950s hormonal supplementation with either estrogen or progesterone was used though there is no experimental evidence in appropriately controlled trials that these are in any way beneficial[36] and subsequent events have shown the association between *in-utero* diethylstilbesterol (DES) exposure and the subsequent development of vaginal adenosis and clear cell adenocarcinoma.

INCOMPLETE ABORTION

The value of an ultrasound examination in cases of early pregnancy bleeding is that it not only establishes the presence of a viable fetus or early pregnancy failure but it also defines the need for subsequent treatment. Conventionally, cases of early pregnancy failure with the demonstrated presence of retained products of conception (Figure 5.3) are classified as cases of incomplete abortion and have been treated by surgical evacuation of the uterus in order to prevent complications such as hemorrhage and endometritis. Due to the frequency of early pregnancy failure these cases form a significant part of the surgical workload in maternity hospitals as well as occupying bed space and consuming significant resources. During 1993, 705 cases of evacuation of retained products of conception were performed in the Coombe Women's Hospital and this comprised 13.4% of the total number of gynecological cases[37].

It has long been suspected that a significant proportion of patients with small amounts of retained products of conception could probably be allowed to pass these products

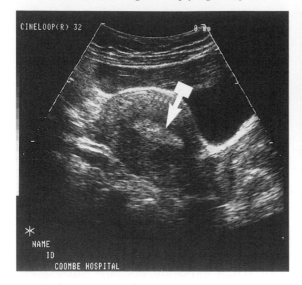

Figure 5.3. Sonogram showing retained products of conception (arrowed).

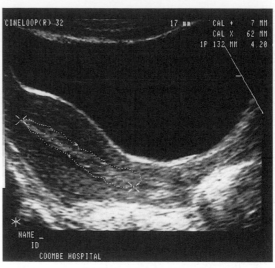

Figure 5.4. Sonogram demonstrating quantitative measurement of retained products of conception.

spontaneously without recourse to surgical evacuation and without any detrimental effects to themselves. Haines *et al.*[38] measured the uterine cavity area after surgical evacuation to define the population who might not need surgical intervention after incomplete abortion and concluded that the measurement limits where this could be considered after ultrasonographic evaluation in cases of early pregnancy included a width of 5 cm and a cavity surface area of 6 cm² on a saggital scan (Figure 5.4). Medical evacuation of the uterus is now an effective alternative to surgery and without its attendant risks. The combination of the progesterone synthesis inhibitor Trilostane, and prostaglandin methyl $F_{2\alpha}$ has been shown effectively to empty the uterus in cases of incomplete and missed abortion[39]. More recently, mifepristone has been used to medically evacuate intrauterine pregnancy[40,41]. Finally, there is evidence to support the further clinical investigation of expectant management in selected cases of incomplete miscarriage[42].

ANEMBRYONIC PREGNANCY

The diagnosis of anembryonic pregnancy is readily made on scan and was described by Donald[43]. Typical findings are a large gestation sac (>20 mm on transabdominal scan and >16 mm on TVS) without fetal echoes (Figure 5.5). The shape of the sac is often irregular and the decidual ring thin. Over the past 20 years the incidence of anembryonic pregnancy in the Coombe Women's Hospital has remained within the range 11–20% of all spontaneous abortions. Occasionally, errors in diagnosis may be made because of suspect dates[32] and in cases where the gestation sac is well formed and round with a good trophoblast ring, re-examination a week later will dispel any doubt. Following a number of instances in which fetal death was erroneously diagnosed at ultrasound examination, the Royal College of Radiologists and the Royal College of Obstetricians and Gynaecologists jointly issued a guidance document[44] on ultrasound examinations in early pregnancy which clearly defines the protocol to be adopted in cases where doubt exists concerning the ultrasonographic findings in cases of bleeding in early pregnancy.

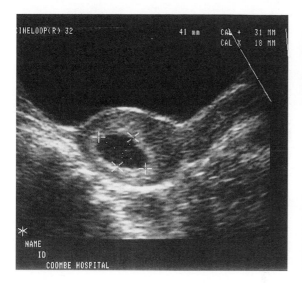

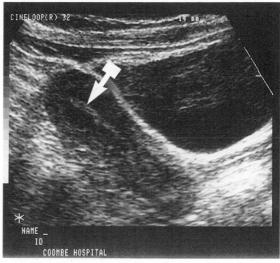

Figure 5.5. Sonogram of an anembryonic pregnancy (blighted ovum).

Figure 5.6. Sonogram showing an empty uterine cavity (arrowed) in a case of complete abortion.

MISSED ABORTION

This condition is characterized by the presence within the gestation sac of a fetus without cardiac activity. It commonly presents in the second trimester and may be associated with a diminution or disappearance in the symptoms of pregnancy. The fetus is frequently smaller than expected for gestation and ultimate fetal demise may be presaged by fetal bradycardia noted at previous examinations[45].

COMPLETE ABORTION

Complete spontaneous expulsion of uterine contents in cases of early pregnancy failure occurs in 8–17% of cases[31]. This is often associated with cessation of pain and a reduction in the volume of vaginal bleeding. The diagnosis is readily confirmed by ultrasonography where the uterine cavity will be seen to be empty (Figure 5.6). The differential diagnosis includes ectopic pregnancy (see Chapter 7) and a non-pregnant uterus with the passage of a decidual cast. In the series reported by Drumm only three of 122 (2.5%) patients who were discharged without evacuation of the uterus after an ultrasonographic diagnosis of complete abortion had to be re-admitted to hospital because of vaginal bleeding and in none of the three cases were products of conception obtained at subsequent curettage.

GESTATIONAL TROPHOBLASTIC DISEASE (HYDATIDIFORM MOLE)

Gestational trophoblastic disease is an uncommon but serious cause of vaginal bleeding in early pregnancy in Europe and the United States. It is more common in South East Asia where an incidence of 1 in 823 viable pregnancies has been reported[46], being most common in women over 45 years old (1 in 72 pregnancies) and teenagers (1 in 311 pregnancies). The incidence in women between 25 and 39 years was 1 in 1150 pregnancies which is similar to the incidence reported from the USA[47] although other authors put the incidence in the US at 1 in 2500 pregnancies with choriocarcinoma occurring in approximately 1 in 500 000 pregnancies[48]. The incidence of molar pregnancy in Dublin is 1 in 512 pregnancies[49].

In gestational trophoblast disease the uterus is typically large for dates[50], although it may also be small for dates[51], and may be filled with vesicular molar tissue with no evidence of embryonic or fetal tissues (complete mole). Such moles usually have a 46,XX chromosome complement[52] with the chromosomes being entirely of paternal origin and arising as a result of fertilization of an ovum with a chromosome which then replicates, maternal chromosomes being absent or inactive. In other cases molar degeneration may be limited to part of the placenta and fetal tissue may be present. Fetuses in cases of partial mole often display the features of triploidy or tetraploidy[53] and it has been suggested that partial moles are the result of fertilization of a normal ovum by two spermatazoa[54]. Complete and partial moles appear to be associated with different etiological factors and whereas complete mole is commoner in pregnant women over the age of 35 years, no such association has been found in the case of partial moles[55].

DIAGNOSIS OF GESTATIONAL TROPHOBLASTIC DISEASE

Hydatidiform mole should be suspected in all cases of early pregnancy bleeding particularly where the patient is in a high risk category. Vaginal bleeding is the commonest presenting complaint and vesicles may have been passed vaginally with the patient usually describing them as 'grapes'. The uterus is more commonly large than small for dates and fetal heart activity will not be present on listening with Doppler. Hyperemesis may be present and pre-eclampsia occurs in 10% of cases[56]. Hydatidiform mole is one of the few conditions causing pre-eclampsia before the 20th week of pregnancy.

The diagnosis of molar pregnancy is usually made by ultrasonography although the typical fluid-filled vesicles do not develop until the 10th week of pregnancy and therefore the diagnosis may be missed in very early pregnancy[57]. Ultrasonography gives the typical 'snowstorm' appearance (Figure 5.7) and ovarian theca lutein cysts may be present, unilateral in 8% of cases and bilateral in 12%[56]. Maternal β-hCG levels are excessively raised and form the basis of a tumor marker for follow-up. Pulmonary, liver and renal metastases may be present. Invasive investigative techniques including amniography, pelvic arteriography and uterine sounding are not now used. In all cases the diagnosis should be confirmed by histopathological examination of tissue. A discussion on the treatment and follow-up of cases of gestational trophoblastic disease is beyond the scope of this chapter.

ABDOMINAL PAIN DUE TO CAUSES OTHER THAN PREGNANCY

Abdominal pain is a common reason for hospital admission in premenopausal women and in 29% of cases no diagnosis is ever made. In a series of 100 consecutive cases admitted to the Mater Hospital in Dublin[58] it was found that 23% of cases were due to histologically confirmed acute appendicitis, 20% were due to

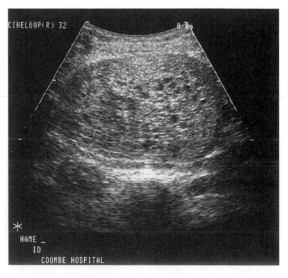

Figure 5.7. Sonogram showing the 'snowstorm effect' of molar pregnancy.

ovarian cysts, 9% to renal tract disorders (urinary tract infection and calculi), 5% to pelvic inflammatory disease and 9% to miscellaneous conditions of the bowel including inflamed Meckel's diverticulum, Crohn's disease, *Enterobius vermicularis* infestation, obstruction secondary to adhesions and gastroenteritis. Overall 30% of all cases were considered to be due to disease of the female reproductive tract.

The problem facing the doctor treating a woman in the reproductive years who presents with abdominal pain is differentiating between those causes associated with pregnancy (miscarriage, ectopic), and other causes unrelated to pregnancy, for a history of amenorrhea or pregnancy is neither always obtained, nor necessarily reliable. The gynecologist will generally consider all such patients to have an ectopic pregnancy until proven otherwise. The availability of a rapid radioimmunoassay (RIA) of maternal serum β-hCG is a particularly valuable test as it will detect pregnancy 8 days after fertilization[59] and in practical terms a negative RIA β-hcG test excludes pregnancy.

In a series of 170 emergency cases admitted to a London teaching hospital the pregnancy test was found to be positive in 75% of cases and the primary reason for admission in 39% of pregnant patients was pelvic pain[60]. Routine sonography of these patients altered management in 33% of cases and the most valuable contribution was to confirm an intrauterine pregnancy in cases of suspected ectopic gestation.

FIBROIDS AND PREGNANCY

Previously asymptomatic fibroids may cause acute pain in pregnancy due to red degeneration (necrobiosis). This may be associated with fever, leukocytosis and the development of a surgical acute abdomen[61]. The diagnosis may be suspected by finding a localized area of exquisite tenderness in the uterus and the presence of a myoma may be confirmed by ultrasonography (Figure 5.8). Areas of cystic

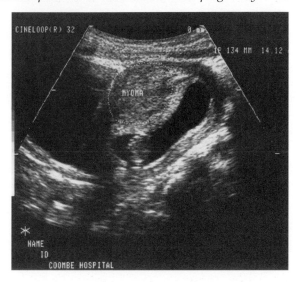

Figure 5.8. Sonogram of a pregnancy in a patient with a uterine myoma.

degeneration may be noted within the fibroid. Conservative treatment is the rule with appropriate analgesia often resulting in the rapid resolution of symptoms. Torsion of a pedunculated subserous fibroid may necessitate laparotomy but the general rule is that myomectomy should not be carried out during pregnancy because of the danger of uncontrollable hemorrhage.

OVARIAN LESIONS

Corpus luteum cysts are common in early pregnancy[62] and are usually less than 6 cm in size (Figure 5.9). Larger cysts may be found and haemorrhage into the cyst may result in a suspicious appearance on ultrasonography. It is generally considered that the corpus luteum of pregnancy secretes progesterone which helps maintain the pregnancy until the placenta takes over at the end of the first trimester and that removal of a corpus luteum cyst, if necessary, should be postponed until the second trimester. More recently, aspiration of simple unilocular ovarian cysts has been performed under ultrasound guidance[63] with

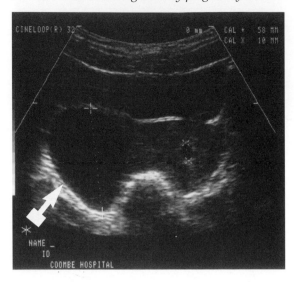

Figure 5.9. Sonogram of a pregnancy in a patient with an ovarian cyst (arrowed).

satisfactory outcome and this is suggested as an alternative treatment for cysts more than 6 cm in diameter that cannot be safely treated conservatively.

Dermoid cysts (benign cystic dermatoma) are the commonest true ovarian neoplasms encountered during pregnancy and may undergo torsion resulting in acute abdominal pain. The ultrasonographic features of dermoid cysts are variable and six different appearances have been described[64] varying from the purely cystic to the densely echogenic, the latter being the most common and being found in a third of all cases. This may make differentiation from malignancy difficult although ovarian malignancy is very uncommon during pregnancy[62].

GASTROINTESTINAL LESIONS

Acute appendicitis is the commonest surgical emergency during pregnancy[65]. Although the diagnosis is often difficult in the latter part of pregnancy due to the displacement of the appendix by the enlarging uterus; in early pregnancy the diagnosis is more likely to be made before perforation of the appendix[66] as the symptoms closely resemble those found in the non-pregnant patient.

Disease of the gall bladder is the second commonest surgical condition requiring treatment in pregnancy[67] affecting approximately 1 in 1000 pregnancies. The management of acute cholecystitis and biliary obstruction during pregnancy is the same as in the non-pregnant patient and the outcome for the fetus appears to be optimal if any surgery required can be performed during the second trimester.

Acute pancreatitis is a less common cause of abdominal pain in pregnancy occurring in 1 in 1100 deliveries[68]. Although it typically occurs in late pregnancy, acute pancreatitis can occur at any gestation and the presentation is the same as in the non-pregnant patient with acute abdominal pain, mainly in the epigastrium and often radiating through to the back. Less common causes of acute abdominal pain in early pregnancy include intestinal obstruction, colonic carcinoma and peptic ulceration.

RENAL DISEASE

Acute pyelonephritis complicates 1–2% of all pregnancies and usually presents as acute loin pain on the affected side accompanied by fever, rigors, dysuria and vomiting. The diagnosis is confirmed by culture of a mid-stream urine sample. Renal colic occurs in approximately 1 in 1500 pregnancies[69], although it is most likely to occur during the second and third trimester or during the puerperium. Colic is equally likely to occur on the right and left sides[70] and there is usually either gross or microscopic hematuria. The diagnosis may be confirmed by modified intravenous urogram. Spontaneous passage of the calculus occurs in up to 50% of cases[71]. Acute urinary retention may occur at the end of the first trimester of pregnancy, often associated with retroversion of the uterus. The diagnosis is usually self-evident as the patient complains of lower abdominal pain due to distension of the bladder and associated anuria of short duration, although, in some patients overflow incontinence may confuse the unwary.

Occasionally, acute abdominal pain in pregnancy may be due to spontaneous rupture of the liver, uterine veins, splenic artery aneurysm or hematoma of the rectus abdominis muscle.

REFERENCES

1. Strobino, B.A. and Pantel-Silverman, J. (1987) First trimester vaginal bleeding and the loss of chromosomally normal and abnormal conceptions. *Am. J. Obstet. Gynecol.*, **157**, 1150–4.
2. Hill, L.M., Guzick, D., Fries, J. *et al.* (1990) Fetal loss rate after ultrasonically documented cardiac activity between 6 and 14 weeks menstrual age. *J. Clin. Ultrasound*, **19**, 221–3.
3. Warren, W.B., Timor Trisch, I., Peisner, D.B. *et al.* (1989) Dating the early pregnancy by the sequential appearance of embryonic structures. *Am. J. Obstet. Gynecol.*, **161**, 747–9.
4. Jeanty, P. and Romero, R. (1984) *Obstetrical Ultrasound*, McGraw–Hill, New York, p. 39.
5. Jauniaux, E., Gavriil, P. and Nicolaides, K.H. (1996) Ultrasonographic assessment of early pregnancy complications, in *Ultrasound and Early Pregnancy* (eds D. Jurkovic and E. Jauniaux), Parthenon, Carnforth, pp. 53–64.
6. Doyle, M.B., DeCherney, A.H. and Diamond, M.P. (1991) Epidemiology and etiology of ectopic pregnancy. *Obstet. Gynecol. Clin. North Am.*, **18**, 1–17.
7. Nordenskjold, F. and Ahlgren, M. (1991) Risk factors in ectopic pregnancy: results of a population based case controlled study. *Acta Obstet. Gynecol. Scand.*, **70**, 575–9.
8. Westrom, L., Bengtsson, L.P.H. and Mardh, P.A. (1981) Incidence, trends and risks of ectopic pregnancy in a population of women. *Br. Med. J.*, **282**, 15–18.
9. Wong-Ho, C., Daling, J.R., Weiss, N.S. *et al.* (1986) IUD use and subsequent tubal ectopic pregnancy. *Am. J. Public Health*, **76**, 536–9.
10. Hughes, G.J. (1979) The early diagnosis of ectopic pregnancy. *Br. J. Surg.*, **66**, 789–92.
11. Martinez, F. and Trounson, A. (1986) An analysis of factors associated with ectopic pregnancy in a human in vitro fertilisation programme. *Fertil. Steril.*, **45**, 79–87.
12. Turner, G. (1989) Ectopic pregnancy, in *Obstetrics* (eds Sir A. Turnbull and G. Chamberlain), Churchill Livingstone, Edinburgh, pp. 443–52.
13. Christensen, H., Thyssen, H.H., Schebye, O., *et al.* (1990) Three highly sensitive 'bedside' serum and urine tests for pregnancy compared. *Clin. Chem.*, **36**, 1686–8.
14. Ferrazzi, E., Garbo, S., Sulpizio, P. *et al.* (1993) Miscarriage diagnosis and gestational age estimation in the early first trimester of pregnancy: transabdominal versus transvaginal sonography. *Ultrasound Obstet. Gynecol.*, **3**, 36–41.
15. Ackerman, T.E., Levi, C.S., Lyons, E.A. *et al.* (1993) Decidual cyst: endovaginal sonographic sign of ectopic pregnancy. *Radiology*, **189**, 727–31.
16. Fleischer, S.C., Pennell, R.G., McKee, M.S. *et al.* (1990) Ectopic pregnancy: features at transvaginal sonography. *Radiology*, **174**, 375–8.
17. Timor-Tritsch, I.E., Yeh, M.N., Peisner, D.B. *et al.* (1989) The use of transvaginal ultrasonography in the diagnosis of ectopic pregnancy. *Obstet. Gynecol.*, **161**, 157–61.
18. De Cherney, A.H. and Diamond, M.P. (1987) Laparoscopic salpingostomy for ectopic pregnancy. *Obstet. Gynecol.*, **71**, 889–92.
19. Wolf, G.C. and Witt, B.R. (1991) Outpatient laparoscopic management of ectopic pregnancy with a local methotrexate injection. *J. Reprod. Med.*, **36**, 489–92.
20. Cust, M.P. and Filshie, G.M. (1991) Modern management of ectopic pregnancy. *Curr. Obstet. Gynaecol.*, **1**, 210–16.
21. Lindblom, B., Hahlin, M. and Sjoblom, P. (1989) *Am. J. Obstet. Gynecol.*, **161**, 397–400.
22. Yeko, T.R., Gorill, M.W., Hughes, L.H. *et al.* (1987) Timely diagnosis of ectopic pregnancy using a single blood progesterone measurement. *Fertil. Seteril.*, **48**, 1048–50.
23. Stovall, T.G. and Ling, F.W. (1993) Ectopic pregnancy – diagnostic and therapeutic algorithms minimising surgical intervention. *J. Reprod. Med.*, **38**, 807.
24. Kirchler, H.Ch., Kolle, D. and Schwegel, P. (1994) Changes in tubal blood flow in evaluating ectopic pregnancy. *Ultrasound Obstet. Gynaecol.*, **2**, 283–8.
25. Yeh, H.-C., Goodman, J.D., Carr, L. *et al.* (1986) Intradecidual sign: A U.S. criterion of early intrauterine pregnancy. *Radiology*, **161**, 463–7.
26. Benson, C.B., Doubilet, P.M. and Laks, M.P. (1993) Outcome of twin gestations following sonographic demonstration of two heart beats

in the first trimester. *Ultrasound Obstet. Gynaecol.*, **3**, 343–5.

27. Cadkin, A.V. and McAlpin, J. (1984) Detection of fetal cardiac activity between 41 and 43 days of gestation. *J. Ultrasound Med.*, **3**, 499–503.

28. Rossavik, J. (1991) *Practical Obstetrical Ultrasound With and Without a Computer*. First Word Publishing Company, Oklahoma, p. 19.

29. Bromley, B., Harlow, B.L., Laboda, L.A. *et al.* (1991) Small sac size in the first trimester as a predictor of poor fetal outcome. *Radiology*, **178**, 375–8.

30. Williams, J.W. (1930) *Obstetrics*, 6th edn. Appleton, New York, p. 768.

31. Drumm, J.E. (1981) The value of ultrasonography in the management of first trimester haemorrhage. *Prog. Obstet. Gynaecol.*, **1**, 30–8.

32. Drumm, J.E. and Clinch, J. (1975) Ultrasound in the management of clinically diagnosed threatened abortion. *Br. Med. J.*, **2**, 424.

33. Levi, C.S., Dashefsky, S.M., Lyons, E.A. *et al.* (1994) First trimester ultrasound: a practical approach, in *Diagnostic Obstetrical Ultrasound* (eds J.P. McGahan and M. Porto), J.B. Lippincot, Philadelphia, pp. 1–25.

34. Achiron, R., Tadmor, O. and Maschiach, S. (1991) Heart rate as a predictor of first trimester spontaneous abortion after ultrasound proven viability. *Obstet. Gynecol.*, **78**, 330–3.

35. Crowther, C. and Chalmers, I. (1990) Bed rest and hospitalisation in pregnancy, in *Effective Care in Pregnancy and Childbirth* (eds I. Chalmers, I.M. Enkin and M.J.N. Keirse), Oxford University Press, Oxford, pp. 624–32.

36. Klopper, A. (1992) Endocrine support of early pregnancy, in *Obstetrics in the 1990s: Current Controversies* (eds T. Chard and M.P.M. Richards), Mac Keith Press, London, pp. 43–64.

37. Coombe Women's Hospital, Dublin (1993) *Annual Clinical Report*.

38. Haines, C.J., Shand, K.L. and Leung, D.Y.L. (1991) Transvaginal sonography of the uterine cavity following curettage for early pregnancy failure. *Ultrasound Obstet. Gynaecol.*, **1**, 417–19.

39. Paraskevaides, E., Prendiville, W., Stuart, B. *et al.* (1992) Medical evacuation of first trimester incomplete abortion and missed abortion. *J. Gynaecol. Surg.*, **8**, 159–63.

40. El Rafaey, H., Rajasekar, D., Abdallah, M. *et al.* (1995) Induction of abortion with mifepristone and oral or vaginal misoprostol. *N. Engl. J. Med.*, **332**, 983–7.

41. Hinshaw, K. (1997) Medical management of miscarriage, in *Problems in Early Pregnancy: Advances in Diagnosis and Management* (eds J.G. Grudzinskas and P.M.S. O'Brien), Royal College of Obstetricians and Gynaecologists, London.

42. Chipchase, J. and James, D. (1997) Randomised trial of expectant versus surgical management of spontaneous miscarriage. *Br. J. Obstet. Gynaecol.*, **104**, 840–1.

43. Donald, I. (1977) Ultrasonic investigations in obstetrics and gynaecology, in *Ultrasonics in Clinical Diagnosis*, 2nd edn (ed. P.N.T. Wells), Churchill Livingstone, Edinburgh, p. 62.

44. Royal College of Radiologists and Royal College of Obstetricians and Gynaecologists (1995) *Guidance on Ultrasound Procedures in Early Pregnancy*.

45. Laboda, L.A., Estroff, J.A. and Benacerraf, B.R. (1989) First trimester bradycardia: a sign of impending fetal loss. *J. Ultrasound Med.*, **8**, 561–3.

46. Teoh, E.-S. (1988) Asian approaches in the treatment of trophoblastic disease. *Obstet. Gynecol. Clin. North Am.*, **15**, 545–64.

47. Teoh, E.-S., Dawood, M.Y., Ratnam, S.S. *et al.* (1971) Epidemiology of hydatidiform mole in Singapore. *Am. J. Obstet. Gynecol.*, **110**, 415–20.

48. Novak, E.R., Jones, G.S. and Jones, H.W. (1970) Trophoblast disease, in *Novaks' Textbook of Gynecology*. Williams & Wilkins, Baltimore, p. 516.

49. Rotunda Hospital (1998) Annual Clinical Report. Rotunda Hospital, Dublin.

50. Szulman, A.E. and Surti, U. (1982) The clinicopathological profile of the partial hydatidiform mole. *Obstet. Gynecol.*, **59**, 597–602.

51. Smith, D.B., O'Reilly, S.M. and Newlands, E.S. (1993) Current approaches to diagnosis and treatment of gestational trophoblastic disease. *Curr. Opin. Obstet. Gynecol.*, **5**, 84–91.

52. Kajii, T. and Ohama, K. (1977) Androgenetic origin of hydatidiform mole. *Nature*, **268**, 633–4.

53. Dehner, L.P. (1980) Gestational and nongestational trophoblastic neoplasia. *Am. J. Surg. Pathol.*, **4**, 43–58.

54. Lawler, S.D., Fischer, R.A. and Dent, J. (1991) A prospective genetic study of complete and partial hydatidiform moles. *Am. J. Obstet. Gynecol.*, **164**, 1270–7.

55. Parazzani, F., Mangili, G., La Vecchia, C. *et al.* (1991) Risk factors for gestational trophoblastic disease: a separate analysis of complete and partial hydatidiform moles. *Obstet. Gynecol.*, **78**, 1039–45.

56. Ratnam, S.S. and Ilancheran, A.H. (1982)

Disease of the trophoblast. *Clin. Obstet. Gynecol.*, **9**, 539–64.

57. Hill, L.M. (1994) Placental abnormalities. *Diagnostic Ultrasound Applied to Obstetrics and Gynecology*, 3rd edn (ed. R. Sabbaggha), J.B. Lippincott, Philadelphia, pp. 308.

58. O'Byrne, J.M., Dempsey, C.B., O'Malley, M.K. *et al.* (1991) Non-specific abdominal pain in premenopausal women. *Ir. J. Med. Sci.*, **160**, 344–6.

59. Wilson, E.A. (1990) The laboratory diagnosis of pregnancy, in *Current Therapy in Obstetrics and Gynecology*, (eds E.J. Quilligan and F.P. Zuspan), W.B. Saunders, Philadelphia, pp. 248.

60. Mould, T.A.J., Byrne, D.L. and Morton, K.E. (1992) The role of ultrasound in gynaecological emergencies. *Ultrasound Obstet. Gynaecol.*, **2**, 121–3.

61. Novak, E.R., Jones, G.S. and Jones, H.W. (1970) Myoma of the uterus, in *Novaks' Textbook of Gynecology*. Williams & Wilkins, Baltimore, p. 324.

62. Fleischer, A.C., Boehm, F.H. and James, A.E. Jr (1985) Sonographic evaluation of pelvic masses and maternal disorders occurring during pregnancy, in *The Principles and Practice of Ultrasonography in Obstetrics and Gynecology*, 3rd edn (eds R.C. Saunders and A.E. James A. Jr), Appleton–Century–Crofts, New York, pp. 435–47.

63. Aboulghar, M., Mansour, R. and Serour, G. (1992) Ovarian cysts during pregnancy: the role of ultrasonically guided transvaginally aspiration. *Ultrasound Obstet. Gynaecol.*, **2**, 349–51.

64. Cohen, L. and Sabbagha, R. (1993) Echo patterns of benign cystic teratomas by transvaginal ultrasound. *Ultrasound Obstet. Gynaecol.*, **3**, 120–3.

65. Levine, W. and Diamond, B. (1961) Surgical procedures during pregnancy. *Am. J. Obstet. Gynecol.*, **81**, 1046–52.

66. Finch, D.R.A. and Lee, E. (1974) Acute appendicitis complicating pregnancy in the Oxford Region. *Br. J. Surg.*, **61**, 129–32.

67. Woodhouse, D.R. and Hayden, B. (1985) Gallbladder disease complicating pregnancy. *Aust. N.Z. J. Obstet. Gynaecol.*, **25**, 233–7.

68. Corlett, R.C. and Mishell, D.R. (1972) Pancreatitis in pregnancy. *Am. J. Obstet. Gynecol.*, **113**, 281–90.

69. Gabert, H.A. and Miller, J.M. (1985) Renal disease in pregnancy. *Obstet. Gynecol. Surv.*, **40**, 449–61.

70. Klein, E.A. (1984) Urological problems in pregnancy. *Obstet. Gynaecol. Surv.*, **39**, 605–15.

71. Lattanzi, D.R. and Cook, W.A. (1980) Urinary calculi in pregnancy. *Obstet. Gynecol.*, **56**, 462–6.

6

MEDICAL UTERINE EVACUATION IN THE MANAGEMENT OF FIRST TRIMESTER MISCARRIAGE

K. Hinshaw

INTRODUCTION

First trimester miscarriage is the commonest complication of pregnancy[1] affecting 10–20% of clinically recognized pregnancies[2,3]. In Italy, an analysis of temporal trends from 1980 to 1991 shows a rise in the incidence of early miscarriage[4]. The use of improved diagnostic techniques over the period of the study, in particular serum human chorionic gonado-trophin (hCG) and transvaginal ultrasonography accounts for some of the rise, but there appears to be a genuine increase in the background incidence of early miscarriage which as yet remains unexplained. Thus, miscarriage is an increasingly common problem and most women who miscarry will be admitted to hospital for further assessment. At present if the pregnancy is confirmed to be non-viable the majority are subsequently offered a routine surgical uterine evacuation. Surgical curettage accounts for three quarters of emergency gynecological operations in Britain[5] where the vast majority of procedures are performed under general anesthesia. It is strange that in modern practice the place of the standard surgical approach has not been questioned and alternative methods of achieving uterine evacuation have rarely been considered. Indeed, things have changed little since Hertig and Livingstone[6] stated that 'treatment becomes a matter of emptying the uterus as quickly and as safely as possible'. The justification for this approach is the concern that retained tissue within the uterus may lead to serious infection or hemorrhage[7]. Although surgical evacuation is a minor procedure it is associated with rare but serious morbidity, including upper tract infection, trauma (cervical laceration, uterine perforation, bowel damage, etc.), intrauterine adhesions and hemorrhage[8]. Large studies of therapeutic abortion, using a similar surgical approach, showed an incidence of serious morbidity of 2.1%[9] and a mortality of 0.5 per 100 000 mainly associated with general anesthesia[10].

In this chapter, alternative 'medical' methods of achieving uterine evacuation are discussed. The principle underlying the medical approach to uterine evacuation is not new. Herbal remedies were given for many years before the nineteenth century to encourage the uterus to expel its contents[11]. Surgical evacuation first gained popularity in the latter half of the nineteenth century, although medical evacuation with ergot or oxytocics emerged for a short time in the earlier part of this century, particularly for infected cases. As general anesthetic techniques developed the surgical approach once more became standard management. Russell[12] reported a large series of 3739 abortions managed conservatively of which the vast majority (90%) were 'spontaneous' (9.1% were 'criminal' and only 0.9% 'therapeutic'). With a combination of careful observation and the use of ergot or

Clinical Management of Early Pregnancy. Edited by Walter Prendiville and James R. Scott. Published in 1999 by Arnold, ISBN 0 340 74100 7

pitocin, surgery was avoided in 94.6% of cases. This approach was even used in cases of septic abortion in order to avoid potentially traumatic intrauterine manipulation.

Medical methods have only re-emerged recently in modern practice and initial work used either prostaglandin, prostaglandin analogs or antiprogesterones alone. Garcea *et al.*[13] described the use of the prostaglandin analog ONO-802 administered vaginally in non-viable pregnancies and Asch *et al.*[14] reported three cases of early anembryonic pregnancy and missed abortion successfully evacuated after a single 600 mg oral dose of the antiprogesterone mifepristone ('Mifegyne'® or 'RU486', Roussel, Uxbridge, UK).

BACKGROUND

MIFEPRISTONE (RU486)

Mifepristone is a steroid derivative of the synthetic progestin norethindrone with an additional hydrophobic side chain which accounts for its antiprogestogenic activity. It acts at the cellular level and is a highly competitive progesterone receptor antagonist which impairs gene transcription and thus protein synthesis[15]. Relative to natural progesterone, it has two to ten times the affinity for the progesterone receptor. In early pregnancy there are several mechanisms which may contribute to the abortifacient effect of mifepristone. Decidual production of prostaglandin is increased and there may also be an increase in the number of gap junctions. This leads to an increased sensitivity of the myometrium to the action of prostaglandin with resulting increased tone and contractility[16]. The decidua starts to breakdown in the 24–48 h after administration and the cervix softens and dilates. Other mechanisms are not as clearly delineated but there may be a direct effect on the corpus luteum leading to luteolysis and reduced progesterone production. The majority of research on mifepristone has focused on its role in first trimester therapeutic

abortion. However, it is now apparent that it has many potential uses throughout pregnancy including reduction in the induction–termination interval during midtrimester termination[17–19], cervical softening prior to vacuum aspiration, labor induction, management of intrauterine fetal death as well as developments in the area of early miscarriage.

THERAPEUTIC MEDICAL ABORTION

Mifepristone has been licenced in the UK since 1991 for therapeutic medical abortion up to 63 days. It is used in combination with the prostaglandin E_1-analog gemeprost ('Cervagem'®, Farillon, Romford, UK) which is given as a single vaginal pessary 36–48 h after mifepristone. This combination has been shown to achieve complete abortion in 94.8% of cases[20] although there may be some fall off in efficacy at gestations >50 days[21]. In a partially randomized comparative study, both medical and surgical abortion techniques showed high levels of patient acceptability[22]. There was evidence of a significantly reduced incidence of upper tract infection after medical abortion. More recently, alternative prostaglandin analogs such as misoprostol have been used in combination with mifepristone. Misoprostol is uterotonic and has advantages over gemeprost, achieving effective rates of abortion with vaginal or combined vaginal–oral administration[18,23]. The combination of mifepristone and misoprostol for early abortion was compared with surgical termination in a randomized controlled trial in developing countries (*n* = 1373). It was found to be safe, efficacious and highly acceptable[24]. The development of similar effective methods of achieving complete uterine evacuation in early miscarriage could have significant implications for developing countries where surgical facilities are not easily accessible.

MISOPROSTOL AND PROSTAGLANDINS

Prostaglandins have a varied role in early pregnancy. From animal studies it is clear that prostaglandin levels rise locally at the site of implantation and are vital for successful implantation[25]. This must occur without a generalized rise in prostaglandin production which would lead to myometrial contractions, spiral arteriolar constriction, decidual break-down and menstruation. Prostaglandin receptors are present in the human cervix[26] and prostaglandin is intimately involved in the process of cervical softening[27] and myometrial contractility. These receptors are sensitive to the presence of both endogenous and exogenous prostaglandin.

The prostaglandin E_1 analog misoprostol ('Cytotec'®, Searle, High Wycombe, UK) is licenced for use in the management of gastro-duodenal ulceration. It has a side-effect profile common to all prostaglandins (i.e. pyrexia, nausea, vomiting and diarrhea). However, its use in therapeutic abortion has been associated with a low and comparable incidence of side effects compared to the 'standard' prostaglandin gemeprost. Misoprostol may be administered orally or vaginally and can be stored at room temperature. Gemeprost has to be refrigerated and is significantly more expensive (1 mg gemeprost = £22.53; 800 μg misoprostol = £1.43)[19]. In a quantitative study of uterine contractility using intrauterine pressure transducers, misoprostol was shown to achieve significant increases in uterine tone and contractility after pretreatment with mifepristone[28]. Further studies have confirmed the effectiveness of misoprostol when compared with gemeprost as a softening agent prior to surgical abortion[29] and in the management of therapeutic medical abortion[18]. As with mifepristone, misoprostol has great potential for use in pregnancy including termination for fetal abnormality[19], induction of labor[30] and prevention of postpartum hemorrhage[31]. Zieman *et al.*[32] have described the pharmacokinetics of vaginal and oral misoprostol. The oral route achieves peak plasma concentrations in 34 min after which there is a rapid fall-off. With vaginal administration peak levels are only

reached after 80 min but levels remain high for 3–4 h. These pharmacokinetic studies mirror the differences observed in clinical practice. The vaginal route is more efficacious when single dosing is used[33], but may prime the cervix and allow effective use of subsequent oral doses in multiple dosing regimens[19].

MEDICAL UTERINE EVACUATION IN EARLY MISCARRIAGE

Medical methods of achieving uterine evacuation have developed from the successful work in the field of therapeutic abortion. These techniques offer several benefits including: improved choice for women who miscarry; avoidance of the risks associated with surgery and anesthesia; a reduction in unsupervised 'out of hours' emergency operating by trainees and the potential for significant economic savings[34]. Economic benefits could result from more effective use of in-patient beds and re-allocation of the time freed up on routine operating lists.

PILOT STUDIES

In our first pilot study, 60 women with a confirmed 'missed abortion' (non-viable fetus) or 'anembryonic pregnancy' (empty gestation sac) were managed using a combination of mifepristone 600 mg followed 36–48 h later by two sequential oral doses of misoprostol (400 μg and 200 μg) 2 h apart[35]. Patients were eligible with a maximum sac diameter less than 60 mm or a fetal crown–rump length less than 55 mm (i.e. less than 12 weeks' gestation or *equivalent size*). Women were allowed home during the 36–48 h 'priming phase'. Their median age was 27 (range 15–44) years and the median duration of amenorrhea was 71 (range 42–110) days. If products of conception were not expelled within 4 h of starting prostaglandin, a transvaginal scan was performed and surgical evacuation offered if a gestation sac was seen. One woman was subsequently found to have an ectopic pregnancy and in three women the treatment failed. A total of 39 (66%) did not require pain relief, 13 (22%) requested oral analgesia and seven (12%) used parenteral narcotics. All women were reviewed and assessed clinically at 10–14 days. Overall the efficacy was 95% (defined as complete evacuation without resort to surgical intervention). Although two women underwent surgical evacuation more than two weeks after treatment, in neither case were products of conception confirmed histologically.

In the second pilot study, 44 women with an 'incomplete abortion' (hemodynamically stable with an open cervical os) received a prostaglandin analog immediately after confirmation of 'retained products of conception'[22]. All women underwent transvaginal ultrasonography and were deemed to have 'retained products' if the anteroposterior diameter of the cavity was >10 mm. Using this criterion Rulin *et al.*[36] have shown a positive predictive value of 69% for the presence of chorionic villi (i.e. histologically confirmed 'products of conception'). The first 20 patients were given the prostaglandin E_2 analog sulprostone. This was voluntarily withdrawn by the manufacturer during the course of the study because of three reported myocardial infarctions (one fatal) in women who were heavy smokers over the age of 40 undergoing therapeutic abortion[37]. The remaining women in our study received a single 400 μg dose of oral misoprostol and were observed for 12–18 h when pelvic examination was repeated. A decision on the need for surgical evacuation was made clinically. Visible 'products' were removed with ovum forceps and the women were discharged if bleeding was settling, to be reviewed at 14 days. One woman was subsequently found to have an ectopic pregnancy and two women required surgical evacuation. Again the overall efficacy was 95%; 11 (26%) used oral analgesia but only two (5%) required parenteral narcotics. The median change in hemoglobin concentration was –2.0 (range +9.0 to –1.7) g/l.

Other exclusion criteria for both studies included: heavy vaginal bleeding, anemia <100 g/l, pyrexia >37.5°C, contraindications to prostaglandin (mitral stenosis, glaucoma, sickle cell anemia, hypertension, severe asthma) or treatment with antiprostaglandins in the previous 24 h. In addition mifepristone was contraindicated in the presence of adrenal insufficiency, long-term steroids or anticoagulant therapy.

MEDICAL VERSUS SURGICAL EVACUATION: A RANDOMIZED CONTROLLED TRIAL

Medical aspects

The previous studies suggested that medical evacuation was a feasible alternative with similar efficacy to that obtained in studies of early medical abortion and we embarked on a prospective partially randomized study[38]. The main pragmatic objective of the study was to compare the efficacy of the new medical methods with the 'gold standard' of surgical uterine evacuation. Preliminary results from this trial will be presented and discussed.

Women who are miscarrying are already emotionally distressed. Medical methods in particular, require intense involvement during the process and from our pilot work we were aware that approximately half the women we approached would not be prepared to be randomized and would express a strong preference for one or other treatment. We chose a patient-centred, partially randomized design[39]: those with a strong preference were allocated to their treatment of choice, whereas those without a preference were allocated to treatment at random. This allows the effect of patient choice on various outcomes to be assessed while maintaining a valid, randomized group for comparison of the two interventions.

A total of 437 women were recruited and formed four study arms (Table 6.1); 54% of women were not prepared to be randomized. Although one third of women preferred surgical evacuation, 20% immediately expressed a

Table 6.1 Study arms by 'preference' or 'randomization'

Study arm		n	%
Preferred medical method	(PM)	86	20
Preferred surgical method	(PS)	151	34
Randomized to medical	(RM)	100	23
Randomized to surgical	(RS)	100	23
Total		437	100

strong preference for the medical option. There were no differences in physical, reproductive or demographic features between the four study arms.

In managing women with an intact intrauterine sac ('missed abortion' or 'anembryonic pregnancy') the dose of mifepristone was reduced to 200 mg. This was confirmed to be as effective as 600 mg in a large study of early medical abortion (n = 1182) published at the start of our trial[40]. The dose of misoprostol was increased to three sequential oral doses 2 h apart (400/600/400 μg). For those with an 'incomplete miscarriage' oral misoprostol was increased to 400/200 μg 2 h apart. Surgical uterine evacuation was undertaken under general anesthesia using suction curettage in cases with an intact intrauterine sac and gentle sharp curettage for 'incomplete abortion'. A total of 399 (91.3%) women attended for review at a median of 15 (SD 3.85) days. At review, 'complete uterine evacuation' was confirmed by clinical history and examination without arranging routine ultrasonography. General practitioners were sent a questionnaire 8 weeks after the miscarriage to record any complications which had not been reported by the patient. The response rate was 97.3%.

Treatment was defined as successful, and evacuation was deemed 'complete', if surgical curettage (or re-curettage) was not required within 8 weeks of initial treatment. The overall efficacy for medical evacuation was 93% (172/186) compared to 98% (247/251) for surgical evacuation (P = 0.004 χ^2). However,

for women with 'incomplete miscarriage' the success rate was 100% for both methods (medical n = 75 and surgical n = 27). In 353 women who had a 'missed abortion' or 'anembryonic pregnancy' the efficacy with medical methods was dependent on both sac size and gestation. Although success rates were always less with medical evacuation, there were no statistical differences at gestations <71 days and with sac diameters <24 mm (Table 6.2). With increasing gestation and sac size, complete uterine evacuation was still achieved in 84 and 86% of cases, respectively.

Somatic symptoms were assessed including the Pain Rating Index in the McGill pain questionnaire[41]. Symptom scores were significantly higher for medical methods at the time of discharge although these differences were not maintained at the time of follow-up. This reflects procedure-related symptomatology and is not unexpected as women were fully conscious throughout medical evacuation. Analgesic use with medical evacuation mirrored symptom scores, with 19 (10.2%) using parenteral opiates compared to 3 (1.2%) for those managed surgically (P < 0.0001 χ^2). However, opiate use was confined to medical evacuation in cases of 'missed abortion' or 'anembryonic pregnancy' only. Analgesic use after discharge, duration of bleeding and fall in hemoglobin were similar for both methods. The mean fall in hemoglobin between treatment and 2 week follow-up was not significantly different after medical or surgical evacuation and was clinically insignificant for most women (mean change –3.9 g/l). There were no differences in the overall time taken to return to work or to normal household activities.

During the 'priming' phase between mifepristone and misoprostol 32% (42/129) of the women undergoing medical evacuation miscarried. This is much higher than the rate associated with early therapeutic medical abortion (1.2%)[20]. It is important for women undergoing medical evacuation to have direct and easy access to the ward if necessary.

Table 6.2 Missed abortion and anembryonic pregnancy: efficacy by gestation and sac diameter

Parameter	Medical (n = 129)	Surgical (n = 224)	P-value (χ^2)
Gestation <71 days			
n	38	69	
No. requiring subsequent curettage	3	2	
'Complete uterine evacuation' rate	92%	97%	0.482
Gestation 71–144 days			
n	70	119	
No. requiring subsequent curettage	10	2	
'Complete uterine evacuation' rate	86%	98%	0.002
Sac diameter <24 mm			
n	34	72	
No. requiring subsequent curettage	2	1	
'Complete uterine evacuation' rate	94%	98%	0.500
Sac diameter 24–77 mm			
n	64	97	
No. requiring subsequent curettage	10	1	
'Complete uterine evacuation' rate	84%	99%	0.001

Estimated gestation was missing for a number of women (i.e. women unsure of last menstrual period). Sac diameter was missing for a number of women.

Consultation rates with family doctors in the six weeks following miscarriage were the same after both methods (40%) with half of the visits being for perceived psychological or psychiatric symptoms. This confirms the vital need for support that many women (and their partners) require after early miscarriage. Clinical evidence of pelvic infection requiring antibiotic prescription was significantly higher after surgical evacuation (13.2% vs 7.1% ($P < 0.001$ χ^2)).

There were three cases of partial molar pregnancy (medical $n = 2$ and surgical $n = 1$). All were appropriately registered and followed-up with serial hCG estimations. Levels of hCG fell rapidly after medical evacuation and did not require surgical intervention. Major complications affected six (1.7%) women. Three women with 'missed abortion' treated medically had an estimated blood loss >500 ml and two required blood transfusion. In the surgical group, a uterine perforation occurred during suction curettage requiring laparotomy and small bowel resection. In another case, a significant cervical tear occurred during suction curettage and required suturing. The final woman was readmitted after surgical evacuation with significant sepsis and pelvic infection which responded to high-dose intravenous antibiotic therapy.

Patient acceptability and psychological aspects

Table 6.3 shows the main reasons why women preferred one or other method at the time of recruitment into the study. Not surprisingly the majority of those choosing medical methods did so because of concerns about surgery or anesthesia. However, more than one third felt it allowed them to be more 'in control' of the process. For those choosing surgery, most did not want to defer 'definitive' treatment.

In order to assess the acceptability of methods, all the women were asked which method they would choose to undergo in the future. The following percentages show those women who would 'choose the same method'

Table 6.3 Reasons for initially choosing medical (PM) or surgical (PS) methods

Reasons	n	%
'Prefer medical' (n = 84)		
Avoidance of general anesthetic or surgery	48	57
'More natural/in control'	30	36
'Prefer surgical' (n = 147)		
Timescale	106	72
Issues of awareness etc	63	43
Avoidance of pain/bleeding	60	41
'Method more effective'	19	13

Women could give more than one reason.

Table 6.4 Relative costs of treating miscarriage: medical versus surgical

Cost per patient	Medical	Surgical	P value
Staff	£125 (12.75)	£119 (12.30)	<0.001
Consumables	£79 (21.74)	£52 (6.80)	<0.001
Operating room	£8 (28.27)	£106 (34.55)	<0.001
Hotel	£134 (71.36)	£120 (78.80)	0.05
Total	£346 (94.71)	£397 (112.91)	<0.001
95% Cl	£333–361	£383–411	

Mean (SD).

in the future: prefer medical, 85%; prefer surgical, 98%; randomized to medical, 85%; randomized to surgical, 99%. Overall, acceptability was significantly less for medical methods ($P < 0.001$ χ^2) although this was not so for 'incomplete miscarriage', nor for gestations less than 71 days in cases of 'missed abortion' or 'anembryonic pregnancy'. It is likely that the symptomatology associated with medical evacuation plays a significant role in how women perceive the overall acceptability of the method.

Psychological dysfunction was assessed using the HAD Scale[42]. This revealed an average 'borderline raised' level of anxiety at the time of miscarriage for all groups, with no differences between medical or surgical arms. Levels had returned to normal for most women by the time they returned for two week review. At discharge, women who were heavy smokers or those with a prior history of psychiatric or psychological dysfunction tended to have high HAD scores and may be a group who require special support. At the two-week review those who reported excessive tiredness or pain were statistically more likely to have maintained a high HAD score.

Economic aspects

A detailed economic analysis was undertaken to estimate the potential cost-benefits to the

NHS[43]. The average costs per patient are given in Table 6.4 and suggest a mean cost-saving of £50 per patient for medical evacuation ($P < 0.001$). However, using the concept of 'opportunity cost' and sensitivity analysis three different scenarios were compared. These differed in the relative amount of human or operating room resource which was released. The extra cost of introducing medical methods ranged from a cost saving of £71 to an additional cost of £47 per patient. In order to fully realize the cost savings it is vital that resources freed by reduced operating room use are fully utilized. This depends on whether surgical evacuations are undertaken on elective lists or on 'out of hours' emergency lists.

OTHER STUDIES

Three further studies have been published evaluating medical evacuation in the management of miscarriage. Within a group of 212 women presenting with inevitable miscarriage, Chung *et al.*[44] defined a group of 132 women with transvaginal scan evidence of 'retained products'. All patients were given a course of up to 5×1 mg gemeprost pessaries; 60 (45.5%) passed 'products' and were discharged home and the remaining 72 (55.5%) underwent repeat scan followed by surgical evacuation. One woman in each arm of the study required repeat curettage at a later date. The low success rate in this study is related to the fact that the authors did not differentiate between cases with an intact sac (i.e. 'missed abortion' and 'anembryonic pregnancy') and those with 'incomplete miscarriage'. Our own work suggests that these two groups require different approaches if high success rates are to be achieved. In the presence of an intact sac, priming with an antiprogesterone before prostaglandin administration will lead to complete evacuation in 89% of cases overall.

In a similar study to the pilot trial undertaken by Henshaw et al.[22], de Jonge et al.[45] randomized 50 women with incomplete miscarriage to surgical evacuation or oral misoprostol. Their success rate in the medical arm was dramatically less than that achieved by Henshaw et al. (13% versus 95%). However, when 'products' were not passed, their management again involved immediate ultrasonographic assessment. Repeat ultrasonography at that stage is very likely to show heterogeneous echoes suggestive of residual tissue and will inevitably lead to intervention. A further period of observation (preferably of more than a week) may have improved their success rate. In our own study only 42% of women undergoing medical evacuation for incomplete miscarriage passed further 'products' in the 6–8 h after misoprostol. As long as bleeding was settling they were discharged home without ultrasonographic assessment and all had stopped bleeding when reviewed at two weeks (efficacy 100%).

Nielsen et al.[46] managed 31 patients with 'missed abortion' with a combination of 400 mg mifepristone followed by a single dose of oral misoprostol (400 µg). Ultrasonography showed that 16 (52%) had an empty uterus six days later, 11 (35%) underwent surgical evacuation for 'retained products' at six days and four (13%) required urgent surgical evacuation for bleeding etc. These results suggest that medical methods may not be as efficacious as we have described. However, only one dose of orally administered misoprostol was given and pharmacokinetic studies would suggest that multiple sequential doses are necessary if the oral route is used[32]. The three oral doses

used in our study were given at 2 h intervals and may well account for the higher success rates.

CONCLUSION

It is time for gynecologists to review the management of early miscarriage[47]. Septic abortion is no longer a common complication and the studies described in this chapter highlight alternative methods of evacuation which warrant further assessment. Indeed several workers are now suggesting an even more conservative approach with no intervention but 'observation alone'[48,49]. In the first study, spontaneous resolution occurred in 79% of cases[48]. Chipchase and James[49] had no failures in a smaller randomized study comparing conservative and surgical approaches ($n = 35$). Medical uterine evacuation and conservative management will not replace, but should complement, the surgical approach increasing the options that we can offer to women who miscarry. Our initial work suggests that at least 20% of women would choose medical evacuation if it were available. Regimens need further refinement in order to increase their efficacy and reduce unwanted side effects. A reduced dose of mifepristone (200 mg) is effective in therapeutic abortion extending into the midtrimester[50] implying that even smaller doses could be used in the management of miscarriage. We have used the oral route for prostaglandin in our initial miscarriage studies but there is increasing evidence that vaginal misoprostol is more effective[32,33,51]. Medical methods could be integrated in the services offered by an 'early pregnancy assessment unit'[52] and should help to avoid unnecessary hospital admission for many women. The methods have the potential to offer economic benefits and to reduce unsupervised 'out of hours' operating by trainees. The majority of women managed medically will avoid a general anesthetic which is still the most frequent cause of death associated with therapeutic termination of pregnancy in the United

States[10]. There are no direct data on conception rates after medical evacuation but expectant management with observation alone has little or no effect on future fertility[49,53]. From a global perspective, medical evacuation may offer a safe and effective alternative to surgery for populations where sepsis is still a major problem. Further clinical research for this extremely common problem should be encouraged.

ACKNOWLEDGMENTS

The study discussed in this chapter was funded by a grant from the Scottish Office Home and Health Department. The author worked under the supervision of Professor Allan Templeton in the University Department of Obstetrics and Gynaecology, Aberdeen, Scotland. The opinions expressed are those of the author.

REFERENCES

1. Smith, N. (1988) Epidemiology of spontaneous abortion. *Contemp. Rev. Obstet. Gynecol.*, **1**, 43–8.
2. Warburton, D. and Fraser, F.C. (1964) Spontaneous abortion risks in man: data from reproduction histories collected in a medical genetics unit. *Hum. Genet.*, **16**, 1–25.
3. Alberman, E. (1992) Spontaneous abortion: epidemiology, in *Spontaneous Abortion: Diagnosis and Treatment* (eds S. Stabile, G. Grudzinkas and T. Chard), Springer-Verlag, London, pp. 9–20.
4. Parazzini, F., Restelli, S., Chatenoud, L. *et al.* (1996) Trend of spontaneous abortions in Italy 1980–1991. *Hum. Reprod.*, **11**, 914.
5. McKee, M., Priest, P., Ginzlet, M. and Black, M. (1992) Can out-of-hours operating in gynaecology be reduced? *Arch. Emerg. Med.*, **9**, 290–8.
6. Hertig, A.T. and Livingstone, R.G. (1944) Spontaneous, threatened and habitual abortion: their pathogenesis and treatment. *N. Engl. J. Med.*, **230**, 797–806.
7. Huisjes, H.J. (1984) Spontaneous abortion. *Curr. Rev. Obstet. Gynaecol.*, **8**, Churchill Livingstone, Edinburgh.
8. Ratnam, S.S. and Prasad, R.N.V. (1990) Medical management of abnormal pregnancy. *Baillières Clin. Obstet. Gynaecol.*, **4**, 361–74.
9. Joint Study of the Royal College of General Practitioners and the Royal College of Obstetricians and Gynaecologists (1985) Induced abortion operations and their early sequelae. *J. R. Coll. Gen. Pract.*, **35**, 175–80.
10. Lawson, H.W., Frye, A., Atrash, H.K. *et al.* (1994) Abortion mortality, United States, 1972 through 1987. *Am. J. Obstet. Gynecol.*, **171**, 1365–72.
11. Taussig, F.J. (1936) *Abortion, Spontaneous and Induced. Medical and Social Aspects*, Mosby, St Louis.
12. Russell, P.B. (1947) Abortions treated conservatively. *South Med. J.*, **40**, 314–24.
13. Garcea, N., Dargenio, R., Panetta, V. *et al.* (1987) A prostaglandin analogue (ONO-802) in treated abortion, intrauterine fetal death and hydatidiform mole: a dose-finding trial. *Eur. J. Obstet. Gynecol. Reprod.*, **25**, 15–22.
14. Asch, R.H., Weckstein, L.N., Balmaceda, J.P. *et al.* (1990) Non-surgical expulsion of early pregnancy: a new application of RU 486. *Hum. Reprod.*, **5**, 481–3.
15. Henshaw, R.C. and Templeton, A.A. (1993) Antiprogesterones. *Prog. Obstet. Gynaecol.*, **10**, 259–79.
16. Brogden, R., Goa, K. and Faulds, D. (1993) Mifepristone – a review of its pharmacodynamic and pharmacokinetic properties, and its therapeutic potential. *Drugs*, **45**, 384–409.
17. Rodger, M.W. and Baird, D.T. (1990) Pretreatment with mifepristone (RU486) reduces the interval between prostaglandin administration and expulsion in second trimester abortion. *Br. J. Obstet. Gynaecol.*, **97**, 41–5.
18. El-Refaey, H., Hinshaw, K. and Templeton, A. (1993) The abortifacient effect of misoprostol in the second trimester. A randomised comparison with gemeprost in patients pre-treated with mifepristone (RU486). *Hum. Reprod.*, **8**, 1744–6.
19. Hinshaw, K., El-Refaey, H., Rispin, R. and Templeton, A. (1995) Mid-trimester termination for fetal abnormality: advantages of a new regimen using mifepristone and misoprostol. *Br. J. Obstet. Gynaecol.*, **102**, 559–60.
20. UK Multicentre Trial (1990) The efficacy and tolerance of mifepristone and prostaglandin in first trimester termination of pregnancy. *Br. J. Obstet. Gynaecol.*, **97**, 480–6.
21. Henshaw, R.C., Naji, S.A., Russell, I.T. and Templeton, A.A. (1994) A comparison of medical abortion (using mifepristone and gemeprost) with surgical vacuum aspiration: efficacy and early medical sequelae. *Hum. Reprod.*, **9**, 2167–72.

22. Henshaw, R.C., Naji, S.A., Russell, I.T. and Templeton, A.A. (1993) Comparison of medical abortion with surgical vacuum aspiration: women's preferences and acceptability of treatment. *Br. Med. J.*, **307**, 714–17.

23. El-Refaey, H. and Templeton, A. (1995) Early pregnancy termination induced by a combination of mifepristone and vaginal misoprostol. *Contraception*, **49**, 111–14.

24. Winikoff, B., Sivin, I., Coyaji, K.J. *et al.* (1997) Safety, efficacy and acceptability of medical abortion in China, Cuba and India: a comparative trial of mifepristone–misoprostol versus surgical abortion. *Am. J. Obstet. Gynecol.*, **176**, 431–7.

25. Smith, S.K. (1992) Prostaglandins and implantation, in *Prostaglandins and the Uterus* (eds J.O. Drife and A.A. Calder), Springer-Verlag, London, pp. 91–9.

26. Crankshaw, D.J., Crankshaw, J., Branda, L.A. and Daniel, E.E. (1979) Receptors for E type prostaglandins in the plasma membrane of non-pregnant myometrium. *Arch. Biochem. Biophys.*, **198**, 70–7.

27. Rådestad, A. (1992) Cervical softening in early pregnancy, in *Prostaglandins and the Uterus* (eds J.O. Drife and A.A. Calder), Springer-Verlag, London, pp. 135–46.

28. Norman, J.E., Thong, K.J., Baird, D.T. (1991) Uterine contractility and induction of abortion in early pregnancy by misoprostol and mifepristone. *Lancet*, **338**, 1233–6.

29. El-Refaey, H., Calder, L., Wheatley, D.N. and Templeton, A. (1994) Cervical priming with prostaglandin E_1 analogues, misoprostol and gemeprost. *Lancet*, **343**, 1207–9.

30. Windrim, R., Bennett, K., Mundle, W. and Young, D.C. (1997) Oral administration of misoprostol for labor induction: a randomised controlled trial. *Obstet. Gynecol.*, **89**, 392–7.

31. El-Refaey, H., O'Brien, P., Morafa, W. *et al.* (1997) Use of oral misoprostol in the prevention of postpartum haemorrhage. *Br. J. Obstet. Gynaecol.*, **104**, 336–9.

32. Zieman, M., Fong, S.K., Benowitz, N.L. *et al.* (1997) Absorption kinetics of misoprostol with oral or vaginal administration. *Obstet. Gynecol.*, **90**, 88–92.

33. El-Refaey, H., Rajasekar, D., Abdalla, M. *et al.* (1995) Induction of abortion with mifepristone (RU 486) and oral or vaginal misoprostol. *N. Engl. J. Med.*, **332**, 983–7.

34. Macrow, P. and Elstein, M. (1993) Managing miscarriage medically. *Br. Med. J.*, **306**, 876.

35. El-Refaey, H., Hinshaw, K., Henshaw, R. *et al.* (1992) Medical management of missed abortion and anembryonic pregnancy. *Br. Med. J.*, **305**, 1399.

36. Rulin, M.C., Bornstein, S.G. and Campbell, J.D. (1993) The reliability of ultrasonography in the management of spontaneous abortion, clinically thought to be complete: a prospective study. *Am. J. Obstet. Gynecol.*, **168**, 12–15.

37. Anonymous (1991) A death associated with mifepristone/sulprostone. *Lancet*, **337**, 969–70.

38. Hinshaw, K., Henshaw, R., Rispin, R. *et al.* (1993) Management of uncomplicated miscarriage – randomised trials are possible. *Br. Med. J.*, **307**, 259.

39. Brewin, C.R. and Bradley, C. (1989) Patient preferences and randomised clinical trials. *Br. Med. J.*, **299**, 313–15.

40. WHO Taskforce on Post-ovulatory Methods of Fertility Regulation (1993) Termination of pregnancy with reduced doses of mifepristone. *Br. Med. J.*, **307**, 532–7.

41. Melzack, R. (1975) The McGill Pain Questionnaire: major properties and scoring methods. *Pain*, **1**, 277–99.

42. Zigmond, A.S. and Snaith, R.P. (1983) The Hospital Anxiety and Depression Scale. *Acta Psychol. Scand.*, **67**, 361–70.

43. Hughes, J., Ryan, M., Hinshaw, K. *et al.* (1996) The costs of treating miscarriage: a comparison of medical and surgical management. *Br. J. Obstet. Gynaecol.*, **103**, 1217–21.

44. Chung, T.K.H., Cheung, L.P., Lau, W.C. *et al.* (1994) Spontaneous abortion: a medical approach to management. *Aust. N.Z. J. Obstet. Gynaecol.*, **34**, 432–6.

45. de Jonge, E.T.M., Makin, J.D., Manefeldt, E. *et al.* (1995) Randomised clinical trial of medical and surgical curettage for incomplete miscarriage. *Br. Med. J.*, **311**, 662.

46. Nielsen, S., Hahlin, M. and Platz-Christensen, J.J. (1997) Unsuccessful treatment of missed abortion with a combination of an antiprogesterone and a prostaglandin E_1 analogue. *Br. J. Obstet. Gynecol.*, **104**, 1094–6.

47. Forbes, K. (1995) Management of first trimester spontaneous abortions. *Br. Med. J.*, **310**, 1426.

48. Nielsen, S. and Hahlin, M. (1995) Expectant management of first-trimester spontaneous abortion. *Lancet*, **345**, 84–6.

49. Chipchase, J. and James, D. (1997) Randomised trial of expectant versus surgical management of spontaneous miscarriage. *Br. J. Obstet. Gynaecol.*, **104**, 840–1.

50. Webster, D., Penney, G.C. and Templeton, A.

(1996) A comparison of 600 and 200 mg mifepristone prior to second trimester abortion with the prostaglandin misoprostol. *Br. J. Obstet. Gynaecol.*, **103**, 706–9.

51. Lawrie, A., Penney, G. and Templeton, A. (1996) A randomised comparison of oral and vaginal misoprostol for cervical priming before suction termination of pregnancy. *Br. J. Obstet. Gynaecol.*, **103**, 1117–19.

52. Bigrigg, M.A. and Read, M.D. (1991) Management of women referred to an early pregnancy assessment unit: care and cost effectiveness. *Br. Med. J.*, **302**, 577–9.

53. Kaplan, B., Pardo, J., Rabinerson, D. *et al.* (1996) Future fertility following conservative management of complete abortion. *Hum. Reprod.*, **11**, 92–4.

F.D. Malone and A.H. DeCherney

DEFINITION

Ectopic pregnancy (eccyesis) refers to the implantation of a fertilized ovum outside the endometrial lining of the uterine cavity. Over 95% of ectopic pregnancies are tubal pregnancies, with rarer cases of ectopic pregnancy being ovarian, cervical and intra-abdominal. Tubal pregnancies are classified by site of implantation, with 80–90% being ampullary, 8–12% isthmic, 5% fimbrial and 1–2% interstitial (cornual). Heterotopic pregnancy refers to the simultaneous presence of both intra- and extrauterine pregnancies.

EPIDEMIOLOGY

Ectopic pregnancy is a remarkable disease in that its incidence continues to increase yet its mortality has decreased dramatically. The exact incidence of ectopic pregnancy is difficult to ascertain as the incidence of spontaneous subclinical resolution of ectopic pregnancy remains uncertain. The incidence of ectopic pregnancy is usually reported as a function of total reported pregnancies, although this ignores the not inconsiderable number of illegal terminations, thereby falsely increasing the apparent rate of ectopic pregnancy.

A fourfold increase in the rate of ectopic pregnancies has been reported in the United States from 1970 to 1987, from 4.5 to 16.8 ectopics per 1000 reported pregnancies[1]. This marked increase in incidence has also been seen in other countries, such as Sweden, where the incidence increased from 5.8 to 11.1 per 1000 reported pregnancies from 1960 to 1979[2].

The exact reason for this apparent epidemic is unclear. There has certainly been a marked increase in the incidence of sexually transmitted diseases and consequent salpingitis recently, but up to 70% of cases of ectopic pregnancy are associated with histologically normal tubes. Other factors accounting for this marked increase include the earlier diagnosis of ectopic pregnancy based on the availability of a highly specific radioimmunoassay for human chorionic gonadotropin (hCG), high resolution transvaginal ultrasonography and more frequent use of diagnostic laparoscopy[3]. The increased role of conservative surgery for ectopic pregnancy, resulting in the survival of more tubes, as well as the increasing use of assisted reproductive techniques, also play a role in today's epidemic of ectopic pregnancy.

Associated factors with this increasing incidence of ectopic pregnancy include increasing incidence with advancing maternal age, increased incidence in black versus white populations[4], (twice as common among blacks as whites in the United States), and increased incidence in lower socioeconomic groups.

Among the 88 000 ectopic pregnancies

Clinical Management of Early Pregnancy. Edited by Walter Prendiville and James R. Scott.
Published in 1999 by Arnold, ISBN 0 340 74100 7

reported in the United States in 1987, there were 30 direct maternal deaths, giving a case fatality rate of 0.3/1000. This is in marked contrast to the 3.5 deaths per 1000 ectopic pregnancies reported in 1970. The case fatality rate remains three times higher for black women than white. The relative risk of dying from ectopic pregnancy is 10 times that of childbirth and 50 times that of legal abortion[4]. Ectopic pregnancy remains the commonest cause of direct maternal death in early pregnancy. The marked reduction in mortality may be the result of earlier diagnosis and the awareness of the existence of high risk groups.

PATHOPHYSIOLOGY

The pathological basis of ectopic pregnancy can be related to abnormalities in the anatomy of the tube, hormonal milieu of the tube, or with the conceptus.

Damage to the fallopian tubal anatomy is usually the result of scarring from infection or previous surgery, resulting in abnormal tubal mucosa with disruption of normal cilia function. Intraluminal adhesions and diverticulum formation results, and this can lead to a delay in the usual 3–4 days taken for normal embryo transport into the uterus. Cilia function is important for embryo transfer. Transection and reversal of a segment of ampulla will result in failure of ovum progression, whereas transection alone without reversal of the segment is usually associated with normal tubal transport. Cilia function alone cannot explain all tubal motility as normal intrauterine pregnancy is possible with Kartagener's syndrome (immotile cilia syndrome). The innervation of the myosalpinx is predominantly adrenergic, with a concentration of fibers at the isthmus, which may act as a sphincter mechanism controlling passage of the embryo into the tube. Cigarette smoking has been associated with an increased incidence of ectopic pregnancy and this may be a result of nicotinic effects on these adrenergic receptors.

There may be a hormonal basis to the timing of retention and release of the embryo from tube to uterus[5]. Elevated estrogen levels, such as after postcoital contraception or ovulation induction, may increase smooth muscle tone in the tubal isthmus, delaying release of the embryo into the uterus. Elevated progestin levels, such as after progestin contraception, reduces overall smooth muscle activity leading to decreased tubal peristalsis and slower progression of the embryo through the tube.

Abnormalities with embryogenesis may also be associated with the development of ectopic pregnancy. Prematurely- or delayed-ovulated ova may implant at abnormal times because of differences in density of the cumulus–corona complex[6]. Blighted ova, with no simultaneous embryo, are more likely to implant in the tube. Increased incidence of chromosomal abnormality in ectopic pregnancy has been disproven as a possible factor in pathogenesis[7].

The natural history of ectopic pregnancy demonstrates that the presence of a normal conceptus and corpus luteum within an abnormal tube results in rapid trophoblast proliferation and rapid rise in hCG and progesterone. As the trophoblast erodes into submucosal vessels hematoma of the tube occurs resulting in pain and marked tubal swelling. hCG and progesterone production decreases, resulting in insufficient support of the corpus luteum and decidua, and eventual decidual shedding. This accounts for the abnormal vaginal bleeding reported by the patient early on in the disease course. Eventually, further tubal enlargement results in tubal rupture and significant intra-abdominal hemorrhage.

Some controversy still exists as to the depth of trophoblastic invasion within the tube. Budowick *et al.*[8] suggested that most ectopics penetrate the tubal mucosa early and that subsequent proliferation was extraluminal. Senterman *et al*[9] subsequently showed that 56% of ampullary ectopics were intraluminal, 7% extraluminal and 37% had mixed intra-

and extraluminal proliferation. Isthmic ectopics, however, are equally distributed between extraluminal and mixed types. This may explain the increased amount of mucosal and muscularis destruction seen with isthmic ectopics, and therefore influences the choice of surgical procedure.

Ectopic pregnancies can progress in a number of directions. Spontaneous resolution has been well described, and therefore forms the basis of expectant management of ectopic pregnancy, although the true incidence of this is uncertain. Tubal abortion occurs when the conceptus is extruded from the fimbriated end of the tube into the peritoneal cavity, where spontaneous resolution or secondary re-implantation can occur. Tubal rupture is the well described outcome of persistent intra-tubal ectopic growth. Progression of pregnancy is a rarer possibility, due to secondary re-implantation of a tubal abortion with subsequent abdominal or ovarian pregnancy, or else due to persistence of interstitial pregnancy, possibly leading to uterine rupture.

ETIOLOGY

Many mechanical and functional causes of ectopic pregnancy have been described, including the following.

Pelvic inflammatory disease (PID)

Pelvic infection with *Neisseria gonorrhea*, *Chlamydia trachomatis* and mixed aerobes–anaerobes result in abnormal cilia function, intraluminal adhesions and fimbrial damage. The incidence of tubal obstruction increases from 13% to 35% to 75% after one, two and three episodes of acute PID, respectively[2]. The epidemic of sexually transmitted diseases as well as the development of new antibiotic regimens (which reduce total tubal occlusion) accounts for some of the increased incidence of ectopic pregnancy, but not all, as 70% of cases of ectopic pregnancy are associated with normal tubal histology.

Previous tubal surgery

There is a 2–7% rate of ectopic pregnancy after prior infertility surgery, such as adhesiolysis, fimbrioplasty, salpingostomy or tubal re-anastomosis[10]. This increased incidence may reflect the underlying disease causing the infertility or it may reflect the surgery itself. The rate of ectopic pregnancy after tubal reconstruction for obstruction is usually higher than the rate for tubal re-anastomosis after sterilization, therefore suggesting that the underlying tubal disease is more important than the actual surgical procedure in predicting future ectopic pregnancy. A 16% rate of repeat ectopic pregnancy is seen after conservative surgery for ectopic pregnancy, and this does not differ significantly from the repeat ectopic rate seen after radical surgery[11], again confirming the greater significance of underlying tubal disease rather than the type of tubal surgery.

Intrauterine contraceptive device (IUD)

Intrauterine conceptions are more effectively prevented than extrauterine conceptions by IUD usage. The relative risk of IUD users developing ectopic pregnancy is lower than the risk for non-contraceptive users. It is clear, therefore, that the presence of an IUD does not predispose to ectopic pregnancy, but when a pregnancy does occur with an IUD in place it is more likely to be ectopic[12]. This risk is greater for progestin-containing IUDs than for copper IUDs.

Progestin birth control

Oral contraceptives containing progestin alone may predispose a woman to an ectopic pregnancy because of the high levels of progestin reducing tubal peristalsis. This is only of significance for pregnancies occurring during progestin pill usage.

Failed sterilization procedure

As with IUD use, the incidence of ectopic pregnancy with previous tubal sterilization is much less than that seen with non-sterilized women, but when the procedure fails the resulting pregnancy is much more likely to be ectopic (pregnancy after laparoscopic tubal cautery has 51% risk of being ectopic)[13].

Termination of pregnancy

An increased risk of ectopic pregnancy has been described after uncomplicated legal terminations of pregnancy[14]. If the termination is associated with endometritis or retained products of conception there is a fivefold increased risk of ectopic pregnancy[15]. The marked increased risk of ectopic pregnancy after illegally procured abortion probably reflects the increased incidence of complications.

Assisted reproductive techniques

An increased rate of ectopic pregnancy (3–5%) is well recognized after IVF–embryo transfer procedures, especially if multiple embryos are used[6]. This is also reflected in the increased rate of heterotopic pregnancy (up to 1%) after such procedures[16]. Figure 7.1 demonstrates a heterotopic pregnancy in a patient after ovulation induction and intrauterine insemination. An increased rate of ectopic pregnancy also exists after ovulation induction with clomiphene and gonadotropins, probably by interfering with the hormonal basis of tubal transport of the embryo. All such infertility patients should therefore be considered to be at high risk for ectopic pregnancy.

Salpingitis isthmica nodosa

This is an unusual condition, of uncertain etiology, in which a nodular thickening of the

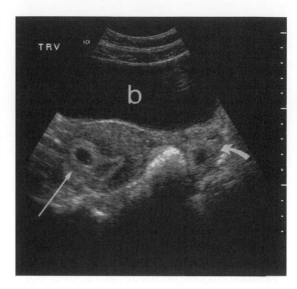

Figure 7.1. Transverse pelvic ultrasound scan through the bladder (b) demonstrating heterotopic intrauterine (straight arrow) and ectopic tubal (curved arrow) pregnancies in a patient following ovulation induction and intrauterine insemination.

isthmus of the tube occurs, with tubal epithelium forming diverticula within the myosalpinx, therefore distorting the tubal anatomy. It occurs in 0.6% of women and is significantly associated with the development of ampullary ectopic pregnancy.

Abnormal tubal anatomy

Anatomic distortion of the tube, with the presence of T-shaped uterus and 'withered tubes' has been described following *in utero* diethylstilbestrol exposure[17]. Tubal fibroids and significant endometriosis may also distort tubal anatomy to such an extent that tubal patency is compromised, and so predispose ectopic pregnancy.

Transmigration of ovum

Theoretically, if both tubes lie close together in the pouch of Douglas an ovum or embryo can pass from one tube into the pouch of Douglas and subsequently implant in the opposite tube. This may explain the 15–25% incidence of corpus luteal presence being on the opposite side to the ectopic. It is uncertain whether this has any etiologic role in the development of ectopic pregnancy.

DIAGNOSIS

HISTORY

Patients with ectopic pregnancy present in one of two distinct groups: those who present with symptoms and signs of abnormal early pregnancy, occasionally with evidence of acute intra-abdominal bleeding, and those who are essentially asymptomatic, but who are in a high risk group and are therefore being followed for the development of normal intrauterine pregnancy. In the latter group the diagnosis and treatment of ectopic pregnancy often precedes the development of any signs or symptoms. Among the group of patients who first present with symptoms, two further subgroups exist: those who present subacutely with non-specific symptoms and signs, and therefore present a diagnostic challenge, and those who present acutely with signs of tubal rupture. Our goal is to accurately diagnose ectopic pregnancy before it proceeds to acute tubal rupture, and in most institutions today a goal of less than 20% incidence of tubal rupture should be attainable.

Abdominal or pelvic pain is the most common presenting symptom, and is reported by 90% of patients. The pain is usually non-specific, sharp or dull, often localized to the affected side, and can be of varying intensity and pattern. Shoulder-tip pain is reported by 20% of patients and may suggest significant intra-abdominal bleeding.

Abnormal vaginal bleeding is present in 50–80% of patients, and is usually the result of poor corpus luteal support of the decidua. The passage of blood suggestive of menses or spontaneous abortion may also be due to the passage of the decidual cast of ectopic pregnancy, further confusing the presentation. When vaginal bleeding occurs it often precedes the pain.

Amenorrhea is an unreliable marker for ectopic pregnancy. Some patients may have up to 12 weeks of amenorrhea before presentation, whereas 10% will have less than 4 weeks of amenorrhea.

Other non-specific symptoms present in 30% of patients include nausea, vomiting, syncope and tenesmus (desire to defecate even though the rectum is empty). One 'classic triad' of pain, bleeding and amenorrhea is seen in only 50% of patients and is unhelpful. Another 'classic triad' of pain, bleeding and the presence of an adnexal mass is even rarer, being present in only 30% of cases.

One of the most significant parts of the patient's history is the elucidation of risk factors for the development of ectopic pregnancy, as this may direct the patient into a diagnostic algorithm prior to re-presentation with tubal rupture.

PHYSICAL EXAMINATION

As with the clinical history of the patient with ectopic pregnancy, the physical examination is mostly non-specific, and is best interpreted in conjunction with background risk factors. Assessment of vital signs is often normal. The patient is rarely febrile (<2%) and when present it is usually a non-specific response to peritoneal irritation by blood. Hypovolemic shock is the presentation of <5% of patients, and orthostatic changes are usually not seen until 15% of blood volume is lost. The quantity of hemoperitoneum does not correlate with tubal rupture, but when hypovolemic shock is seen 75% of such patients will have >1000 ml of intra-abdominal blood. Hypotension is not necessarily associated with tachycardia as the prolonged presence of intraperitoneal blood can cause a parasympathetic response and subsequent bradycardia.

Abdominal signs of bleeding include muscle rigidity, distention and, in severe cases, a blue periumbilical discoloration (Cullen's sign).

Abdominal tenderness can be found in 90% of patients, with or without rebound or involuntary guarding.

Bimanual examination usually shows a soft blue enlarged cervix consistent with pregnancy. Blood is visible at the vaginal vault in 60% of patients, and an enlarged uterus from decidual proliferation is present in 15% of patients. The presence of an enlarged tender adnexal mass is noted in 30–50% of cases, and can be due to either an ectopic pregnancy or an enlarged corpus luteum. Cervical motion tenderness is noted in 60% of patients and is usually worse on motion in the anteroposterior direction, in contrast to PID, which is classically worse with motion from side-to-side. Tenderness specifically in the posterior fornix may be due to the diseased tube occupying the pouch of Douglas.

INVESTIGATIONS

Complete blood count

As with all causes of acute hemorrhage, the hematocrit or hemoglobin level may not correlate well with the volume of blood lost or with blood pressure. Most patients will therefore present with minimal hematological changes, and a mild leucocytosis can be noted in 50% of cases.

Urinary hCG

Highly sensitive and rapid enzyme-linked immunoassays (ELISA) are now available, which pick up all patients with hCG >20 mIU/ml (IRP), and 95% of patients with hCG 5–20 mIU/ml. The false negative rate should be <1%[18], and therefore a negative qualitative urinary hCG effectively rules out pregnancy. False negative hCG results may occur in very early pregnancy, renal failure or with very dilute urine, whereas false positive results have been reported with the nephrotic syndrome.

Serum beta hCG

Today's highly sensitive radioimmunoassays (RIA) for the beta subunit of hCG in serum represent the gold standard for determining trophoblastic activity. A positive RIA can now be expected 7–10 days after ovulation, and will detect hCG levels as low as 5–10 mIU/ml (IRP). Care must be taken in interpreting published literature on hCG assays, as two different standards have been reported. The first standard reported is conversely known as the Second International Standard (SIS), and is based on relatively non-homogeneous assay material. The more commonly used standard today, and that which is used throughout this chapter, is known as the First International Reference Preparation (IRP). It consists of much more homogeneous assay material and its values are roughly twice the SIS values.

Quantitative hCG values in ectopic pregnancy are typically lower than those seen with viable intrauterine pregnancies, but are of little value in differentiating ectopic from non-viable intrauterine pregnancies. Serial evaluation of hCG has been classically used for following abnormal early pregnancies even though prospective studies have failed to confirm the predictive value of such testing[19]. Patients with non-viable pregnancies often show a plateau or even a fall in hCG on serial determinations. The half-life of hCG in serum is 24 h and the doubling time for hCG during the first 6 weeks of normal pregnancy is 1.98 days[20], usually reaching a peak by 10 weeks. An increase of <66% over 2 days is 87% predictive of either ectopic or non-viable intrauterine pregnancy, although up to 15% of viable intrauterine pregnancies have an abnormal doubling time.

The main use of hCG measurement now is to assess the viability of a pregnancy and to signal the optimum time for ultrasonography. The discriminatory zone is the level of hCG at which a gestational sac should be visible on ultrasonography, either transabdominal or transvaginal.

Serum progesterone

A single serum progesterone level determination (by RIA) is an inexpensive, rapid method of assessing pregnancy viability[21]. It is of little value in differentiating ectopic from non-viable intrauterine pregnancy. A value <5 ng/ml is 100% sensitive at predicting non-viable pregnancy, and if the diagnosis of ectopic is still in doubt, such patients could be offered curettage to differentiate ectopic from non-viable intrauterine pregnancy. A value >25 ng/ml is 98.5% sensitive in excluding ectopic pregnancy[22]. Values of 5–25 ng/ml are less helpful, however, as significant overlap exists between viable and non-viable pregnancies, although if hCG is >50 000 mIU/ml in this group ectopic pregnancy is effectively excluded. The main use of a single serum progesterone assay is to aid in rapid triage of patients into high and low risk groups, and may allow for the non-laparoscopic diagnosis of ectopic pregnancy, therefore allowing medical management. Less than 25% of ectopics present with progesterone <5 ng/ml, thus limiting its efficacy.

Other laboratory parameters

A number of other laboratory assessments have been described in evaluating ectopic pregnancy. Maternal serum alphafetoprotein has been reported elevated with ruptured ectopic pregnancy and with abdominal pregnancy, although the wide range of values minimizes its clinical usefulness. Other parameters noted to be elevated in ectopic pregnancy include secretory endometrial protein, estradiol, creatine kinase and pregnancy-associated protein-A, although none of these seems to have clinical application at this time.

Culdocentesis

This involves the transvaginal aspiration of blood from the pouch of Douglas, a positive result requiring at least 5 ml of non-clotted blood with a hematocrit of at least 15%. A negative tap is the aspiration of serous fluid, whereas failure to aspirate any fluid is considered non-diagnostic. A positive culdocentesis with a positive pregnancy test is 99% predictive of ectopic pregnancy[23]. False positives can occur from a hemorrhagic corpus luteum, tubal reflux of blood and any other cause of intraperitoneal bleeding.

It is not a reliable test for ectopic pregnancy as 10% of ectopics have a negative tap, and a positive tap is not diagnostic of tubal rupture as an unruptured ectopic can have a positive tap. Its main role is as a rapid evaluation for the presence of significant intraperitoneal bleeding and therefore allowing the patient to proceed more rapidly to definitive surgical exploration. In other less critical situations its role has been superseded by transvaginal ultrasonography which is highly efficient at diagnosing even small amounts of blood in the pouch of Douglas.

Ultrasonography

The main role of transabdominal ultrasonography (TAUS) is to exclude the presence of an intrauterine pregnancy, therefore raising the suspicion of ectopic pregnancy. With the advent of high frequency transvaginal ultrasonography (TVUS) with color and pulsed Doppler duplex capabilities, we are now in a position to positively identify ectopic pregnancy in many cases.

TAUS can clearly demonstrate an intrauterine pregnancy by 4 weeks' gestational age (6 weeks from LMP), whereas TVUS can confirm intrauterine pregnancy by 3 weeks' gestational age (5 weeks from LMP). A gestational sac appears as a regular, anechoic double ring, (generated by decidua capsularis and parietalis), with a highly echogenic border. It usually has an eccentric location, and subsequently develops a yolk sac at 6 mm sac diameter, and an echogenic fetal pole by 9 mm sac diameter. A pseudogestational sac is seen in 10–20% of ectopics, and is generated by the

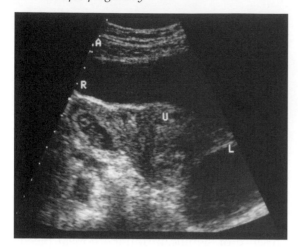

Figure 7.2. Right-sided unruptured ampullary tubal ectopic pregnancy with measurable crown–rump length. A, anterior; R, right adnexa; U, uterus; L, left adnexa.

decidual cast, often being distorted in shape, centrally located, with only a single surrounding ring. Figures 7.2 and 7.3 demonstrate a tubal ectopic pregnancy with identifiable cardiac activity.

In most cases the precise gestational age will be uncertain, and therefore the interpretation of ultrasonographic findings will depend on correlation with the serum hCG level. For TAUS, the discriminatory zone, above which all intrauterine pregnancies should be visible, has been established at 6500 mIU/ml[20]. For TVUS, the discriminatory zone is 1400–2000 mIU/ml[22,24]. The precise discriminatory zone varies with each institution, depending on the expertise of the sonographer, the ultrasound technology available, and the hCG reference standard being used. With multiple gestations the discriminatory zone is generally several hundred mIU/ml higher.

TVUS has greatly improved our ability to positively diagnose ectopic pregnancy without laparoscopy, with up to 90% of ectopics being visualized by transvaginal color Doppler sonography[22]. TVUS is performed at higher frequencies than TAUS (6–9 MHz, versus 3–5 MHz for TAUS), giving better resolution, but reduced depth of vision. Doppler ultrasonography is based on the principle that the frequency of sound is altered with movement

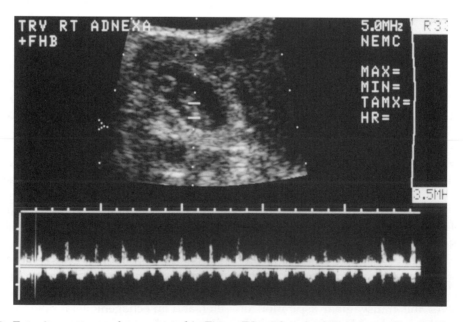

Figure 7.3. Ectopic pregnancy demonstrated in Figure 7.2, with pulsed Doppler confirming the presence of cardiac activity.

of red blood cells towards or away from the probe. Cells moving away from the beam reflect a lower frequency of sound, whereas cells moving towards the beam reflect a higher frequency. Color and Doppler duplex systems can then be applied to illustrate direction and velocity of flow, as well as resistance or impedance characteristics in a vascular bed.

This now allows us preoperatively to differentiate ectopic pregnancy, completed abortion and incomplete abortion[25]. Completed abortions generally show no corpus luteal flow, no intrauterine sac and low intrauterine flow. Incomplete abortions generally show good corpus luteal flow, increased intrauterine flow with enhanced venous drainage, and some intrauterine peritrophoblastic blood flow. Ectopic pregnancies also show good corpus luteal flow, but no intrauterine sac, low intrauterine flow with a high-resistance arterial pattern, and with high velocity, low impedance flow at the placental bed in the adnexa. Adnexal cardiac activity is seen in only 25% of ectopics on TVUS. In the pregnant patient without an intrauterine sac, visualization of a complex adnexal mass on TVUS is over 80% predictive of an ectopic, and the added presence of free fluid in the pouch of Douglas is over 90% predictive.

Uterine curettage

Uterine curettage revealing decidual tissue with no evidence of trophoblastic villi is highly suggestive of ectopic pregnancy. Visualization of villi can be attempted in the operating room by flotation in saline and examination with magnification for the typical frond-like appearance. Frozen section can also be used to confirm the diagnosis, although its accuracy has not been confirmed. One non-laparoscopic algorithm for the diagnosis of ectopic pregnancy relies on curettage in the presence of a serum progesterone <5 ng/ml, with absent villi and a stable hCG, as being diagnostic of ectopic pregnancy, therefore allowing medical management[22]. This approach is, however, not relevant for most ectopics as less than 25% of all ectopics present with serum progesterone values <5 ng/ml.

Diagnostic laparoscopy

When a definitive preoperative diagnosis of ectopic pregnancy cannot be established, diagnostic laparoscopy can be used to rule out other conditions that exist in the differential diagnosis. With today's advances in TVUS and color Doppler flow, accurate preoperative diagnosis is becoming more common so that laparoscopy is more likely to be reserved for definitive surgical management rather than for diagnosis. A characteristic blue swelling along the tube is typical of unruptured ectopic pregnancy. Figure 7.4 demonstrates the unruptured tubal ectopic pregnancy seen in Figures 7.2 and 7.3. Unlike the direct correlation between serum hCG and sonographic findings, no clear correlation exists between serum hCG levels and laparoscopic appearance of the ectopic. A definite danger exists of missing an ectopic pregnancy on diagnostic laparoscopy if performed at very low serum hCG levels.

Diagnostic laparoscopy for ectopic pregnancy requires two absolute prerequisites – an operator skilled in diagnostic and operative laparoscopy, and the immediate availability of operative laparoscopy or laparotomy equipment if needed. Standard laparoscopic techniques should be applied. General anesthesia with good muscle relaxation is required. The patient should be placed in the dorsal lithotomy position, with one arm secured at the patient's side. An indwelling urethral catheter should be in place. If the diagnosis is in doubt, and a desired intrauterine pregnancy is potentially present, the uterus should not be instrumented and a sponge stick placed in the vaginal vault can be used for uterine manipulation.

Standard CO_2 needle insufflation or non-insufflation with an abdominal wall lifting device can be used for the procedure. Once a 10 mm trocar has been placed through the

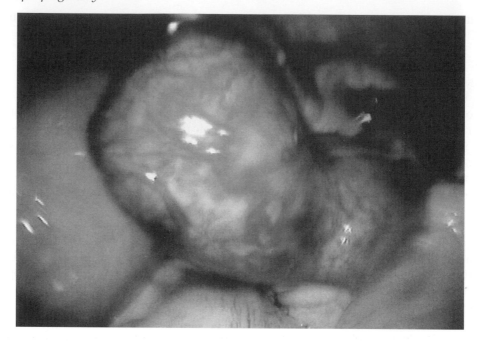

Figure 7.4. Laparascopic appearance of the right-sided unruptured ampullary tubal ectopic pregnancy demonstrated in Figures 7.2 and 7.3.

umbilicus, a camera with video capability is placed and steep Trendelenburg is performed. Once the diagnosis of ectopic pregnancy is confirmed and laparoscopic management is planned, a uterine manipulator, a 5 mm suprapubic trocar and a 5 mm lateral trocar are placed (with care taken to avoid the inferior epigastric vessels). The subsequent operative technique is described later.

DIFFERENTIAL DIAGNOSIS

Normal viable intrauterine pregnancy

This will be confirmed by a single serum progesterone >25 ng/ml, serum hCG >50 000 mIU/ml or an intrauterine pregnancy with cardiac activity visible on ultrasonography.

Spontaneous abortion

Since vaginal bleeding and pelvic pain are the commonest presenting symptoms of both conditions, a reliable diagnosis of viable intrauterine pregnancy is often difficult to achieve. Spontaneous abortion pain is often midline, occurring before bleeding, whereas ectopic pregnancy pain is often unilateral, occurring after bleeding. If the patient has no desire to continue pregnancy, uterine curettage should clarify the diagnosis by providing trophoblastic villi. As noted, TVUS can now more accurately differentiate both conditions.

Ovarian cyst

First trimester ovarian cysts are common, and most arise from the corpus luteum. Pain can occur after rupture, torsion or hemorrhage into a cyst. Cysts in pregnancy are mostly unilateral and resolve spontaneously. Rupture of a cyst may follow intercourse, abdominal trauma or bimanual pelvic examination. TVUS, as described, should help differentiate the two conditions, although laparoscopy may occasionally be needed.

Pelvic inflammatory disease (PID)

Acute salpingitis, tubo-ovarian abscess and hydrosalpinx can mimic the clinical presentation of ectopic pregnancy, as they can produce similar pelvic pain and a palpable adnexal mass with cervical motion tenderness. PID pain, however, is usually bilateral, with other obvious features of infection. A negative pregnancy test usually ends the dilemma, although laparoscopy may be needed to confirm the diagnosis in the rare cases of PID occurring in pregnancy.

Acute appendicitis

The pain of acute appendicitis classically begins at the umbilicus, subsequently localizing to McBurney's point, and is often associated with nausea, vomiting and anorexia. Right iliac fossa tenderness with rebound, involuntary guarding, Rovsing's sign (right sided pain after pressing on the left), psoas sign (pain on hyperextending the hip), and obturator sign (pain on passive internal rotation of the hip), should all be assessed. Acute appendicitis presenting during pregnancy is notoriously difficult to diagnose early, as most classical features of the disease do not apply. In suspect cases laparoscopy should be performed.

Ovarian hyperstimulation syndrome

The risk of ectopic pregnancy is increased among infertile patients treated with ovulation induction agents, and these patients are also at risk for developing ovarian hyperstimulation syndrome. This syndrome usually presents with bilateral lower abdominal pain and obvious abdominal distention, 5–7 days after gonadotropin administration. It is usually a self-limiting condition requiring supportive measures with hydration and analgesia until the symptoms resolve (within 10 days if not pregnant, or 20 days if pregnant). Since bimanual examination and laparoscopy are best

avoided with this syndrome, ultrasonography is the mainstay of diagnosis.

Adnexal torsion

Torsion of adnexal structures is rare, but is more common in pregnancy, often presenting with non-specific pain which can be acute but intermittent. It usually occurs with a background of abnormal adnexal structures, such as ovarian cyst, pedunculated leiomyoma, hydrosalpinx or even a tubal ectopic pregnancy. Color Doppler ultrasonography and laparoscopy are usually required for accurate diagnosis.

Endometriosis

Pelvic pain from endometriosis is non-specific, associated with menstrual irregularity and often coexists with a pelvic mass, such as an endometrioma. The similarity with the presentation of ectopic pregnancy can therefore be quite marked, although all symptoms of endometriosis should improve with pregnancy. The diagnosis of ectopic pregnancy should be assumed in such cases, with hCG and ultrasonography obtained early.

MANAGEMENT

EXPECTANT MANAGEMENT

With the increasing early diagnosis of asymptomatic ectopic pregnancy in high risk groups, we are undoubtedly picking up cases of ectopic pregnancy which would otherwise have resolved spontaneously, either by tubal resorption or tubal abortion. It should, therefore, be possible to follow select cases of ectopic pregnancy expectantly.

Such patients should be completely asymptomatic, hemodynamically stable, with an initial serum hCG <1000 mIU/ml and the hCG level should be persistently falling. An unruptured tubal pregnancy <4 cm in diameter, without cardiac activity should be confirmed by ultrasonography. All patients should be well informed of the symptoms of tubal rupture, and they should be reliable to comply with regular follow-up. The diagnosis should be clear before laparoscopy, as if this is required for diagnosis there is no reason to defer definitive surgical management at that time.

Follow-up should be with weekly serum hCG levels, and frequent TVUS. Six weeks of follow-up is usually required to achieve two sequential negative hCG levels. The resorption of the tubal mass itself may take several months. Up to 25% of all ectopic pregnancy patients will be eligible for expectant management, with 72% successful spontaneous resolution, and 28% requiring surgery (most will be conservative procedures)[26]. Failure of expectant management is noted by plateauing or rising hCG levels, or by the development of symptoms. Expectant management should probably be confined to prospective clinical trials until its true benefits and disadvantages have been elucidated.

MEDICAL MANAGEMENT

The ability to treat ectopic pregnancy with an entirely non-surgical approach is quite attractive, as it removes the anesthesia and surgical complications of laparoscopic management, with an eventual goal of better fertility at less cost. Indeed, some authors now suggest that ectopic pregnancy is a medical rather than a surgical disease[27]. Two approaches are possible – systemic chemotherapy with methotrexate and salpingocentesis with a variety of agents. Medical management should not be used if laparoscopy is required for diagnosis, as there is no reason to defer definitive surgery at that time.

Systemic methotrexate

Methotrexate is a folate antagonist which inhibits dihydrofolate reductase, preventing thymidylate incorporation into DNA, therefore inhibiting rapidly growing cells, such as trophoblasts. Its usefulness against trophoblastic tissue in the management of hydatidiform mole and choriocarcinoma has been known for some time. Methotrexate use has been associated with significant side effects, including bone marrow suppression, liver and renal toxicity, stomatitis, gastrointestinal (GI) tract ulceration, diarrhea, pneumonitis, photosensitive dermatitis and anaphylaxis. These side effects appear to be rare at doses used for ectopic pregnancy, although some regimens have included leucovorin (folonic acid, citrovorum factor) which reduces methotrexate toxicity.

Selection criteria for patients eligible for systemic methotrexate include hemodynamic stability, no evidence of tubal rupture or intra-abdominal hemorrhage, TVUS-confirmation of an ectopic pregnancy <4 cm in greatest diameter, persistent hCG titers, with no evidence of active renal or liver disease. The patient should want to preserve future fertility and should be available for close follow-up. The presence of fetal cardiac activity or serum hCG levels >1500 mIU/ml are not absolute contraindications to methotrexate use, although they may be associated with a less successful outcome[28].

A simple out-patient protocol involves a single intramuscular administration of methotrexate without leucovorin rescue[29]. Baseline laboratory evaluation includes hCG level determination, complete blood count, aspartate aminotransferase, creatinine and blood type. A single 50 mg/m^2 intramuscular dose of methotrexate is given, followed by hCG evaluation at days 4 and 7, and then weekly until resolution. If hCG levels decrease <15% between days 4 and 7, or if weekly titers plateau, a second 50 mg/m^2 dose is given. No other laboratory parameters are required if the patient remains asymptomatic. No further pelvic examinations are performed, and patients are advised to avoid sun exposure and folate-containing supplements, and contraception is continued for 2–3 months. Abdominal pain is common 3–4 days after methotrexate administration and may be due to tubal abortion. Such pain usually lasts <12 h, and repeat TVUS may be needed to differentiate it from pain due to tubal rupture. hCG titers may increase by day 4, but most will show a significant decline by day 7, with full resolution appearing by 3–6 weeks.

Other protocols for systemic methotrexate have been described, using up to four doses of intramuscular or intravenous methotrexate, at doses of 1 mg/kg, given on alternate days with four doses of leucovorin at 0.1 mg/kg. Oral methotrexate protocols have also been used, at doses of 0.3 mg/kg daily for 4 days. Similar follow-up to that described for single-dose methotrexate is required.

A prospective study of 120 patients using the single-dose methotrexate protocol revealed 94.2% successful resolution, with 3.3% of patients requiring a second dose of methotrexate, with mean time to resolution being 5 weeks[29]. The failure rate was 5.8%, all requiring subsequent surgical management. Almost 60% of patients develop abdominal pain after treatment. Subsequent tubal patency was confirmed in 82.3% of cases, and there was a 79.6% subsequent pregnancy rate, with 87.2% being intrauterine and 12.8% being repeated ectopic pregnancies. Minimal methotrexate toxicity was encountered.

These results compare favorably with the multiple-dose protocols[30], with more toxicity being encountered with the multiple-dose protocols. There would, therefore, appear to be little justification for the more costly and more toxic multiple-dose protocols at this time.

Salpingocentesis

Salpingocentesis involves the direct injection of toxic agents into the tubal gestational sac, by laparoscopy, TVUS-guided needle, or hysteroscopic tubal cannulation. Agents used have included methotrexate, prostaglandins $F_{2\alpha}$ and E_2, hyperosmolar glucose and potassium chloride. The impetus for using such measures was to allow local injection of high dose agents, such as methotrexate, without the potentially serious systemic toxicity. It has now become clear, however, that circulating levels of methotrexate are similar after local and systemic injection, so that no obvious benefit of local injection is now apparent[31].

A review of 295 patients treated with local methotrexate showed 83% successful resolution, with 88% subsequent tubal patency and 67% subsequent pregnancy rate[32]. Methotrexate instillation by hysteroscopic cannulation has also been associated with an 87% success rate[33]. Direct prostaglandin injection with PGE_2 or $PGF_{2\alpha}$ may be associated with significant systemic toxicity, such as cardiac arrhythmia, pulmonary edema, hypertension and severe GI upset. A prospective comparison of laparoscopic injection of 50% glucose versus prostaglandins has suggested excellent results for glucose, but less success and more toxicity for prostaglandins[34]. Successful case reports have appeared of direct injection of 20% potassium chloride solution for tubal ectopics[35].

It is unclear whether local injection of relatively large volumes of fluid actually damages the tubal mucosa, and may potentially compromise future fertility. Given the success and simplicity of single-dose systemic methotrexate, there appears to be little reason to recommend the more complicated salpingocentesis techniques, although large-scale prospective randomized trials are still pending.

SURGICAL MANAGEMENT

The surgical management of ectopic pregnancy has undergone considerable change in the last 10 years. The earlier diagnosis of unruptured ectopics in patients desiring future fertility has converted surgical management from a radical into a conservative approach, and from laparotomy into laparoscopy. Conservative surgical strategies include linear salpingostomy, segmental resection and fimbrial expression, whereas radical strategies usually involve total salpingectomy. From a purely surgical viewpoint, salpingectomy is the 'gold standard' procedure, as it best guarantees hemostasis and total trophoblast removal. Today, however, the choice of procedure depends on a number of other factors.

1. Future fertility plans: If no further pregnancies are planned there is no reason to avoid definitive salpingectomy, whereas in patients desiring future pregnancies, it is reasonable to try to preserve the tube in an effort to maximize future fertility.
2. Site of ectopic pregnancy: Linear salpingostomy has been suggested for ampullary ectopics as such pregnancies are predominantly intraluminal, whereas segmental resection has been suggested for isthmic ectopics, as the pregnancy is more likely to have extraluminal spread. Further reviews, however, suggest little impact on future fertility by the site of the ectopic[36].
3. Size of ectopic pregnancy: The upper limit of ectopic pregnancy suitable for laparoscopic management is uncertain. It is predominantly a function of operator skill and experience. The larger the ectopic, the more difficulty may be encountered in removal from the abdomen at laparoscopy, and the more likely hemorrhage from the tubal bed will be seen. The upper limit for an experienced laparoscopist approaches 5–6 cm, whereas for a less experienced operator, 3 cm is probably a suitable upper limit[11].
4. State of fallopian tube: Although tubal rupture is not an absolute contraindication to conservative surgery, the more severely damaged the tube, the more likely a salpingectomy will be needed. If meticulous microsurgical technique is used for debridement of a ruptured tube, reasonable outcome can be expected with conservative surgery[37].
5. Hemodynamic status of patient: The only absolute contraindication to laparoscopic management is the presence of hypovolemic shock. Since this is a rare occurrence (<5% of ectopics), most patients can at least be considered for a conservative approach.
6. Adnexal adhesions: The presence of extensive adnexal adhesions may make a laparoscopic approach impossible, although, in general, this will be a function of operator experience. The presence of ipsilateral tubal adhesions significantly reduced the future intrauterine pregnancy rate from 67.5% to 45.7%, whereas the presence of contralateral adhesions reduced the future intrauterine pregnancy rate from 75.5% to 21.3%[36]. Repeat ectopic pregnancy rate increased from 9.7% in those with a patent contralateral tube to 21.3% in those with a non-functional contralateral tube. Because of such a significantly increased risk of repeat ectopic pregnancy, such cases may require radical, rather than conservative, surgery.
7. Economic considerations: Laparoscopic management is clearly associated with reduced hospital stay[38], reduced hospital costs, reduced recovery time and more rapid return to a normal life style. Such cost savings will drive future ectopic pregnancy management away from routine laparotomy[39].

Linear salpingostomy

This is the conservative surgical approach of choice for unruptured ampullary ectopic pregnancies. It involves opening the tube, removing the ectopic and allowing the tube to heal by secondary intention. There is rarely a role for linear salpingotomy, in which the tube is closed primarily after ectopic removal. A similar intrauterine pregnancy rate is obtained with either salpingostomy or salpingotomy after 2 years, but pregnancy occurs more quickly when primary closure is avoided[40].

Once a laparoscopic approach has been deemed feasible, a standard three-trocar laparoscopic set-up is performed (as described earlier). A vasopressin solution, (0.25 IU/ml), is then injected into the antimesenteric border of the tube over the ectopic, via a spinal needle through the abdominal wall. This gives a local vasoconstricting effect, resulting in excellent hemostasis, which appears to be persistent after the local effect has worn off. Vasopressin should not be injected into the mesosalpinx routinely, as it contributes little to overall hemostasis, but can give significant systemic toxicity.

The antimesenteric tubal incision can be made using laser (CO_2, argon, krypton or Nd:YAG with sapphire tip), unipolar needle electrocautery or electrocautery scissors. The choice of laser type is influenced by the necessity for hemostasis. The CO_2 beam penetrates 0.1 mm into tissue with only 0.5 mm of lateral damage, but gives poor hemostatis. Other laser types give better hemostasis, but at the expense of broader tissue scatter and damage.

Grasping forceps should then be used to gently lift ectopic tissue from its implantation site, avoiding vigorous removal as this will lead to significant hemorrhage and tubal necrosis. Tissue can then be removed through the 10 mm trocar with an endopouch or Semm spoon forceps, or else via a culdotomy or mini-laparotomy incision. Care should be taken not to drop any tissue over loops of bowel, as secondary reimplantation can occur. The implantation site and entire pelvis should be thoroughly lavaged to confirm hemostasis and lack of residual trophoblastic tissue. A similar method of salpingostomy can be performed via a pfannensteil incision if laparotomy is required.

Close postoperative follow-up is required for such conservative surgery, as this approach is not intended to remove all trophoblastic tissue, with minimal residual tissue usually undergoing spontaneous degeneration. Weekly serum hCG levels should be done as with medical management, and if levels plateau or rise, further surgical management or medical management may be needed. Serum hCG should be <20% of preoperative levels by 72 h postoperatively, with an average of 24 days required for complete resolution[11]. Rhesus immunoglobulin should be considered for all rhesus-negative patients to prevent rhesus sensitization. A dose of 50 ug should be sufficient for 8–12 week gestations, or 300 ug for gestations greater than 12 weeks. It is unclear if rhesus sensitization is a significant issue for pregnancies under 8 weeks' gestational age.

Reproductive outcome after conservative laparoscopic surgery has been well documented, with 95% successful resolution seen after salpingostomy performed either at laparoscopy or laparotomy[41,42]. Fertility outcome studies reveal 58–67% intrauterine pregnancy rate and 12–16% repeat ectopic pregnancy rate after linear salpingostomy[11,36].

Segmental resection

Because of the increased likelihood of extraluminal trophoblastic spread and consequent tubal damage with isthmic ectopic pregnancy, segmental resection has been recommended rather than linear salpingostomy[43]. A more recent review, however, suggests similar fertility outcome with salpingostomy or segmental resection for isthmic ectopic pregnancy[36]. Segmental resection can also be used for some cases of ruptured ampullary ectopic pregnancy.

Laparoscopic segmental resection can be performed using electrocautery, with the isthmus being removed 1 cm lateral to the uterotubal junction. Subsequent reanastomosis is usually performed 3–5 months later, as friable and edematous tubal ends can make primary anastomosis difficult. Reanastomosis is performed with standard microsurgical techniques, using an operating microscope and interrupted 6-0 or 7-0 delayed-absorbable extramucosal sutures. Laparoscopic tubal reanastomosis is also currently undergoing investigation.

Fimbrial expression

'Milking' of a distal ectopic pregnancy to the fimbriated end of the tube is contraindicated as it is associated with a high incidence of persistent and recurrent ectopic pregnancy[44]. If an ectopic is minimally attached at the fimbriated end of the tube it may be acceptable to gently dislodge it from the fimbriae without resorting to linear salpingostomy.

Salpingectomy

The indications for salpingectomy include repeated ectopic pregnancies in the same tube with significant tubal damage, uncontrolled intra-abdominal hemorrhage from tubal rupture, and completion of childbearing. Salpingectomy can be performed easily at both laparoscopy and laparotomy. At laparoscopy an endoscopic stapling device, loop ligatures or bipolar electrocautery can be used to excise the tube from the uterus and mesosalpinx. Care should be taken to remove the specimen in its entirety, without spillage of trophoblast into the abdominal cavity.

At laparotomy a standard salpingectomy can easily be performed through a pfannensteil incision, with care taken to ligate the meso-tubarian artery at both ends in order to secure hemostasis at the uterine–ovarian vascular anastomosis. There is no necessity to perform a routine cornual resection during a salpingectomy as it can lead to significant hemorrhage and it may predispose uterine rupture at future pregnancy. Such routine cornual resection does not protect against future interstitial pregnancy[45]. Complete reperitonealization of the exposed cornu of the uterus after salpingectomy using a modified Coffey procedure (suturing of round and broad ligaments over the exposed cornu) may protect against future development of an interstitial pregnancy.

There is no logical reason to perform an oophorectomy during a salpingectomy, unless the ovary has been significantly involved with the ectopic. Prophylactic oophorectomy does not influence subsequent ectopic pregnancy rates and it reduces the number of ova available for assisted reproduction[44]. During salpingectomy care should be taken not to displace the ovary from its normal anatomic position, as this may interfere with future ovum retrieval.

FERTILITY OUTCOME AFTER SURGERY

There is still no overall agreement as to which is the most appropriate surgical procedure for preservation of fertility potential following ectopic pregnancy. The effect of the procedure on fertility potential is confounded by such factors as underlying disease, prior history of infertility, prior history of ectopics and status of both fallopian tubes. Studies evaluating fertility outcome can only be assessed by stratification for these variables.

It would appear that fertility outcome is equally excellent with both conservative and radical surgery if there is no evidence of tubal disease or background infertility. It is, therefore, difficult to make an argument against conservative surgery in such cases. The situation is less clear with a background of tubal disease, with some authors arguing in favor of conservative surgery in an attempt to preserve fertility, whereas others argue in favor of salpingectomy to reduce the risk of recurrent ectopic pregnancy.

A recent review of the literature on this topic suggested a better chance of intrauterine pregnancy without a corresponding significant increase in the risk of repeat ectopic pregnancy when a conservative approach is used – 54% intrauterine pregnancy rate and 18% repeat ectopic pregnancy rate for conservative surgery, and 24% intrauterine pregnancy rate and 13% repeat ectopic pregnancy rate for radical surgery[41].

The dilemma of when to stop offering a conservative surgical approach and to proceed with radical surgery has recently been addressed, with the development of a scoring system to assess the balance between potential intrauterine pregnancy versus potential ectopic pregnancy[36,41]. The factors that significantly alter fertility outcome include prior ectopics, prior adnexal surgery or inflammation, presence of adnexal adhesions and the status of the fallopian tubes, with each factor given a statistical weighting and coefficient to allow calculation of a therapeutic scoring system (Table 7.1). With a score of 1–4, conservative laparoscopic salpingostomy should be performed as the likelihood of an intrauterine pregnancy is high in the absence of significant tubal factors. With a score of 5, radical laparoscopic salpingectomy should be performed as there is a significant risk of homolateral ectopic recurrence. With a score of 6–11, radical laparoscopic salpingectomy with contralateral tubal sterilization should be performed as the risk of recurrent ectopic is high and the likelihood of successful intrauterine pregnancy is probably less than with assisted reproduction.

Until definitive large-scale prospective randomized trials are performed comparing conservative versus radical surgery for ectopic pregnancy scoring systems such as this may be of help in incorporating an individual patient's risk factors into an appropriate management plan.

SPECIAL SITUATIONS

PERSISTENT ECTOPIC PREGNANCY

Continued growth of trophoblastic tissue occurs after conservative surgical management in 5% of cases, after systemic methotrexate in 6% of cases and after expectant management in 28% of cases. The importance

Table 7.1 Scoring system for fertility outcome after ectopic pregnancy [36]

Risk factor	Score
One prior ectopic	2
Each extra ectopic	1
Prior adhesiolysis	1
Prior tubal microsurgery	2
Solitary tube	2
Previous salpingitis	1
Homolateral adhesions	1
Contralateral adhesions	1

of careful, weekly follow-up of serum hCG is therefore obvious. Persistent ectopic pregnancy usually presents as non-specific pelvic pain, or a failure of post-therapeutic serum hCG to fall appropriately. Persistence after conservative surgery should be treated by radical surgery or systemic methotrexate, whereas persistence after expectant management can be treated by either medical or surgical methods.

INTERSTITIAL PREGNANCY

Pregnancy in the uterine cornu or interstitial tube is rare, accounting for <2% of all ectopics. Often symptoms occur late, (after 12 weeks), and it can result in massive intra-abdominal hemorrhage if trophoblasts erode into the uterine–ovarian vascular anastomosis. Examination may suggest an asymmetrically enlarged uterus. Laparotomy will be needed for management in many cases because of extensive bleeding, and over 50% of such cases may require a hysterectomy, with cornual resection being successful in the remaining cases. For unruptured interstitial pregnancies, methotrexate is probably the treatment of choice. Cornual resection may place the patient at significant risk for uterine rupture during a future pregnancy but even conservative surgery does not necessarily protect against uterine rupture.

ABDOMINAL PREGNANCY

Abdominal pregnancy is usually a result of secondary reimplantation of a tubal abortion, although rare cases of primary abdominal pregnancy are possible. The incidence of abdominal pregnancy is quoted as 1 in 7000 to 10 000 births. It presents later than a tubal ectopic, often with abdominal pain during fetal movement and atypical vaginal bleeding. Examination may reveal a dilated but uneffaced cervix, with easily palpable fetal parts and a fundus palpable separate from the fetus. Ultrasonography may often miss the diagnosis, and occasional cases are first diagnosed at cesarean section. There is a 75–95% fetal mortality and up to 20% maternal mortality. Fetal prognosis is worse if membranes rupture, and 50% of fetuses have significant structural abnormalities.

Management should involve early surgical intervention if the diagnosis is made before 24 weeks or if there is membrane rupture, whereas expectant in-patient management has been described for select cases diagnosed after 24 weeks[46]. At surgery, the placenta should be left in place, as life-threatening hemorrhage can occur if it is disturbed. Methotrexate should not be used for a retained placenta, as the rapid necrosis can become superinfected, resulting in significant sepsis.

OVARIAN PREGNANCY

This is a rare condition, with most cases being secondary to tubal abortion, or associated with the presence of an IUD. It may present as a hemorrhagic corpus luteum, and can be difficult to diagnose, even at laparoscopy. The hemorrhagic area should be resected, and in most cases the remainder of the ovary can be preserved. Confirmation of the diagnosis requires normal fallopian tubes with obvious ovarian tissue within the gestational sac.

CERVICAL PREGNANCY

This is the rarest form of ectopic pregnancy, occurring in 1 per 16 000 births. It often presents as painless vaginal bleeding, with an open cervix which is larger than the uterine corpus. Visible tissue in the os may suggest an inevitable abortion or cervical neoplasm. Severe hemorrhage can occur during curettage for presumed inevitable abortion. Treatment of choice is methotrexate prior to hemorrhage (using the single dose protocol as described earlier), but if the patient presents with significant hemorrhage, hemostasis can be attained by placement of a cerclage, ligation of the cervical branches of the uterine arteries, selective

arterial embolization or tamponade of bleeding surfaces[47,48]. Persistent hemorrhage will often require a hysterectomy for definitive control.

For the great majority of tubal ectopic pregnancies a standard management protocol will allow the minimum of unnecessary intervention with maximum efficiency, safety and patient satisfaction. Such an algorithm is here detailed.

REFERENCES

1. Centers for Disease Control (1988) Ectopic pregnancy surveillance, United States, 1970–1987. *MMWR*, **39**(SS-4), 9.
2. Westrom, L., Bengtsson, L.P. and Mardh, P.A. (1988) Incidence, trends and risks of ectopic pregnancy in a population of women. *Br. Med. J.*, **282**, 15–18.
3. Ory, S.J. (1992) New options for diagnosis and treatment of ectopic pregnancy. *JAMA*, **267**, 534–7.
4. Dorfman, S.F. (1987) Epidemiology of ectopic pregnancy. *Clin. Obstet. Gynecol.*, **30**, 173–80.
5. Lavy, G. and DeCherney, A.H. (1987) The hormonal basis of ectopic pregnancy. *Clin. Obstet. Gynecol.*, **30**, 217–24.
6. Doyle, M.B., DeCherney, A.H. and Diamond, M.P. (1991) Epidemiology and etiology of ectopic pregnancy. *Obstet. Gynecol. Clin. North Am.*, **18**, 1–17.
7. Elias, S., LeBeau, M., Simpson, J.L. *et al.* (1981) Chromosomal analysis of ectopic human conceptuses. *Am. J. Obstet. Gynecol.*, **141**, 698–703.
8. Budowick, M., Johnson, T.R., Genadry, R. *et al.* (1980) The histopathology of the developing tubal ectopic pregnancy. *Fertil. Steril.*, **34**, 169–71.
9. Senterman, M., Libodh, R. and Tulandi, T. (1988) Histopathologic study of ampullary and isthmic tubal ectopic pregnancy. *Am. J. Obstet. Gynecol.*, **159**, 939–41.
10. Soules, M.R. (1986) Infertility surgery, in *Reproductive Failure* (ed. A.H. DeCherney), Churchill Livingstone, New York, p. 117.
11. Thornton, K.L., Diamond, M.P. and DeCherney, A.H. (1991) Linear salpingostomy for ectopic pregnancy. *Obstet. Gynecol. Clin. North Am.*, **18**, 95–109.
12. Xiong, X., Buekens, P. and Wollast, E. (1995) IUD use and the risk of ectopic pregnancy: a

meta-analysis of case-control studies. *Contraception*, **52**, 23–34.

13. McCausland, A. (1980) High rate of ectopic pregnancy following laparoscopic tubal coagulation failures: Incidence and etiology. *Am. J. Obstet. Gynecol.*, **136**, 97–101.

14. Parazzini, F., Ferraroni, M., Tozzi, L. *et al.* (1995) Induced abortions and risk of ectopic pregnancy. *Hum. Reprod.*, **10**, 1841–4.

15. Chung, C.S., Smith, R., Steinhoff, P.G. *et al.* (1982) Induced abortion and ectopic pregnancies in subsequent pregnancies. *Am. J. Epidemiol.*, **115**, 879–87.

16. Molloy, D., Hynes, J., Deambrosis, L.V. *et al.* (1990) Multiple sited (heterotopic) pregnancy after in vitro fertilisation and gamete intrafallopian transfer. *Fertil. Steril.*, **53**, 1068–71.

17. DeCherney, A.H., Cholst, I. and Naftolin, F. (1981) Structure and function of the fallopian tubes following exposure to diethylstilbestrol (DES) during gestation. *Fertil. Steril.*, **36**, 741–5.

18. Christensen, H., Thyssen, H.H., Schebye, O. *et al.* (1990) Three highly sensitive 'bedside' serum and urine tests for pregnancy compared. *Clin. Chem.*, **36**, 1686–8.

19. Shepherd, R.W., Patton, P.E., Novy, M.J. *et al.* (1990) Serial beta hCG measurements in the early detection of ectopic pregnancy. *Obstet. Gynecol.*, **75**, 417–20.

20. Kadar, N., Caldwell, B.V. and Romero, R. (1981) A method of screening for ectopic pregnancy and its indications. *Obstet. Gynecol.*, **58**, 162–6.

21. al-Sebai, M.A., Kingsland, C.R., Diver, M. *et al.* (1995) The role of a single progesterone measurement in the diagnosis of early pregnancy failure and the prognosis of fetal viability. *Br. J. Obstet. Gynecol.*, **102**, 364–9.

22. Stovall, T.G. and Ling, F.W. (1993) Ectopic pregnancy – diagnostic and therapeutic algorithms minimising surgical intervention. *J. Reprod. Med.*, **38**, 807–12.

23. Romero, R., Copel, J.A., Kadar, N. *et al.* (1985) Value of culdocentesis in the diagnosis of ectopic pregnancy. *Obstet. Gynecol.*, **65**, 519–22.

24. Fossum, G.T., Davajan, V. and Kletzky, O.A. (1988) Early detection of pregnancy with transvaginal ultrasound. *Fertil. Steril.*, **49**, 788–91.

25. Emerson, D.S., Cartier, M.S., Altieri, L.A. *et al.* (1992) Diagnostic efficacy of endovaginal color doppler flow imaging in an ectopic pregnancy screening program. *Radiology*, **183**, 413–20.

26. Ylostalo, P., Cacciatore, B., Korhonen, J. *et al.* (1993) Expectant management of ectopic pregnancy. *Eur. J. Obstet. Gynecol. Reprod. Biol.*, **49**, 83–4.

27. Buster, J.E. and Carson, S.A. (1995) Ectopic pregnancy: new advances in diagnosis and treatment. *Curr. Opin. Obstet. Gynecol.*, **7**, 168–76.

28. Corson, G.H., Karacan, M., Qasim, S. *et al.* (1995) Identification of hormonal parameters for successful systemic single-dose methotrexate therapy in ectopic pregnancy. *Hum. Reprod.*, **10**, 2719–22.

29. Stovall, T.G. and Ling, F.W. (1993) Single-dose methotrexate: an expanded clinical trial. *Am. J. Obstet. Gynecol.*, **168**, 1759–65.

30. Ory, S.J. (1991) Chemotherapy for ectopic pregnancy. *Obstet. Gynecol. Clin. North Am.*, **18**, 123–34.

31. Schiff, E., Shalev, E., Bustan, M. *et al.* (1992) Pharmacokinetics of methotrexate after local tubal injection for conservative treatment of ectopic pregnancy. *Fertil. Steril.*, **57**, 688–90.

32. Carson, S.A. and Buster, J.E. (1993) Current concepts: ectopic pregnancy. *N. Engl. J. Med.*, **329**, 1174–81.

33. Risquez, F., Forman, R., Maleika, F. *et al.* (1992) Transcervical cannulation of the fallopian tube for the management of ectopic pregnancy: prospective multicenter trial. *Fertil. Steril.*, **58**, 1131–5.

34. Lang, P., Weiss, P.A. and Mayer, H.O. (1989) Local application of hyperosmolar glucose solution in tubal pregnancy. *Lancet*, **ii**, 922–3.

35. Robertson, D.E., Smith, W., Moyle, M.A. *et al.* (1987) Reduction of ectopic pregnancy by injection under ultrasound control. *Lancet*, **i**, 974–5.

36. Pouly, J.L., Canis, M., Chapron, C. *et al.* (1991) Multifactorial analysis of fertility after conservative laparoscopic treatment of ectopic pregnancy in a series of 223 patients. *Fertil. Steril.*, **56**, 453–60.

37. DeCherney, A.H., Polan, M.L., Kort, H. *et al.* (1980) Microsurgical techniques in the management of tubal ectopic pregnancy. *Fertil. Steril.*, **34**, 324–7.

38. Vermesh, M., Silva, P.D., Rosen, G.F. *et al.* (1989) Management of unruptured ectopic gestation by linear salpingostomy: a prospective randomized clinical trial of laparoscopy versus laparotomy. *Obstet. Gynecol.*, **73**, 400–4.

39. Gray, D.T., Thorburn, J., Lundorff, P. *et al.* (1995) A cost-effectiveness study of a randomised trial of laparoscopy versus

laparotomy for ectopic pregnancy. *Lancet*, **345**, 1139–43.

40. Tulandi, T. and Guralnick, M. (1991) Treatment of tubal ectopic pregnancy by salpingectomy with or without tubal suturing and salpingectomy. *Fertil. Steril.*, **55**, 53–5.

41. Chapron, C., Pouly, J.L., Wattiez, A. *et al.* (1993) Laparoscopic management of tubal ectopic pregnancy. *Eur. J. Obstet. Gynecol. Reprod. Biol.*, **49**, 73–9.

42. DiMarchi, J.M., Kosasa, T.S., Kobara, T.Y. *et al.* (1987) Persistent ectopic pregnancy. *Obstet. Gynecol.*, **70**, 555–8.

43. DeCherney, A.H. and Boyers, S.P. (1985) Isthmic ectopic pregnancy: segmental resection as the treatment of choice. *Ferti. Steril.*, **44**, 307–12.

44. Timonen, S. and Nieminen, U. (1967) Tubal pregnancy, choice of operative method of treatment. *Acta Obstet. Gynecol. Scand.*, **46**, 327–9.

45. Kooi, S. and Kock, H.C. (1993) Surgical treatment for tubal pregnancies. *Surg. Gynecol. Obstet.*, **176**, 519–26.

46. Hage, M.L., Wall, L.L. and Killam, A. (1988) Expectant management of abdominal pregnancy. A report of 2 cases. *J. Reprod. Med.*, **33**, 407–10.

47. Van de Meerssche, M., Verdonk, P., Jacquemyn, Y. *et al.* (1995) Cervical pregnancy: three case reports and a review of the literature. *Hum. Reprod.*, **10**, 1850–5.

48. Marston, L.M., Dotters, D.J. and Katz, V.L. (1996) Methotrexate and angiographic embolization for conservative treatment of cervical pregnancy. *South. Med. J.*, **89**, 246–8.

TERMINATION OF PREGNANCY IN THE FIRST TRIMESTER

8

C.M. Paterson

BACKGROUND TO UNWANTED PREGNANCY

Pregnancy, whether planned or unplanned, often results in great happiness but, if unwanted, can cause great emotional, social and physical stress. Pregnancies are likely to be unwanted if the woman lacks the resources to care for a child, and, particularly, if she does not have the support of her partner. Unplanned pregnancy occurs when problems in the relationship make sexual intercourse unpredictable and when contraception is difficult to obtain or when its use is not part of the couple's tradition[1].

In 1996 89% of abortions in England and Wales were performed at less than 13 and 40% at less than 9 weeks' gestation[2]. Only 1.1% of all abortions in England and Wales are performed for fetal abnormalities[2] and the majority of these are in the second trimester, although more might be performed in the first trimester as earlier methods of diagnosing fetal abnormality are developed.

CURRENT LEGAL STATUS

The reasons for which abortion can be legal varies between countries and can be divided into four major groups: (1) only to save the life of the pregnant woman; (2) only on medical grounds; (3) social factors in addition to health and (4) abortion on request. In addition when abortion is allowed it is often only permitted in the first trimester. Even where the law is more liberal many medical practitioners limit the service that they offer to less than 13 weeks' gestation. Legally, abortion is available on request in the United States, although in practice there are large geographical areas with no provision. In England, Wales and Scotland it is allowed on broad social grounds but two registered medical practitioners must certify in good faith that the operation is being performed for grounds specified within the 1967 Abortion Act, as amended in 1990.

Neither a woman nor the doctor is compelled under any law to accept or to perform an abortion against their wishes, but doctors who are opposed to abortion on religious or ethical grounds have a moral obligation to declare their position to women who consult them and to offer referral to another doctor who does not share their views.

ASSESSMENT FOR ABORTION

All women requesting abortion should be offered counseling, medical assessment and information.

COUNSELING

Abortion counseling should be directed at ascertaining what a woman really wants, ensuring that she is aware of the alternatives to

Clinical Management of Early Pregnancy. Edited by Walter Prendiville and James R. Scott.
Published in 1999 by Arnold, ISBN 0 340 74100 7

abortion, helping her to take ultimate responsibility for her decision and to avoid serious regrets. The amount of support a woman needs will depend on her reason for requesting abortion, her educational level and her social support network. Allen[3] describes interviews with women who had just had an abortion and 56% said that as soon as they suspected that they were pregnant they wanted an abortion, but 16% initially wished to continue with the pregnancy. The rest were undecided. Most women attending an abortion assessment clinic have already discussed the situation with their partner, family and/or peers, and have decided on their course of action, but a small proportion are still undecided and wish to discuss all options with a counselor.

Within our district pregnancy advisory clinic about 40% of women elect to see a counselor, and those who prefer not to are offered the opportunity to contact a counselor postabortion if they wish.

MEDICAL ASSESSMENT

Medical assessment should cover confirmation of gestation, fitness for anesthesia, and rhesus typing. It is rarely necessary to perform ultrasonography to confirm gestational age. Even when the last menstrual period (LMP) is uncertain or unknown clinical assessment is usually sufficient, although scanning may be indicated to exclude ectopic pregnancy, or where gestation would influence the method of abortion, or the choice of surgeon. Although it is likely that pregnancies ended at very early gestations do not have the ability to provoke a rhesus antibody response in the mother, Thong *et al.*[4] demonstrated significant changes in the maternal levels of placental hormones and α-fetoprotein following early medical abortion and concluded that it was important to give all rhesus-negative women anti D following an abortion.

There has been considerable debate about the prevention of postabortal sepsis. Some centers give antibiotic prophylaxis, usually a tetracycline but occasionally metronidazole (or both) to all women, others screen all women and treat as indicated, and some selectively screen women thought to be at risk of infection. All these strategies reduce postabortal sepsis and the one used generally depends on the time available between assessment and abortion and the resources available.

A recent review of published data[5] suggests that the routine use of periabortal antibiotics may prevent up to half of all cases of postabortal infection.

INFORMATION

The woman should be given information about the methods of abortion available in relation to gestation and local facilities. If all options are available the differences between medical and surgical abortion should be discussed, and for surgical abortion the type of anesthesia. When the method of abortion has been decided the process (both administrative and medical) should be clearly explained to the woman and this explanation should be backed up by written leaflets. Although the woman should be reassured that a planned abortion is generally a safe and straightforward procedure, possible important complications should be discussed. With surgical abortion these include the possibility of uterine damage and subsequent laparotomy and the risks associated with anesthesia. All abortions also carry the risk of, and problems associated with, pelvic infection and/or retained products of conception. Women should also be aware of the rare occurrence of failed abortions, or unrecognized ectopic pregnancy, especially at very early gestations. The rates of occurrence of complications should be derived locally.

METHODS OF ABORTION

Abortion in the first trimester may be surgical or medical. In the majority of women this can be offered as a day-care procedure. Surgical abortion may be performed under either local or general anesthesia depending on the preference of the woman and her surgeon, and the resources available. Inhalational anesthetic gases which are associated with uterine bleeding should be avoided.

SURGICAL ABORTION

Abortions have been performed for thousands of years. Dilatation and curettage has been documented since the time of the Egyptian Middle Kingdom 4000 years ago, however, since the late 1960s vacuum aspiration has been recognized as the method of choice throughout the world after its reintroduction by Wu and Wu in China in 1958[6]. This method involves the insertion of a cannula through the cervix and application of negative pressure, either mechanical or manual, to remove the products of conception. At gestations of 8 or more weeks this usually involves dilatation of the cervix which should be performed using tapered dilators rather than straight-sided Hegar dilators. An experienced operator using transparent suction cannulae can usually recognize the products of conception, but if there is any doubt the aspirate should be examined for a fetal sac, chorionic villi or fetal parts.

There is some concern about the risk of failed surgical abortion at early gestations and at less than 6 weeks the failure rate is 2.9 times higher than that at 7–12 weeks[7]. This failure may not be diagnosed at the time, and it should also be remembered that the absence of a gestational sac may indicate an ectopic pregnancy.

Cervical preparation is rarely necessary in multiparous women having a termination of pregnancy in the first trimester but may be beneficial in young nulliparous women, either at very early gestations of less than 7 weeks, or at 10–12 weeks' gestation when the cervix may need to be dilated to ≥10 mm. Preparation may also be helpful where there is distortion of the anatomy such as following cone biopsy or laser treatment of the cervix, or where there are multiple or large fibroids.

The most widely used method of preparation in the first trimester in England and Wales is the prostaglandin E_1 analog gemeprost. However, there have recently been publications comparing this with the less expensive, more stable, analog misoprostol[8] and with the oral antigestagen mifepristone[9] showing that all these are effective. Intracervical tents such as laminaria (seaweed), hypan (a hydrophilic polyacrylonitrile polymer) and lamicel (a polyvinyl alcohol foam sponge impregnated with magnesium sulfate) may also be used. These all work by absorption of fluid, so that they expand and dilate the cervix over a period of time. The maximum effect with laminaria is observed at 24 h[10], but both hypan[11] and lamicel[12] are effective within 3 h and are more suitable for day care surgery.

Surgical abortion is a common and safe operation. Complications associated with this procedure include rare anesthetic reactions, cervical tears and uterine perforation, rarely with damage to other pelvic organs, pelvic sepsis, partial retention of products of conception and failed abortion. Early complications have been reviewed by Heisterberg and Kringlebach[13] and in a report of 170 000 cases by Hakim-Elahi *et al.*[14]. Daling *et al.*[15] found no increase in tubal infertility in relation to prior induced abortion and Frank *et al.*[16] found no difference in the birthweight or gestation of babies born to mothers who had a previous abortion when compared to those of mothers whose previous pregnancy ended in childbirth. There was also no difference in the incidence of non-viable pregnancy between the groups. However, most studies demonstrate that experienced operators have the lowest complication rates.

MEDICAL ABORTION

In 1970 it was demonstrated that prostaglandins could be used to induce abortion in the first trimester]17], but the high dose required was associated with unacceptable gastrointestinal side effects. One of the most important advances in abortion provision has been the synthesis of the orally active progesterone antagonist mifepristone (RU486), a derivative of norethisterone[18]. Mifepristone binds with high affinity to progesterone receptors blocking the action of endogenous progesterone. It also binds to the glucocorticoid and weakly to androgen receptors. Progesterone is essential for the establishment and maintenance of pregnancy and any substance which antagonizes this action will cause a pregnancy to fail[19]. Early studies demonstrated that with varying dose regimens mifepristone induced complete abortion in 60–85% of women depending on gestation[20]. When a single dose of mifepristone is followed 48 h later by a dose of prostaglandin the complete abortion rate is over 95% at gestations up to 63 days, with a 1% continuing pregnancy rate[21].

Hausknecht[22] published a series of 178 women who had an early medical abortion induced using a combination of the cytotoxic agent methotrexate followed by vaginal misoprostol. Although 14% of women required a second dose of misoprostol, overall 96% had a successful abortion. Although there were some reservations about the long-term safety of methotrexate this combination could offer medical abortion to women in areas where mifepristone is not available.

Indications

Mifepristone is currently licensed in Great Britain for the termination of pregnancies of less than 63 days' gestation at a dose of 600 mg followed by 1 mg vaginal gemeprost 48 h later.

Contradindications and risks

Mifepristone appears to be a very safe drug. Nausea, vomiting, faintness and skin rashes have been reported in a minority of patients[23], but most contraindications to medical abortion relate to the concomitant use of a prostaglandin. There have been reports of adverse cardiac effects, one of which was fatal[24], but these have usually been associated with the rapidly absorbed intramuscular administration of the prostaglandin sulprostone. There has also been a report of cardiac arrest following use of a prostaglandin pessary[25]. Medical abortion is therefore contraindicated in women at risk of cardiac disease and smokers over the age of 35 years. It should not be used in women with renal or hepatic impairment as these might delay metabolism or excretion of the drugs. Prostaglandins may also cause bronchospasm and should not be used in women with asthma or chronic obstructive airways disease. As mifepristone is an antiglucocorticoid it should not be used in women on long-term steroid therapy. It would be prudent to avoid medical abortion in women with bleeding disorders.

Dose

There have been many publications relating to the optimal dose of mifepristone, and the best dose, formulation and route of administration of the prostaglandin. Mifepristone has a long half-life (20 h) and can therefore be given as a single dose. The World Health Organization (WHO), in a large randomized double blind multicentre trial, demonstrated that, in conjunction with gemeprost 1 mg, a single dose of 200 mg of mifepristone was as effective as the currently recommended 600 mg dose[26]. The current recommended dose of prostaglandin, 1 mg gemeprost vaginally, has also been challenged. El-Refaey *et al.*[27] looked at the combination of 600 mg mifepristone with 800 μg of misoprostol, the orally active prostaglandin analog, given vaginally or orally and achieved a 95% complete abortion rate with vaginal administration, compared to 87% when given orally. Penney *et al.*[28] gave 200 mg of mifepristone with 800 μg of vaginal misoprostol and also achieved success rates of 95% at less than

49 days' gestation but a slightly lower rate of 93% at 49–63 days.

Procedure

After counseling, medical assessment and confirmation of gestation the woman should be given a dose of mifepristone and told that she may continue normal activities for the next 48 h. In most women who are sure of the date of their last menstrual period clinical assessment of gestation is adequate, but if there is doubt, or suspicion of an ectopic pregnancy, an ultrasound scan should be performed. The woman should be advised to eat before taking the tablets in order to reduce the risk of vomiting. If the mifepristone is vomited within 2 h of ingestion the dose should be repeated. The woman should be told that 35% of women have vaginal bleeding, and in 3 in 100 women the abortion will occur before admission for prostaglandin administration. She should be reassured that this is usually neither alarming nor dangerous and given a 24 h contact telephone number to ring if she is concerned, or if the bleeding is significantly heavier than a period. She should be advised against using non-steroidal anti-inflammatory drugs which inhibit prostaglandin synthetase and could theoretically reduce the efficacy of the regimen.

She should be admitted to a day-care unit, with access to resuscitation and operating facilities, 36–48 h later for administration of a prostaglandin. Thong *et al.*[29] asked women their preferred accommodation in the day-care unit and found that 87% of women randomized to a sitting room and allowed to wear their day clothes and 80% of women randomized to a ward bed and night clothes would prefer accommodation in the sitting room. However, about one third of the women treated in the sitting room requested to lie on a bed at some time after the prostaglandin administration therefore bed, couches or fully reclining chairs should be available. We treat women in a small sitting room with reclining armchairs which is satisfactory but occasionally women transfer

to a ward bed if they require parenteral analgesia. Although women desire privacy, many find the support of other women having the same procedure helpful, and in Thong's study 46% of women would have liked the company of a friend or partner. Thong also found that 10% of women overall required parenteral analgesia (diamorphine), 2% in the women treated with misoprostol and 18% in the women given gemeprost; 52% of women did not request any analgesia.

The onset of uterine contractions and vaginal bleeding after the administration of prostaglandin is variable. All women should be asked to use a commode so that products of conception can be seen as soon as passed. If the products are not seen by 4 h a vaginal examination should be performed and if present they should be removed from the cervical os or vagina with sponge forceps. If the passage of products is not confirmed by 8 h we allow the patient to go home and arrange an ultrasound scan five days later. The women sometimes report passing tissue at home but the majority are unaware of this. Only two of our patients in a series of 300 have had an ongoing pregnancy when scanned.

All women are seen two weeks after discharge in the family planning clinic and if they are still bleeding an ultrasound scan is performed. Few of these show significant retained products of conception, the evacuation rate is 4%.

COMPARISON OF MEDICAL AND SURGICAL METHODS

PATIENT PREFERENCE

Henshaw *et al.*[30] published a patient centered partially randomized trial where 363 women presenting for abortion at less than 63 days' gestation were given written information on both surgical and medical abortion and asked if they were willing to be allocated to a method of abortion at random. A total of 189 women agreed to random selection – 94 to medical abortion and 95 to vacuum aspiration; 72 women said they preferred surgical abortion, and 84 asked for vacuum aspiration. Reasons given for preferring medical abortion included fear of surgery or anesthesia, a feeling that the medical process was more 'natural', and a preference for the slower timescale and awareness of the procedure. Vacuum aspiration was chosen because women wished to be unconscious and unaware of the procedure, they thought the timescale of medical abortion was too slow or they were worried about the effect of the drugs. The acceptability of both methods was high when chosen by the woman but when randomized to the method only 74% of women would have a repeat medical abortion whereas 87% of those having vacuum aspiration would use the same method again.

The other important variable was gestation. Only one woman at less than 49 days gestation would not use the medical method in the future.

Urquhart and Templeton[31] looked at psychiatric morbidity 2 days before and one month after for women having medical and surgical abortions and found no difference between the two groups.

MEDICAL OUTCOME

At less than 50 days' gestation there is little to choose between the two methods of abortion in terms of efficacy, pain, vaginal bleeding and recovery time[32]. However, there is a reduction in acceptability and an increase in bleeding and the failure rate at increasing gestations with medical abortion, whereas there is no reduction in efficacy or acceptability with the surgical method.

CONTRACEPTION

All women who have had an abortion should be offered contraceptive counseling and be taught about postcoital contraception and how to access it. During the stressful period surrounding an abortion and the uncertainty of future sexual activity it may be difficult to make long-term contraceptive plans, however women should be aware that they may ovulate as early as 10 days after an abortion and be offered at least short-term cover until they are sure of their future plans. The oral contraceptive pill may be started on the evening of operation or completed medical abortion. Depo progestogen preparations may be given before discharge. An intrauterine contraceptive device can be inserted at the time of surgical termination of pregnancy. Long-term (e.g. Norplant) or permanent (e.g. sterilization) contraception is probably best delayed until the woman has fully recovered from her abortion, and the woman advised to use condoms or oral contraception in the interim. A diaphragm can be fitted or checked after the first menstrual period.

FOLLOW-UP

All women should be given a 24 h contact number when they leave the hospital or clinic, and advised to contact a physician if they have persistent heavy vaginal bleeding, uterine cramps, an offensive vaginal discharge or a fever. They should also be given a follow-up appointment within two weeks to see a family planning trained doctor. This visit allows the woman to discuss any aspect of the abortion or its aftermath, physical or emotional. It is also an opportunity to discuss whether she is happy with her chosen method of contraception, understands how to use it and where to get further supplies and knows about emergency contraception.

PSYCHOLOGICAL MORBIDITY

Most studies have found increased psychiatric morbidity in women with an unwanted pregnancy. Dagg[33] reviewed 225 papers and found that abortion-related stress is greatest before the abortion and wanes afterwards when the majority of women feel a sense of relief. He also found that when abortion is denied women may be resentful for many years and children born in these circumstances may have a variety of interpersonal and occupational difficulties. Gilchrist[34] in a prospective cohort study of 13 261 women with an unplanned pregnancy found that rates of reported psychiatric disorder were no higher after termination of pregnancy than after childbirth. Women with a previous history of psychiatric disorder were most at risk regardless of the outcome of the pregnancy.

The situation is different in women having abortions for fetal abnormality. It might be thought that these women would be relieved to have fetal abnormality diagnosed early enough to have the option of abortion. However, there are many reasons why, for these women, relief is not the predominant emotion, not least the fact that most of these pregnancies are wanted and termination means the rejection of a wanted child. Iles[35] discussed the psychological sequelae of termination of pregnancy for fetal abnormality and found that morbidity was higher in those women whose fetus had a less serious abnormality and might have survived, and in those who had their pregnancy terminated later in the second trimester.

CONCLUSION

Up to 63 days' gestation abortion may be medical or surgical. After this, vacuum aspiration, with or without cervical preparation is the method of choice. Up to 56 days' gestation medical abortion is probably the safest method for women who have no medical contraindications as this removes the risks associated with anesthesia or surgical trauma. Although there is still a 1% risk of failed abortion this is less likely to be missed than after a very early surgical termination of pregnancy. Surgical abortion, especially in nulliparous women, is probably best reserved for those with a gestation greater than 49 days. Both methods are acceptable to women, particularly if she has chosen the method herself.

There is no evidence to suggest that an uncomplicated abortion has any adverse effect on future reproductive performance, and most studies suggest that there is more psychological morbidity in women who have been refused abortion than in those who have access to legal, safe abortion on request.

REFERENCES

1. Paintin, D.B. (1991) in *Abortion – an Introduction* (P. Diggory) Birth Control Trust, London, p. 3.
2. ONS (1997) *Population and Health Monitor* Series AB, no. 93, Office for National Statistics, London.
3. Allen, I. (1985) *Counselling services for Sterilisation, Vasectomy and Termination of Pregnancy*, no. 641, Policy Studies Institute, London.
4. Thong, K.J., Norman, J.E. and Baird, D.T. (1993) Changes in the concentration of alpha-fetoprotein and placental hormones following 2 methods of medical abortion in early pregnancy. *Br. J. Obstet. Gynaecol.*, **100**, 1111–14.
5. Sawaya, G.F., Grady, D., Kerlikowska, K. and Grimes, D.A. (1996) Antibiotics at the time of induced abortion: the case for universal prophylaxix based on a meta-analysis. *Obstet. Gynecol.*, **87**, 884–90.
6. Diggory, P. (1991) *Abortion – An Introduction*, Birth Control Trust, 16 Mortimer St, London W1N 7RD, p. 17–18.
7. Kaunitz, A.M., Rovira, E.Z., Grimes, D.A. and Schulz, K.F. (1985) Abortions that fail. *Obstet. Gynecol.*, **66**, 533–7.
8. El-Refaey, H., Calder, L., Wheatley, D.N. and Templeton, A. (1994) Cervical priming with prostaglandin E$_1$ analogue, misoprostol and gemeprost, *Lancet*, **343**, 1207–9.
9. Carbonne, B., Brennand, J.E., Maria, B. *et al.* (1995) Effects of gemeprost and mifepristone on the mechanical properties of the cervix prior to first trimester termination of pregnancy. *Br. J. Obstet. Gynaecol.*, **102**, 553–8.
10. Eaton, C.J., Cohn, F. and Bollinger, C.C. (1972) Laminara tent as a cervical dilator prior to aspiration-type therapeutic abortion. *Obstet. Gynecol.*, **39**, 533–7.
11. Darney, P.D. and Dorwood, K. (1987) Cervical dilatation before first trimester elective abortion: a controlled comparison of meteneprost, laminara and hypan. *Obstet. Gynecol.*, **70**, 397–400.

12. Norstrom, A., Bryman, I. and Hansson, H.A. (1988) Cervical dilatation by lamicel before first trimester abortion: a clinical and experimental study. *Br. J. Obstet. Gynaecol.*, **95**, 372–6.

13. Heisterberg, L. and Kringelbach, M. (1987) Early complications after induced first trimester abortion. *Acta Obstet. Gynecol. Scand.*, **66**, 201–4.

14. Hakim-Elahi, E., Tovell, H.M.M. and Burnhill, M.S. (1990) Complications of first trimester abortion: a report of 170,000 cases. *Obstet. Gynecol.*, **76**, 129–35.

15. Daling, J.R., Weiss, N.S., Voigt, L. *et al.* (1995) Tubal infertility in relation to prior induced abortion. *Fertil. Steril.*, **43**, 389–94.

16. Frank, P.I., McNamee, R., Hannaford, P.L. *et al.* (1991) The effect of induced abortion on subsequent pregnancy outcome. *Br. J. Obstet. Gynaecol.*, **98**, 1015–24.

17. Karim, S.M.M. and Filshie, G.M. (1970) Therapeutic abortion using prostaglandin F2alpha. *Lancet*, **i**, 157–9.

18. Baird, D.T. (1993) Antigestogens. *Br. Med. Bull.*, **49**, 73–87.

19. Csapo, A.L. and Pulkkinen, M. (1978) Indispensability of the human corpus luteum in the maintenance of early pregnancy. *Obstet. Gynecol.*, **33**, 69–81.

20. Van Look, P.F.A. and Bydgeman, M. (1989) Antiprogestational steroids: a new dimension in fertility regulation. *Oxford Rev. Reprod. Biol.*, **11**, 1–60.

21. UK Multicentre Trial (1990) The efficacy and tolerance of mifepristone and prostaglandin in first trimester termination of pregnancy. *Br. J. Obstet. Gynaecol.*, **97**, 480–6.

22. Hausknecht, R. (1995) Methotrexate and misoprostol to terminate early pregnancy. *N. Engl. J. Med.*, **333**, 537–40.

23. Rodger, M.W. and Baird, D.T. (1990) Pretreatment with mifepristone (RU486) reduces interval between prostaglandin administration and expulsion in second trimester abortion. *Br. J. Obstet. Gynaecol.*, **97**, 41–5.

24. Anonymous (1991) A death associated with mifepristone/sulprostone. *Lancet*, **337**, 969–70.

25. Kaira, P.A., Litherland, D., Sallomi, D.F. *et al.* (1989) Cardiac standstill induced by prostaglandin pessaries. Lancet, **i**, 1460–1.

26. World Health Organization Task Force on Post-Ovulatory Methods of Fertility Regulation (1993) Termination of pregnancy with reduced doses of mifepristone. *Br. Med. J.*, **307**, 532–7.

27. El-Refaey, H., Rajasekar, D., Abdalla, M. *et al.* (1995) Induction of abortion with mifepristone and oral or vaginal misoprostol. *N. Engl. J. Med.*, **332**, 983–7.

28. Penney, G.C., McKessock, L., Rispin, R. *et al.* (1995) An effective low cost regime for early medical abortion. *Br. J. Family Planning*, **21**, 5–6.

29. Thong, K.J., Dewar, M.H. and Baird, D.T. (1992) What do women want during medical abortion? *Contraception*, **46**, 435–42.

30. Henshaw, R.C., Naji, S.A., Russell, I.T. and Templeton, A.A. (1993) Comparison of medical abortion with surgical vacuum aspiration: women's preferences and acceptability of treatment. *Br. Med. J.*, **307**, 714–17.

31. Urquhart, D.R. and Templeton, A.A. (1991) Psychiatric morbidity and acceptability following medical and surgical methods of induced abortion. *Br. J. Obstet. Gynaecol.*, **98**, 396–9.

32. Henshaw, R.C., Naji, S.A., Russell, I.T. and Templeton, A.A. (1994) A comparison of medical abortion (using mifepristone and gemeprost) with surgical vacuum aspiration: efficacy and early medical sequelae. *Hum. Reprod.*, **9**, 2167–72.

33. Dagg, P.K.B. (1991) The psychological sequelae of theraputic abortion – denied and completed. *Am. J. Psychiatr.*, **148**, 578–85.

34. Gilchrist, A.C., Hannaford, P.C., Frank, P. and Kay, C.R. (1995) Termination of pregnancy and psychiatric morbidity. *Br. J. Psychiatr.*, **167**, 243–8.

35. Iles, S. (1989) The loss of early pregnancy. *Baillieres Clin. Obstet. Gynecol.*, **3**, 769–90.

IMMUNOLOGY OF RECURRENT MISCARRIAGE: ETIOLOGY, DIAGNOSIS, THERAPY AND PROGNOSIS

9

J.A. Hill

Spontaneous abortion causes significant emotional distress for couples desiring children. Loss of a clinically recognized pregnancy before 20 weeks of gestation occurs at a frequency of 15%[1,2]. In an estimated 70% of human conceptions fetal viability is not achieved with approximately 50% lost prior to the first missed menses[3]. The actual rate of early pregnancy loss after implantation may exceed the number of recognized pregnancies and may be as high as 31%[4]. Recurrent abortion, traditionally defined as the occurrence of three or more clinically detectable pregnancy losses before the 20th week of gestation, occurs in approximately 1 in 300 pregnant women[4,5]. Search for causation is recommended after two consecutive pregnancy losses. It is especially recommended for couples without a successful pregnancy where fetal heart activity had been identified, couples where the woman is older than 35 years of age and couples having difficulty conceiving[5–7]. The calculated risks for recurrent abortion based on epidemiological surveys are 24% after one abortion, 30% after two, 35% after three, and approximately 40% after four consecutive clinical losses[1]. Many instances of recurrent spontaneous abortion have identifiable etiologies such as parental chromosomal anomalies[8]. Non-genetic causes of recurrent abortion are difficult to ascribe, although numerous associations have been made with maternal muellerian[9], endocrinologic[10,11], infectious[12,13] and antiphospholipid antibody[14,15] abnormalities. Conventional diagnostic tests used in the evaluation of individuals with recurrent abortion include peripheral blood karyotype analysis, hysterosalpingography, thyroid function studies, a luteal phase endometrial biopsy, cervical cultures, and antiphospholipid antibody determinations. However, the cause of abortion remains unknown in 40–60% of couples experiencing recurrent pregnancy loss[16–18]. Immunologic etiologies have been proposed for many couples with otherwise unexplained recurrent abortion. However, the majority of these theories have not withstood rigorous analysis and are no longer commonly accepted[6,19].

The immunologic aspects of recurrent abortion are the most promising and controversial to diagnose and treat. The purpose of this chapter is to provide an up-to-date analysis of immunologic recurrent abortion, discussing the potential etiologies that may be treated and those that as yet cannot. Also outlined are the diagnostic tests and therapies that are potentially useful and effective and others that are neither. This information should be helpful to both practitioners and investigators interested in the problem of recurrent spontaneous abortion.

Clinical Management of Early Pregnancy. Edited by Walter Prendiville and James R. Scott.
Published in 1999 by Arnold, ISBN 0 340 74100 7

IMMUNOLOGIC HYPOTHESES FOR RECURRENT ABORTION

Maternal acceptance of the fetal–placental, semiallograft is one of the most intriguing and perplexing phenomena in nature. Speculation has arisen that pregnancy loss may be caused by impaired maternal immune tolerance to the semiallogenic conceptus since the developing embryo and trophoblast are immunologically foreign to the maternal host because of their paternally inherited gene products and tissue-specific differentiation antigens (reviewed in ref. 20). Four antibody-mediated hypotheses have been proposed for recurrent spontaneous abortion (Table 9.1). Of these four proposed humoral immune mechanisms, antiphospholipid antibodies remain the only scientifically well substantiated humoral immune cause for pregnancy loss.

Antiphospholipid antibodies are IgG and IgM autoantibodies with specificity for negatively charged phospholipid. The antiphospholipid antibodies most commonly associated with recurrent pregnancy loss are anticardiolipin and antiphosphatidylserine. Antiphospholipid antibodies are also characterized by prolonged phospholipid-dependent coagulation tests *in vitro* known as lupus anticoagulant tests (aPTT, Russel viper venom time), and thrombosis *in vivo*, thrombocytopenia and fetal

Table 9.1 Proposed immunologic factors in recurrent spontaneous abortion

Humoral mechanisms
1. Antiphospholipid antibodies
2. Antisperm antibodies
3. Antitrophoblast antibodies
4. Blocking antibody deficiency

Cellular mechanisms
1. TH1 cellular immune response to reproductive antigens (embryo/trophoblast–toxic factors/cytokines)
2. TH2 cytokine, growth factor and oncogene deficiency
3. Suppressor cell and factor deficiency
4. Major histocompatibility antigen expression

loss. The association of antiphospholipid antibodies with one or more of these characteristic clinical features has been termed the antiphospholipid syndrome[15]. Direct pathologic evidence for placental vascular damage is limited in clinical cases of recurrent abortion as not all women with the antiphospholipid syndrome and recurrent abortion have placental infarctions or evidence of maternal surface abruption and hemorrhage[21]. Similarly, although the extent of placental pathology appears insufficient to explain fetal death in many cases of antiphospholipid antibody-positive women, other placentas show these characteristic lesions, yet the mother has no hematologic evidence of antiphospholipid antibodies[22]. Therefore, although substantial clinical evidence exists for the antiphospholipid syndrome being involved in recurrent abortion, the direct pathologic evidence remains equivocal. The presence of antiphospholipid antibodies during pregnancy is a major risk factor for adverse pregnancy outcome[23]. Obstetric complications in addition to recurrent spontaneous abortion in the first or second trimester include: premature labor; premature rupture of membranes; stillbirth; intrauterine growth retardation; and pre-eclampsia[14]. The incidence of the antiphospholipid syndrome in women experiencing recurrent abortion varies between studies. In our series of 300 couples evaluated for recurrent pregnancy loss, the incidence of antiphospholipid antibodies using standardized assays was 3%[18] which was similar to the 4.8% reported by others[24]. Other series of women with recurrent abortion have reported higher percentages, 11–48%[25–28]. However not all of these studies used standardized assays or they considered low positive values to be significant. These percentages like all percentages of potential etiologies for recurrent abortion vary according to physician referral patterns.

Pathophysiologic mechanisms responsible for adverse fetal outcome in women with antiphospholipid antibodies are poorly defined. Most proposed mechanisms involve inhibition of vascular endothelial prostacyclin production leading to vasoconstriction and thrombosis[28]. This mechanism, although, plausible has not been uniformly confirmed pathologically[29]. Other pathophysiologic mechanisms proposed to explain antiphospholipid antibody-mediated abortion include: interception of signal transduction processes by antibody binding to phospholipid epitopes on second messenger molecules[30]; platelet damage due to antiphospholipid antibody causing platelet binding to vascular endothelium resulting in platelet aggregation and local thrombosis[31]; and impaired fibrinolytic activity through antiphospholipid interference with protein C activation[32,33]. *In vitro* evidence using the trophoblast-derived choriocarcinoma cell line BeWo, has indicated that antibody against phosphatidylserine, especially the IgM isotype can inhibit syncytial trophoblast formation[34].

Spontaneous abortion has been shown to occur in animals immunized against sperm to produce antisperm antibodies[35]. Women with antisperm antibodies in their serum have been reported to be at increased risk for spontaneous abortion[36–38]. However, this work has been challenged by others who could not confirm this association[39,40]. In our series we found antisperm antibodies in cervical mucus of only 2 of 300 women with recurrent abortion[18]. Therefore, antisperm antibodies appear unlikely as a significant cause of recurrent abortion.

The hypothesis that antitrophoblast antibodies are involved in recurrent abortion has also been proposed but not unequivocably substantiated. Reports associating antithyroid antibodies in 31% of women with recurrent abortion[41,42] may represent an epiphenomenon in women with abortion or generalized non-specific autoantibody activation[43]. We tested the hypothesis that antithyroid antibodies may recognize shared epitopes on trophoblast, but our results indicated that there was no cross-reactivity. It appears unlikely that antithyroid antibodies are a causative factor in pregnancy loss. Individuals with antithyroid antibodies, however, are at increased risk for developing hypothyroidism which may contribute to pregnancy loss.

The hypothesis that maternal blocking antibody deficiency is a cause of recurrent pregnancy loss has received much attention since its proposal by Rocklin *et al.* in 1976[44]. The foundation of this controversial theory involved three suppositions: (1) there is an antifetal, maternal cell-mediated immune response that develops in all pregnancies that must be blocked; (2) blocking antibodies develop in all successful pregnancies that prevent this maternal, antifetal, cell-mediated immune response; and (3) in the absence of blocking antibodies, abortion of the fetus always occurs. Unfortunately, these suppositions have not been unequivocally validated[45]. There is no direct pathologic evidence that an antifetal, maternal immune response occurs in all pregnancies either with or without purported blocking antibodies. There is also no direct evidence that blocking antibodies occur in all successful pregnancies to prevent this presumed antifetal immune response. A specific, verifiable assay to detect the proposed immunoglobulin effectors has also not been defined.

Mixed lymphocyte culture (MLC) reactivities between maternal responder and paternal stimulator cells were originally used to determine whether blocking activity in response to uncharacterized serum factors existed. Rocklin *et al.*[44] were the first to associate the absence of a serum blocking factor with recurrent abortion. This work was later extended by others [46,47]. This hypothesis began to be questioned when women with successful pregnancies were found who did not produce serum factors capable of mixed lymphocyte culture inhibition[48] and when not all successfully pregnant women were found to make antibodies against paternal human lymphocyte antigens[49]. Further doubt concerning the relevance of MLC reactivities in spontaneous abortion remains since purported blocking factors could be the consequence rather than the cause of pregnancy success and other pregnancy-related serum factors such as steroid hormones or cytokines may be responsible for the observed effects. The fact that agammaglobulinemic women and mice are able to reproduce successfully[50] renders any theory concerning the necessity of an antibody for pregnancy success untenable.

It has also been proposed that human leukocyte antigen (HLA) dissimilarity is required for successful gestation, based on the belief that HLA heterogeneity facilitated blocking antibody production[44]. This hypothesis failed to consider the fact that genetically identical mice have been successfully bred for generations. Similarly, early studies[44–47] which were of limited size, retrospective and without population-based controls, reporting an association between parental HLA profiles and recurrent abortion, were later disproven by population-based control studies in Hutterites which demonstrated that HLA heterogeneity was not an essential requirement for successful pregnancy[51].

A novel HLA-linked antigen system termed TLX was proposed to explain pregnancy loss based on polyclonal rabbit antisera that was cross-reactive with trophoblast and lymphocytes[52]. This hypothesis stated that sharing of TLX antigens that were proposed to be crosslinked with HLA antigens caused the inability to produce maternal blocking antibodies. As previously mentioned, blocking antibodies have never been adequately characterized. Recent data indicate that rather than defining a new alloantigen system, TLX is CD46, a complement receptor[53] which is found on a wide variety of cells including trophoblast, lymphocytes and spermatozoa[54], thus explaining the cross-reactive nature of the antisera that originally defined TLX and contributed to the misconception that this antiserum defined a new alloantigen system.

Neither human nor animal studies support the concept that an intact maternal immune system is necessary for maintaining normal pregnancy. The possibility exists, however, that immune mechanisms may be involved in pregnancy failure.

Four cellular immune mechanisms have been proposed to explain immunologic pregnancy loss (Table 9.1). An abnormal T helper 1 (TH1) cellular immune response is the most recent hypothesis proposed for immunologic reproductive failure[18,55–61]. This hypothesis states that the conceptus may be a target of local, cell-mediated, immune responses culminating in abortion. In affected women, trophoblast, sperm, microbial or other antigens may activate maternal immune and inflammatory cells (macrophages, T-lymphocytes and natural killer cells) to produce a cellular immune response mediated by the TH1 cytokines, interferon(INF)-gamma and tumor necrosis factor (TNF) which have been shown to inhibit *in vitro* embryo development and trophoblast growth and function[62–64]. TNF-α may also mediate intravascular thrombous formation[65]. Depending on the individual series, comprising a total of over 2000 women, approximately 50% of women with otherwise unexplained recurrent spontaneous abortion have been found to have evidence of an abnormal TH1 cellular immune response to trophoblast antigens, whereas less than 3% of women with normal reproductive histories have cellular immunity to these same trophoblast antigens[8,55,60,61]. In contrast to TH1 immunity to trophoblast in women with unexplained recurrent abortion, evidence also indicates that a majority of women with normal reproduction make a TH2 immune response involving the cytokines interleukin(IL)-4 and IL-10 to the same trophoblast antigens that women with recurrent abortion respond to with TH1 immunity[62]. These data provide evidence for a new, non-major histocompatibility-related mechanism for reproductive failure. More studies are needed to validate this hypothesis. Of interest, another study has reported higher levels of TNF and IL-2, another TH1 cytokine, in serum samples from women with unexplained recurrent abortion than in controls. Unfortunately, however, cause-versus-effect phenomena were not addressed in this study[66]. Schust and Hill[67] were unable to substantiate the hypothesis that serum cytokine levels are predictive of pregnancy outcome.

The finding that intravenous or intraperitoneal bacterial lipopolysaccharide injection in mice mediates abortion through TNF production provides further evidence for a non-specific TH1-mediated etiology for abortion[68]. IFN-γ and TNF-α injected directly into mice may also cause abortion[69]. Other immunologic cytokines have also been implicated in murine pregnancy loss. IL-2 administration early in murine pregnancy has been reported to cause abortion[70]. IL-2 may mediate abortion by inducing T-cell and NK-cell activation and proliferation which could have cytotoxic effects via cell–cell contact, or through the secretion of IFN-γ which can interfere with murine embryo development[62,71], implantation events, and trophoblast outgrowth[63,64]. IL-2 can also directly stimulate decidual macrophages, further amplifying TNF secretion which adversely affects murine reproductive events. Thus, by both direct and indirect effects, TH1 cytokines may interfere with reproductive events depending on the specific cytokines secreted, their concentrations, and differentiation stage of potential reproductive target tissues. Further evidence for bidirectional cytokine effects in murine pregnancy comes from two studies. In one, TH2 cytokines were found in the decidua of successful pregnancies[72] and in the other TH1 cytokines predominated in decidual tissues of CBA/J × DBA/2 aborting mice[68]. This mouse model may provide an infection-mediated mechanism involving TH1 immunity since some investigators have reported that treating CBA/J × DBA/2 mice with tetracycline abrogates fetal resorption in this model[74].

In women, infections with mycoplasma and chlamydia have also been associated with recurrent abortion and other adverse pregnancy outcomes[75,76] potentially through a cellular immune-mediated mechanism. These infections may activate TH1 immunity leading to chronic non-infectious persistence of these organisms in the upper genital tract of women with reproductive failure despite eradication of culture-positive organisms in the uterine cervix[77]. We propose that local endometrial activation of TH1 immunity by sexually transmitted pathogens may provide mechanisms for reproductive failure in women with occult (non-culturable) mycoplasma or chlamydia. New molecular biology techniques involving DNA primer pairs specific for conserved regions of potentially infectious organisms have been developed enabling detection of as few as one copy of DNA pathogen per 10^5 host cells by polymerase chain reaction (PCR)[78]. An improvement of the PCR assay has been devised called the ligase chain reaction (LCR) which allows detection of as few as 10 molecules of target DNA[79]. Thus, LCR appears to be the most sensitive tool for detecting occult or persistent pathogens that are otherwise unculturable[80]. Further work is needed to elucidate the potential immunopathologic mechanisms responsible for infection-mediated immunologic abortion.

Other immunologic cytokines, growth factors and oncogenes are involved in mammalian development[81,82]. The absence of the cytokine, colony stimulating factor-1 (oncogene c-*fms*), has been theorized to contribute to abortion in mice[83]. However, this same cytokine has been shown to cause rather than prevent abortion in some mouse strains[84]. The absence of transforming growth factor beta and epidermal growth factor have also been shown to cause abortion in mice[85,86]. The oncogene c-*mos* can cause mitotic arrest[87]. Aberrant expression of this oncogene during oocyte or embryo development could theoretically lead to pregnancy failure. The majority of studies regarding deficiencies in cytokines, growth factors and oncogenes have been performed in mice and other laboratory animals. Many of these same factors, however, have been identified in human pregnancy, and the absence of these factors have been theorized to lead to spontaneous abortion in women[85,88]. Further work is needed in humans to validate these theories and to identify the responsible factors and their possible mechanism of action in causing abortion.

Suppressor cell and factor deficiency is another cellular immune mechanism proposed for recurrent abortion. The concept of suppressor cells and their existence is a controversial topic in immunology. The hypothesis of suppressor cell and factor deficiency as a cause of pregnancy loss was based on the finding of suppressor immune cell deficiency in abortion-prone CBA/J × DBA/2 mice prior to pregnancy loss[89]. Extrapolation of data derived from non-primate animal models to humans must be cautiously interpreted because of inherent anatomical, morphological, endocrinological and immunological differences between species. However, support for the theory that deficient suppressor cells/factors are involved in human abortion comes from the observation of decidual suppressor cell deficiency in endometrial biopsies from women with failing chemical pregnancies following *in vitro* fertilization and embryo transfer[90], and also from one report of three women with a missed abortion between 2 and 11 weeks of gestation[91]. The fact that in this study 3 of 15 women having elective pregnancy termination were also found to have evidence of suppressor cell/factor deficiency compromises this hypothesis. Evidence from our own laboratory, in support of suppressor cell/factor deficiency, indicates that decidual macrophage and lymphocyte function which are normally suppressed during human pregnancy are enhanced in cases of spontaneous abortion. However, all these findings do not necessarily indicate causality, as all the observations in support of suppressor cell/factor deficiency being a cause of spontaneous abortion may simply reflect the effects of spontaneous abortion rather than its cause. Similarly, the factors and cells involved in this theory have not been precisely defined nor have their specificities been determined. Larger, better controlled studies are needed before this theory can be substantiated.

Normal human syncytiotrophoblast does not express major histocompatibility complex (MHC) class I or II antigens (reviewed in ref. 92) except for a truncated form of class I on cytotrophoblast termed HLA-G[93,94]. Due to the absence of classic MHC determinants, trophoblast cannot be a classical immunogen for maternal sensitization or serve as a target for MHC-directed cytotoxic T cells. Human trophoblast is also resistant to natural killer cell attack. As previously described, non-MHC-related mechanisms may be involved in reproductive failure such as TH1-mediated immunity, but MHC-related mechanisms cannot. The TH1 cytokine interferon-γ has been shown to induce major histocompatibility complex antigen expression on placental tissues derived from human trophoblast and human trophoblast cell lines *in vitro*[95,96]. If MHC determinants were to be expressed *in vivo*, then cytotoxic T-cell attack could occur potentially culminating in abortion. This theory, although plausible and supportable by *in vitro* experiments, nevertheless, appears unlikely as a major factor for abortion, as recent studies[97] indicate no difference in MHC expression between placentas from women experiencing recurrent, sporadic, or elective abortions.

Normal human placentas are also replete with complement regulatory and binding proteins that are thought to protect pregnancy from complement-mediated attack]53]. The hypothesis has been suggested that if trophoblast does not express these regulatory proteins then abortion might occur through complement mediation[98]. Experimental evidence does not support this hypothesis, as trophoblasts from elective terminations, sporadic and recurrent spontaneous abortions clearly express complement regulatory and binding proteins[97].

IMMUNOLOGIC EVALUATION OF RECURRENT ABORTION

Investigative measures potentially useful in the evaluation of recurrent spontaneous abortion are listed in Table 9.2. Laboratory assessment of potential immunological causes should include antiphospholipid antibody determinations for cardiolipin and phosphatidylserine both IgG and IgM, together with a test for lupus anticoagulant (aPTT or Russell viper venom time)[99,100].

A complete blood cell count and platelet count should be obtained as thrombocytosis has been associated with recurrent abortion[101]. Blood type and rhesus factor determinations and rubella immune status should also be part of the routine evaluation.

Antisperm antibody determinations in the woman's serum and mid-cycle cervical mucus are unnecessary as the incidence of a positive result is very low (<1%) and its clinical significance questionable.

Additional work is needed before diagnostic capabilities are clinically available to assess potential TH1 cellular immunity, suppressor cell or factor, and other cytokine, growth factor and oncogene mechanisms of recurrent pregnancy loss. Rapid advances in cellular and molecular immunology and reproductive biology are occurring. New diagnostic tests for TH1 cellular immunity in recurrent abortion are being actively pursued and may be clinically available in the near future.

There is no place in the modern medical management of recurrent abortion for ascertainment of antinuclear antibody (ANA) titers, antipaternal cytotoxic antibodies, HLA profiles, MLC reactivities or autoantibody titers other than to cardiolipin and phosphatidylserine (Table 9.3).

ANA titers should not be obtained because these antibodies are heterogeneous, and occur commonly and non-specifically in the general population. Their presence is often transitory and an association of recurrent abortion with subclinical autoimmunity as reflected by a positive ANA titer is at best controversial and speculative[102,103]. There is also no substantive value in obtaining antipaternal cytotoxic antibodies as they are rarely demonstrable before 28 weeks of gestation and usually disappear between pregnancies[104]. One small published series[105] showed that antipaternal cytotoxic antibodies were associated with spontaneous abortion; however, a larger series[106] reported that 10% of 50 women whose pregnancies ended in spontaneous

---

Table 9.2 Evaluation of recurrent spontaneous abortion

A. History
B. Physical
C. Laboratory
    1. Parental peripheral blood karyotype
    2. Hysterosalpingogram followed by hysteroscopy/laparoscopy if indicated
    3. Luteal phase endometrial biopsy
    4. Thyroid function tests (TSH, T4)
    5. Antiphospholipid antibodies (cardiolipin, phosphatidylserine)
    6. Lupus anticoagulant (a PTT or Russel viper venom)
    7. Complete blood count with platelets
    8. Antisperm antibodies (cervical mucous, peripheral serum)[*]
    9. Cervical cultures (*Mycoplasma, Chlamydia*, Beta streptococcus)[*]
    10. TH1 embryotoxic cytokines to reproductive antigens[†]
    11. LH testing/ultrasound assessment for PCOS[†]

[*]Last resort; [†]Experimental.
Adapted from Hill [6].

Table 9.3 Investigative measures of no benefit in the clinical evaluation of recurrent spontaneous abortion

---

A. Antinuclear antibodies
   1. Association with recurrent pregnancy loss controversial
   2. No difference between women with presumed and unknown etiologies for their abortions
   3. Commonly and non-specifically occur in the general population
   4. Heterogeneous
   5. May be transitory
   6. Clinical significance in reproduction not established

B. Antipaternal cytotoxic antibodies
   1. Present in 32% of 256 women achieving a successful pregnancy as compared to 10% of 50 women whose pregnancy ended in a spontaneous abortion
   2. Rarely demonstrable before 28 weeks' gestation
   3. Positive values during pregnancy usually disappear between pregnancies

C. Parental HLA profiles
   1. Reports suggesting an association with recurrent abortion have generally been of limited size, retrospective and without population-based controls
   2. Prospective, population-based control studies in Hutterites have conclusively demonstrated that HLA heterogeneity is not an essential requirement for successful pregnancy
   3. Animal studies also do not support the concept that MHC heterozygosity is required for successful gestation since inbred animal strains have been maintained for generations

D. MLC reactivities
   1. Not all women with presumed immunologic pregnancy loss have evidence of suppressed MLC reactivity with their partners since spontaneous abortion can occur in the presence of 'blocking activity'
   2. Not all women with successful pregnancies produce serum factors capable of inhibiting MLC reactions since viable pregnancies can occur in the absence of 'blocking activity'
   3. Causal relationships not addressed as MLC hyporesponsiveness may represent an effect of abortion or differences resulting from multiple live births rather than being the cause of recurrent abortion
   4. Interpretation of 'blocking activity' in maternal serum depends on the equation used for calculating MLC results

E. Autoantibodies other than cardiolipin and antiphosphatidylserine
   1. Association with recurrent pregnancy loss controversial
   2. Commonly and non-specifically occur in general population
   3. May be transitory

---

abortion were positive for antipaternal cytotoxic antibodies, whereas 32% of 256 women achieving successful pregnancies also had positive values. Therefore, the presence of antipaternal cytotoxic antibodies is not a useful screening test for either the diagnosis or prognosis of recurrent abortion[104,106,108]. Assessment of parental HLA profiles in the evaluation of recurrent abortion is also not clinically justified[92,109,110].

Assessment of mixed lymphocyte culture (MLC) reactivity between partners with recurrent abortion looking for purported 'blocking antibodies' also cannot be clinically justified as the results of these tests reflect the number and duration of prior pregnancies rather than serving as a marker for recurrent abortion and their presence is not necessarily predictive of pregnancy outcome[45,108,110,111].

Until more information is known, the

routine clinical assessment of antiphospholipid antibodies other than to cardiolipin and phosphatidylserine or other autoantibodies is not clinically justified, except under a specific study protocol following informed consent.

IMMUNOTHERAPY PROPOSED FOR RECURRENT ABORTION

Both immunostimulating and immunosuppressive therapies have been proposed for recurrent abortion (Table 9.4) depending on whether the maternal immune system was thought to be hypo- or hyperresponsive to paternal–fetal antigen stimulation[6,19]. Immunostimulation in the form of immunization with leukocytes[112,113], trophoblast membrane vesicle extracts[115] and seminal plasma[115] has been performed based on the controversial theory of blocking antibody deficiency as a cause of recurrent pregnancy loss. The scientific rationale for immunization therapy as previously discussed has been disputed by numerous investigators[6,19,108,110,111]. There are also clinical risks in administering viable leukocytes to healthy women, such as sensitization to HLA or other leukocyte antigens, or to platelet or blood group antigens[116]. Other transfusion-related risks are potentially increased, notably after third-party immunization, such as cytomegalovirus (CMV) or human immunodeficiency virus (HIV) transmission by viable leukocytes. The variation in live-born delivery rates for control groups in randomized immunotherapy studies[117,119] has readdressed attention towards the strength of the 'placebo effect' in immunotherapeutic studies for recurrent abortion[19]. Meta-analysis results derived from the published double-blind, placebo-controlled trials, which have not all supported efficacy, indicate a relative risk of 1.0, suggesting that paternal leukocyte immunization does not influence pregnancy outcome[120]. Two independent meta-analyses published together by the Recurrent Miscarriage Immunotherapy Trailist Group

sponsored by the American Society for Reproductive Immunology (ASRI) concluded, 'that paternal leukocyte immunization appears to be useful therapy, but the treatment is effective in only a small proportion of women in partnerships with unexplained recurrent spontaneous abortion. From the two analyses it appears that about 11 patients had to be immunized to achieve one additional birth'[121]. Although there may have been statistical evidence of efficacy in the ASRI sponsored study, the vast majority of successful pregnancy outcomes in women (92%) were not attributable to leukocyte immunization[121]. Whether the additional 8% successful pregnancy rate achieved in leukocyte-immunized patients in the ASRI study was clinically relevant remains uncertain. The ASRI study found that approximately 60% of untreated women had a successful pregnancy outcome[121] which is in agreement with epidemiological data indicating a 50–60% chance of successful pregnancy in untreated women with as many as four consecutive spontaneous abortions[1]. The ASRI study also reported a 2.1% complication rate among immunized patients which was significantly more than among controls. Maternal autoimmune complications occurred in three women and a 'transfusion reaction' occurred in six[121]. These complications are particularly concerning since they have the potential for lethality. The authors conceded that the newborns were not subjected to 'formal long-term surveillance' which must be performed before this therapy can be considered safe. Indeed, two infants born of immunized women had thrombocytopenia at birth[121]. This may have been due to alloimmunization resulting from platelets or platelet antigens in the paternal leukocyte preparation. Reported complications resulting from immunization therapy, together with the relative paucity of neonatal follow-up studies, led to the conclusion that it is premature to consider that paternal leukocyte immunization is either safe or effective.

There are still many unresolved variables in

Table 9.4 Immunotherapies proposed for recurrent spontaneous abortion

---

A. Immunostimulation not substantiated
   1. Leukocyte transfusions
   2. Trophoblast vesicle fluid transfusions
   3. Seminal plasma suppositories
B. Immunosuppression not substantiated
   1. Intravenous immunoglobulin – anti-idiotype binding of idiotypes on T-cell receptor, FC receptor blockage, inactivation of complement, inhibit B-cell function, increase suppressor T-cell function.
   2. Phasmopheresis – removal of autoantibodies
   3. Corticosteroids – suppresses a myriad of immune/inflammatory responses
   4. Aspirin – suppresses platelet adhesiveness and inflammatory responses
   5. Heparin – suppresses platelet aggregation
   6. Progesterone – suppresses macrophage phagocytosis and lymphocyte proliferation
   7. Pentoxifyline – suppresses macrophage activation
   8. Cyclosporin A – suppresses immune responsiveness
   9. Nifedipine – may affect macrophage function

Adapted from Hill [6].

this highly controversial area. There is also substantial pressure from both patients and their health care providers for beneficial treatment. A growing number of financially lucrative immunotherapy clinics have appeared; however, there is still no clinical or laboratory method to identify a specific individual who may benefit from such therapy. As Relman[122] stated: 'The ethical duty of every physician is to be sure that the tests and procedures he or she uses are worth the money, inconvenience, and risks involved.' Although many therapies have been adopted in clinical medicine without proof of prior efficacy, given the increasing awareness of escalating health care costs, it is hard to justify the use of a potentially dangerous and expensive therapy for recurrent miscarriage that at best will be effective in only 1 of 11 women treated. Therefore, the ASRI *ad hoc* Ethics Committee appointed by the society's president, Dr Joan Hunt, was unable to condone the routine clinical use of paternal leukocyte immunization for recurrent spontaneous abortion and recommended, 'that diagnostic procedures to identify recurrent aborting couples for leukocyte immunization, and the immunotherapy itself, should only be given following informed consent approved by the local human experimentation insti-

tutional review board in an appropriately controlled trial'[123].

Other immunostimulating therapies have been proposed for recurrent abortion. Trophoblast vesicle fluid transfusions were attempted to mimic fetal cell contact with maternal blood[114]. A randomized, double-blind, placebo-controlled trial using this therapy reported no difference in pregnancy outcome between trophoblast vesicle fluid, placebo and no treatment[114]. Third-party seminal plasma suppositories have also been advocated as an immunotherapy for recurrent abortion[115]. The rationale for such action remains elusive and its efficacy unsubstantiated.

Because of the low treatment effect with immunization therapy, alternative immunomodulating therapies have been sought for unexplained recurrent abortion. Immunosuppressive therapy has been advocated for many women suffering recurrent pregnancy loss believed due to adverse humoral (autoimmune) or cellular (alloimmune) immune responses to the developing conceptus[6,19]. Corticosteroids have been recommended for pregnancy loss due to antiphospholipid antibodies[124], although not all investigators have found these agents to be effective in preventing fetal loss in women with antiphospholipid antibodies[124]. The potential adverse side effects of corticosteroids also temper their use in treating presumed immunologic reproductive failure. Low dose aspirin and heparin are currently recommended in the treatment of autoimmune reproductive failure in women with antiphospholipid antibodies[126]. Safe, immunosuppressive agents are still needed to treat reproductive failure believed due to immune activation.

The 21-carbon molecule, progesterone, is essential for the maintenance of pregnancy[127]. Progesterone has been called 'nature's immunosuppressant'[128], since concentrations attained at the maternal–fetal interface (10^{-5} M) are capable of inhibiting immune function including macrophage phagocytosis, lymphocyte proliferation and cytotoxic natural killer and T-cell activity[129]. Progesterone may also mediate the release of immunosuppressive factors during pregnancy[130]. Increased concentrations of progesterone have been reported to be secreted by trophoblast from pre-eclamptic pregnancies and have been shown to suppress TH1-cytokine (IL-2)-activated mononuclear cell cytotoxicity[131]. Progesterone or one of its synthetic derivatives has been used since the 1950s for a variety of pregnancy-related disorders including as an antiabortifacient agent[132]. The use of progesterone during pregnancy was based on the potential endocrinologic benefit it may afford[132]. Meta-analysis of the data obtained from trials using inconsistent and often unspecified dosages of progestational agents during pregnancy have not revealed a therapeutic benefit for their use[133], except in cases of luteal insufficiency[134], although, these data are also controversial. In all but one of these previous studies, progesterone therapy did not begin until after 7 weeks of gestation. The one study that began progesterone therapy before conception initiated therapy three days after the LH surge during a conception cycle. This study reported that the therapy was efficacious in preventing a repeat abortion, but was uncontrolled[134]. The tenuous association of the synthetic progestogens with teratogenicity have limited their use in treating reproductive disorders. The natural, 21-carbon molecule, progesterone, however, has no teratogenic potential and only minor maternal side effects including: tiredness, fluid retention and delayed menses if taken and maintained after ovulation. Depression may occur in less than 1% of individuals taking progesterone. Intrauterine levels of progesterone, approaching potentially immunosuppressive levels (10^{-5} M), have been obtained using 100 mg vaginal suppositories but not with equivalent dosages given intramuscularly[135]. Progesterone receptors within the endometrium and decidua should ensure that higher levels are retained in these tissues than in the peripheral circulation. Use of potentially local (intrauterine), immunosuppressive doses of progesterone beginning in the luteal phase of a conception cycle has never been tested in a prospective, randomized, double-blind, placebo-controlled trial in the treatment of unexplained recurrent pregnancy loss. Such a study is needed before its routine clinical use can be justified.

Other uncontrolled immunomodulating approaches have been used to treat women with unexplained recurrent spontaneous abortion. The use of intravenous immunoglobulin in the treatment of recurrent abortion in women with antiphospholipid syndrome[136] was based on reports of efficacy with its use in immunohematologic disorders and autoimmune disease[137]. Intravenous immunoglobulin has also been used to treat unexplained recurrent pregnancy loss[138,139,139a], however, these studies have been of limited sample size, have included women with only two prior losses or patients with limited evaluations, and have neither been randomized nor placebo controlled. There have now been four studies performed throughout the world claiming to be placebo controlled. The results have not unequivocally substantiated efficacy. None of the studies testing potential efficacy have prestratified study participants by age and number of prior losses before randomization. This is critical since these two factors are independently associated with spontaneous abortion[141,142]. The specific rationale for the use of intravenous immunoglobulin in previous studies has not been clear, although known immunoregulating actions of immunoglobulin include: anti-idiotype binding to idiotypes on the T-cell receptor; blockade of Fc receptors on antigen presenting cells; inactivation of complement components; enhanced T-suppressor cell function; down-regulation of B-cell function, inhibition of natural killer activity and TH1-cytokine production[137]. Therefore, intravenous immunoglobulin may be beneficial in treating unexplained recurrent abortion in cases where associated TH1-immunity to trophoblast may be involved. Properly designed studies addressing this possibility have not as yet been adequately performed.

Rapid advances in molecular immunology and transplantation biology will undoubtedly enable the formulation and availability of new, more effective treatment modalities for couples experiencing immunologic reproductive failure. Therapeutic options may include antigen-specific immunotherapy and tolerance induction brought about by anti-immune cell antibodies, growth factors, cytokines and anticytokines.

Treatment modalities are needed for recurrent spontaneous abortion. However, the rationale for therapy, must be scientifically well founded and the therapy itself must be more innocuous than the disease[142]. A compilation of studies to date concerning immunotherapy for recurrent abortion[143] reveals no significant difference between current and past therapies and placebo (Table 9.5). Very few of these studies were well designed. Twelve criteria are needed to test the therapeutic efficacy of agents proposed in the treatment of recurrent abortion (Table 9.6). A moratorium should be placed on the publication of retrospective, non-randomized, non-placebo controlled trials of therapies in inadequate numbers of patients with fewer than three spontaneous abortions who were not prestratified by maternal age and number of prior pregnancy losses before being randomized for therapy. The strength of placebo effects should not be underestimated in immunotherapeutic studies concerning recurrent spontaneous abortion as 'tender loving care' has been reported to be efficacious in 80–85% of women experiencing pregnancy loss even after four consecutive previous pregnancy losses[17].

PROGNOSIS

Epidemiologic studies indicate that the probability of completing a successful pregnancy even after four consecutive spontaneous

Table 9.5 Summary of immunotherapies

Treatment	No. individuals treated	Success (%)
Paternal leukocyte immunization	822	73
Third party leukocyte immunization	79	75
Trophoblast membrane infusion	79	57
Intravenous immunoglobulin	69	68
Seminal plasma suppositories	44	55
Progesterone controls	225	75
Autologous leukocyte immunization	101	60
Intralipid infusion	20	70
Psychotherapy	135	85
Saline alone	32	67
No treatment	304	58

Adapted from Johnson and Ramsden [144].

Table 9.6 Criteria needed to test therapeutic efficacy

1. Understand the underlying mechanism involved in reproductive failure
2. Scientifically sound rationale for using a particular therapy
3. Power calculation to ensure adequate number of subjects needed to test efficacy
4. Exclusion of patients with less than three spontaneous abortions
5. Prospective
6. Prestratification by maternal age and number of prior pregnancy losses before randomization and therapy
7. Randomized
8. Double-blinded
9. Placebo-controlled
10. No other concomitant therapy given
11. Follow-up to ensure maternal–fetal safety
12. Karotype analysis of all abortions

Adapted from Hill [6].

abortions is 50–60%[1,2,141,144–146]. The majority of these epidemiologic studies considered neither potential underlying causes for spontaneous abortion nor maternal age. The prognosis for successful pregnancy depends on the cause of previous spontaneous abortions. The probability of a successful pregnancy for couples found to have an immunologic etiology may range between 40 and 90%. Viable pregnancy rates between 70% and 90% have been reported for women receiving therapy for antiphospholipid syndrome[147,148]. An abnormal resistance index as measured with color Doppler ultrasonography in women with the antiphospholipid syndrome has been reported to predict pregnancies with poor fetal outcome[149]. In a study of 200 pregnant women with a history of two or more pregnancy losses, we were unable to predict pregnancy outcome using Doppler flow ultrasonography[150]. Measurement of TH1 immunity in the form of immune cell secretion of embryotoxic factors has been reported to predict pregnancy outcome in women with a history of unexplained recurrent abortion having a positive and negative predictive value of 0.76 and 0.86, respectively. Of 56 women found to be positive in early pregnancy, 40 (71%) miscarried and 16 (29%) delivered a viable infant. Of 85 women found to be negative for embryotoxic factors in early pregnancy, only 11 (13%) had a subsequent spontaneous abortion whereas 74 (87%) delivered a viable infant[55]. The live birth rate after documentation of fetal cardiac activity between 5 and 6 weeks from last menses in women with two or more unexplained spontaneous abortions has been reported to be approximately 77%[7].

CONCLUSION

Recurrent spontaneous abortion is a frustrating problem not only for couples experiencing pregnancy loss but also for their health care providers. This frustration often leads to the recommendation of therapies with little scientific rationale resulting in significant emotional and financial costs to the couple who are experiencing reproductive failure and to unnecessary increases in health care expenditures. The ethical duty of every physician is to be sure that the tests and procedures he or she uses are worth the money, inconvenience and risks involved[122].

A caring empathetic attitude on the part of the physician toward the couple experiencing pregnancy loss is prerequisite for healing. The acknowledgement to couples of the pain and suffering they have experienced because of their losses and the resulting stress within themselves and within their relationships with each other, friends and family may act as a catharsis which will facilitate their ability to incorporate their experience of loss into their lives rather than their lives into their experience of loss[6].

Understanding the immunologic mechanisms potentially involved in reproductive failure together with a caring and empathetic attitude toward the couple will enable amelioration of the emotional distress they face and will facilitate a rational, scientific assessment ultimately leading to appropriate management.

REFERENCES

1. Warburton, D. and Fraser, F.C. (1963) Spontaneous abortion rate in man: data from reproductive histories collected in a medical genetics unit. *Am. J. Hum. Genet.*, **16**, 1–28.

2. Alberman, E. (1988) The epidemiology of repeated abortion, in *Early Pregnancy Loss: Mechanisms and Treatment*, Springer-Verlag, New York, pp. 9–17.

3. Edmonds, D.K., Lindsay, K.I. and Miller, J.F. (1982) Early embryonic mortality in women. *Fertil. Steril.*, **38**, 447–53.

4. Wilcox, A.J., Weinberg, C.R., O'Connor, J.F. *et al.* (1990) Incidence of early loss of pregnancy. *N. Engl. J. Med.*, **319**, 189–94.

5. Stirrat, G.M. (1990) Recurrent miscarriage: its definition and epidemiology. *Lancet*, **336**, 673–5.

6. Hill, J.A. (1994) Sporadic and recurrent spontaneous abortion. *Curr. Prob. Obstet. Gynecol. Fertil.*, **17**, 115–62.

7. Laufer, M.R., Ecker, J.L. and Hill, J.A. (1994) Pregnancy outcome following ultrasound detected fetal cardiac activity in women with history of multiple spontaneous abortion. *J. Soc. Gynecol. Invest.*, **2**.

8. Portnoi, M.F. Joye, N., Vanden Akker, J. *et al.* (1988) Karyotypes of 1142 couples with recurrent abortion. *Obstet. Gynecol.*, **72**, 31–4.

9. Munich, J.R. and Behrman, S.T. (1978) Obstetric outcome before and after uteroplasty in women with uterine anomalies. *Obstet. Gynecol.*, **52**, 63.

10. Jones, G.E.S. and Delfs, E. (1951) Endocrine patterns in term pregnancies following abortion. *JAMA*, **146**, 1212.

11. Winikoff, D. and Malinek, M. (1975) The predictive value of thyroid 'Test Profile' in habitual abortion. *Br. J. Obstet. Gynaecol.*, **82**, 760.

12. Craea, E., Botez, D., Ioanid, L. *et al.* (1981) Genital mycoplasmas and chlamydia in infertility and abortion. *Arch. Roum. Pathol. Exp. Microbiol.*, **40**, 107.

13. Kunsdin, R.B., Driscoll, S.G. and Ming, P.L. (1967) Strain of mycoplasma associated with human reproductive failure. *Science*, **157**, 1573.

14. Branch, D.W., Scott, J.R., Kochenour, N.K. *et al.* (1985) Obstetric complications associated with the lupus anticoagulant. *N. Engl. J. Med.*, **313**, 1322.

15. Harris, E.N. (1986) Syndrome of the black swan. *Br. J. Rheumatol.*, **26**, 324–6.

16. Tho, P.T., Byrd, J.R. and McDonough, P.G. (1979) Etiologies and subsequent reproductive performance of 100 couples with recurrent abortion. *Fertil. Steril.*, **32**, 389.

17. Stray Pederson, B. and Stray Pederson, S. (1984) Etiologic factors and subsequent reproductive performance in 195 couples with a prior history of habitual abortion. *Am. J. Obstet. Gynecol.*, **148**, 140–6.

18. Hill, J.A., Polgar, K., Harlow, B.L. and Anderson, D.J. (1992) Evidence of embryo- and trophoblast-toxic cellular immune response(s) in women with recurrent spontaneous abortion. *Am. J. Obstet. Gynecol.*, **166**, 1044–52.

19. Hill, J.A. (1992) Immunologic mechanisms of pregnancy maintainance and failure: a critique of theories and therapy. *Am. J. Reprod. Immunol.*, **22**, 33–42.

20. Hill, J.A. and Anderson, D.J. (1988) The embryo as an immunologic target in infertility and recurrent abortion, in *Perspectives in Immunoreproduction: Conception and Contraception* (eds S. Mathur and C.M. Fredericks), Hemisphere, New York, pp. 261–77.

21. Hanley, J.G., Gladman, D.D., Rose, T.H. *et al.* (1988) Lupus pregnancy: a prospective study of placental changes. *Arthritis Rheum.*, **31**, 358.

22. Lockshin, M.D., Druzin, M.L., Goei, S. *et al.* (1985) Antibody to cardiolipin as a predictor of fetal distress or death in pregnant patients with systemic lupus erythematosus. *N. Engl. J. Med.*, **313**, 152.

23. Out, H.J., Bruinse, H.W., Christians, C.M.L. *et al.* (1991) Histopathological findings in placentae from patients with intrauterine fetal death and antiphospholipid antibodies. *Eur. J. Obstet. Gynecol. Reprod. Biol.*, **41**, 179.

24. Branch, D.W. and Scott, J.R. (1990) Clinical implication of anti-phospholipid antibodies: The Utah experience, in *Phospholipid-binding Antibodies* (eds E.N. Harris, T. Ener, G.R.V. Hughes and R.A. Anderson), CRC Press, Boca Raton, FL, pp. 335–46.

25. Unander, A.M., Narberg, R., Hahn, L. *et al.* (1985) Anticardiolipin antibodies and complement in ninety-nine women with habitual abortion. *Am. J. Obstet. Gynecol.*, **156**, 114.

26. Edelman, P., Rouquette, A.M., Verdy, E. *et al.* (1986) Autoimmunity, fetal losses, lupus anticoagulant: beginning of systemic lupus erythematosus or new autoimmune entity with gynaeco-obstetrical expression. *Hum. Reprod.*, **1**, 295.

27. Howard, M.A., Firkin, B.G., Healy, D.L. *et al.* (1987) Lupus anticoagulant in women with multiple spontaneous miscarriage. *Am. J. Hematol.*, **26**, 175.

28. Carreras, L.O., Vermylen, J., Spitz, B. *et al.* (1981) 'Lupus' anticoagulant and inhibition of prostacyclin formation in patients with repeated abortion, intrauterine growth retardation, and intrauterine deaths. *Br. J. Obstet. Gynaecol.*, **88**, 890.

29. Dudley, D.J., Mitchell, M.D. and Branch, D.W. (1990) Pathophysiology of antiphospholipid antibodies: absence of prostaglandin-mediated effects on cultured endothelium. *Am. J. Obstet. Gynecol.*, **162**, 953.

30. Gleicher, N., Harlow, L., Zilberstein, M. (1992) Regulatory effect of antiphospholipid antibodies on signal transduction: a possible model for autoantibody-induced reproductive failure. *Am. J. Obstet. Gynecol.*, **167**, 637–42.

31. Harris, E.N., Asherson, R.A., Gharavi, A.E. *et al.* (1985) Thrombocytopenia in SLE and related disorders: association with anticardiolipin antibodies. *Br. J. Haematol.*, **59**, 227.

32. Carlou, R., Tobelem, G., Soria, C. *et al.* (1986) Inhibition of protein C activation by endothelial cells in the presence of lupus anticoagulant. *N. Engl. J. Med.*, **314**, 1193.

33. Freyssinet, J.M., Gauchy, J. and Cazemare, J.P. (1986) The effect of phospholipids on the activation of protein C by the human thrombin–thrombomodulin complex. *Biochem. J.*, **238**, 151.

34. Lyden, T.W., Ng, A.K. and Rote, N.J. (1992) Modulation of phosphatidyl-serine epitope expression on BeWo cells during forskolin treatment. *Am. J. Reprod. Immunol.*, **27**, 24.

35. Menge, A.C. (1970) Immune reactions and infertility. *J. Reprod. Fertil.*, **10**, 171–87.

36. Jones, W.R. (1974) The use of antibodies developed by infertile women to identify relevant antigens, in *Immunological Approaches to Fertility Control* (ed. E. Diczfalusy), Karolinska Institute, Stockholm, pp. 376–404.

37. Haas, G.G., Kubota, K., Quebbeman, J.F. *et al.* (1986) Circulating antisperm antibodies in recurrently aborting women. *Fertil. Steril.*, **45**, 209–15.

38. Witkin, S.S. and Chaudry, A. (1989) Association between and recurrent spontaneous abortions and circulating IgG antibodies to sperm tails in women. *J. Reprod. Immunol.*, **15**, 151–8.

39. Juger, S., Kremer, J. and De Wilde-Janssen, I.W. (1984) Are sperm immobilizing antibodies in cervical mucus an explanation for a poor postcoital test? *Am. J. Reprod. Immunol.*, **5**, 56–60.

40. Clarke, G.W. and Baker, H.W.G. (1993) Lack of association between sperm antibodies and recurrent spontaneous abortion. *Fertil. Steril.*, **59**, 463–4.

41. Stagnaro-Green, A., Roman, S.H., Cobin, R.H. *et al.* (1990) Detection of at-risk pregnancy by means of highly sensitive assays for thyroid autoantibodies. *JAMA*, **264**, 1422–5.

42. Pratt, D., Novotny, M., Kaberlein, G. *et al.* (1993) Antithyroid antibodies and the association with non-organ specific antibodies in recurrent pregnancy loss. *Am. J. Obstet. Gynecol.*, **168**, 837–41.

43. Gleicher, N., El-Roeiy, A., Confino, E. *et al.* (1989) Reproductive failure because of autoantibodies: unexplained infertility and pregnancy wastage. *Am. J. Obstet. Gynecol.*, **160**, 1376–80.

44. Rocklin, R.E., Kitzmiller, J.L., Carpenter, C.B. *et al.* (1976) Maternal–fetal relation: absence of an immunologic blocking factor from serum of women with chronic abortions. *N. Engl. J. Med.*, **295**, 1209.

45. Sargent, I.L., Wilkins, T. and Redman, C.W.G. (1994) Maternal immune responses to the fetus in early pregnancy and recurrent miscarriage. *Lancet*, **ii**, 1099–104.

46. Beer, A.E., Quebberman, J.F., Ayers, J.W.I. *et al.* (1981) Major histocompatibility complex antigens, maternal and paternal immune responses and chronic habitual abortion in humans. *Am. J. Obstet. Gynecol.*, **141**, 987–99.

47. McIntyre, J.A. and Faulk, W.P. (1983) Recurrent spontaneous abortion in human pregnancy: results of immunogenetical, cellular and humoral tests. *Am. J. Reprod. Immunol.*, **4**, 165–70.

48. Rocklin, R.E., Kitzmiller, J.L. and Garvey, M.R. (1982) Maternal–fetal relation: further characterization of an immunologic blocking factor that develops during pregnancy. *Clin. Immunol. Immunopathol.*, **22**, 305–15.

49. Amos, D.B. and Kostyn, D.D. (1980) HLA: a central immunological agency of man. *Adv. Hum. Genet.*, **10**, 137–41.

50. Rodger, C. (1985) Lack of a requirement for a maternal humoral immune response to establish and maintain successful allogenic pregnancy. *Transplant*, **40**, 372–5.

51. Ober, C.L., Martin, A.O., Simpson, J.L. *et al.* (1983) Shared HLA antigens and reproductive performance among Hutterites. *Am. J. Hum. Genet.*, **35**, 994–1004.

52. McIntyre, J.A., Faulk, W.P., Verhulst, S.T. *et al.* (1983) Human trophoblast–lymphocyte cross-relative (TLX) antigens define a new alloantigen system. *Science*, **222**, 1135–7.

53. Purcell, D.F.J., McKenzie, I.F.C., Lublin, D.M. *et al.* (1990) The human cell surface glycoproteins Hu Ly-M5, membrane co-factor protein (MCP) of the complement system, and trophoblast leukocyte common (TLX) antigen are CD46. *Immunology*, **70**, 155–61.

54. Anderson, D.J., Michaelson, J.S. and Johnson, P.M. (1989) Trophoblast/leukocyte common antigen is expressed by human testicular germ cells and appears on the surface of acrosome-reacted sperm. *Biol. Reprod.*, **41**, 285–93.

55. Ecker, J.L., Laufer, M.R. and Hill, J.A. (1993) Measurement of embryotoxic factors is predictive of pregnancy outcome in women with a history of recurrent abortion. *Obstet. Gynecol.*, **81**, 84–7.

56. Hill, J.A. and Anderson, D.J. (1988) Cell-mediated immune mechanisms in recurrent spontaneous abortion, in *Contraceptive Research for Today and the Nineties* (ed. G.P. Talwar), Springer-Verlag, New York, pp. 171–80.

57. Anderson, D.J. and Hill, J.A. (1988) Cell-mediated immunity in infertility. *Am. J. Reprod. Immunol. Microbiol.*, **17**, 22–30.

58. Anderson, D.J., Hill, J.A., Haimovici, F. and Berkowitz, R.S. (1991) Adverse effects of immune cell products in pregnancy, in *Molecular and Cellular Immunobiology of the Maternal Fetal Interface* (eds T. Gill and T. Wegmann), Oxford Press, New York, pp. 207–18.

59. Hill, J.A. (1992) Evidence of a new non-MHC related etiology for immunologic recurrent abortion, in *Reproductive Immunology, Serono Symposia Publ.* (eds F. Dondero and P.M. Johnson), New York, Raven Press, **97**, 235–41.

60. Yamada, H., Polgar, K. and Hill, J.A. (1994) Evidence of cell-medicated immunity to trophoblast antigens in women with recurrent spontaneous abortion. *Am. J. Obstet. Gynecol.*, **170**, 1339–44.

61. Hill, J.A., Anderson, D.J. and Polgar, K. (1995) An abnormal TH1 cellular immune response to trophoblast antigens in women with recurrent spontaneous abortion. *JAMA*, **273**, 1933–6.

62. Hill, J.A., Haimovici, F. and Anderson, D.J. (1987) Products of activated lymphocytes and macrophages inhibit mouse embryo development in vitro. *J. Immunol.*, **132**, 2250–4.

63. Haimovici, F., Hill, J.A. and Anderson, D.J. (1991) The effects of soluble products of activated lymphocytes and macrophages and blastocyst implantation events in vitro. *Biol. Reprod.*, **44**, 69–75.

64. Berkowitz, R.S., Hill, J.A., Kurtz, C.B. *et al.* (1988) Effects of products of activated leukocytes (lymphokines and monokines) on the growth of malignant trophoblast cells in vitro. *Am. J. Obstet. Gynecol.*, **158**, 199–203.

65. Shiomura, K., Manda, T., Mukumoto, S. *et al.* (1988) Recombinant human tumor necrosis factor-alpha: thrombus formation is a cause of antitumor activity. *Int. J. Cancer*, **41**, 243.

66. Mallmann, P., Mallman, R. and Krebs, D. (1991) Determination of tumor necrosis factor alpha and interleukin-2 in women with idiopathic recurrent miscarriage. *Arch. Gynecol. Obstet.*, **249**, 73–8.

67. Schust, D.J. and Hill, J.A. (1996) Correlation of serum cytokine and adhesion molecule determinations with pregnancy outcome. *J. Soc. Gynecol. Invest.*, **3**, 259–61.

68. Gendron, R.L., Nestel, F.P., Lapp, W.S. and Baines, M.G. (1990) Lipopolysaccharide-induced fetal resorption in mice is associated with the intrauterine production of tumor necrosis factor-alpha. *J. Reprod. Fertil.*, **90**, 395–402.

69. Chaouat, G., Menu, E., Clark, D.A. *et al.* (1990) Control of fetal survival in CBA/JX DBA/2 mice by lymphokine therapy. *J. Reprod. Fertil.*, **89**, 447–58.

70. Tezabwala, B.U., Johnson, P.M. and Rees, R.C. (1989) Inhibition of pregnancy viability in mice following IL-2 administration. *Immunology*, **67**, 115–19.

71. Polgar, K., Yacono, P.W., Golan, D.E. and Hill, J.A. (1996) Immune interferon gamma (IGN-γ) inhibits translational mobility of a plasma membrane protein in preimplantation stage mouse embryos: a T-Helper 1 mechanism for immunologic reproductive failure. *Am. J. Obstet. Gynecol.*, **174**, 282–7.

72. Lin, H., Mosman, T.R., Guilbert, L. *et al.* (1993) Synthesis of T-helper 2-type cytokines at the maternal–fetal interface. *J. Immunol.*, **151**, 4562–73.

73. Tangri, S., Wegmann, T.G., Lin, H. and Raghupathy, K. (1994) Maternal antoplacental

reactivity in natural immunologically-mediated fetal resorptions. *J. Immunol.*, **152**, 4903–11.

74. Hamilton, M.S. and Hamilton, B.C. (1987) Environmental influences on immunologically associated spontaneous abortion in CBA/J mice. *J. Reprod. Immunol.*, **11**, 237–41.

75. Quinn, P.A., Petric, M., Barkin, M. *et al.* (1987) Prevalence of antibody to *Chlamydia trachomatis* in spontaneous abortion and infertility. *Am. J. Obstet. Gynecol.*, **156**, 291–6.

76. Witkin, S.S. and Ledger, W.J. (1992) Antibodies to *Chlamydia trachomatis* in sera of women with recurrent spontaneous abortions. *Am. J. Obstet. Gynecol.*, **167**, 135–9.

77. Beatty, W.L., Byrne, G.I. and Morrison, R.P. (1993) Morphological and antigenic characterization of interferon-gamma mediated persistent *Chlamydia trachomatis* infection in vitro. *Proc. Natl. Acad. Sci. USA*, **90**, 3998–4002.

78. Pollard, D.R., Tyler, S.D., Ng, C.W. and Rozee, K.R. (1989) A polymerase chain reaction protocol for the specific identification of chlamydia sp. *Mol. Cell. Probes*, **3**, 383–9.

79. Laffler, T.G., Carrino, J.J. and Marshall, R.L. (1993) The ligase chain reaction in DNA based diagnosis. *Ann. Biol. Clin.*, **51**, 821–6.

80. Dille, B.J., Butzen, C.C. and Birkenmeyer, L.G. (1993) Amplification of *Chlamydia trachomatis* DNA by ligase chain reaction. *J. Clin. Microbiol.*, **31**, 729–31.

81. Hunt, J.S. (1989) Cytokine networks in the uteropacental unit: macrophages as pivotal regulatory cells. *J. Reprod. Immunol.*, **16**, 1–17.

82. Simmen, F.A. and Simmen, R.C.M. (1991) Peptide growth factors and proto-oncogenes in mammalian conceptus development. *Biol. Reprod.*, **44**, 1–5.

83. Wegmann, T.G. (1988) Maternal T cells promote placental trophoblast growth and prevent spontaneous abortion. *Immunol. Lett.*, **17**, 297–302.

84. Tartakovsky, B. (1989) CSF-1 induces resorption of embryos in mice. *Immunol. Lett.*, **23**, 65–70.

85. Clark, D.A. (1989) Cytokines and pregnancy. *Curr. Opin. Immunol.*, **1**, 1148–52.

86. Tsutsum, I. and Oka, T. (1987) Epidermal growth factor deficiency during pregnancy causes abortion in mice. *Am. J. Obstet. Gynecol.*, **156**, 241–4.

87. Zhao, X., Singh, B. and Batten, B.E. (1991) The role c-mos protooncogene in mammalian meiotic maturation. *Oncogene*, **6**, 43–9.

88. Kauma, S.W., Ackerman, S.C., Eirman, D. *et al.* (1991) Colony stimulating factor-1 c-fms expression in human endometrial tissues and placenta during the menstrual cycle and early pregnancy. *J. Clin. Endocrinol. Metab.*, **73**, 746–51.

89. Clark, D.A., Chapat, A. and Tutton, D. (1986) Active suppression of host-versus-graft reaction in pregnant mice. VII: Spontaneous abortion of allogeneic CBA/J, DBA/2 fetuses in the uterus of CBA/J mice correlates with deficient non-T cell suppressor cell activity. *J. Immunol.*, **136**, 1668–75.

90. Nobel, C. (1984) Malimplantation – a cause of failure after IVF and GIFT. *Am. J. Reprod. Immunol.*, **6**, 56–7.

91. Daya, S., Clark, D.A., Derlin, C. *et al.* (1985) Preliminary characterization of two types of suppressor cells in the human uterus. *Fertil. Steril.*, **44**, 778–85.

92. Johnson, P.M. (1990) MHC region genetics and trophoblast antigen expression in human pregnancy, in *The Molecular and Cellular Immunobiology of the Maternal Fetal Interface* (eds T. Wegmann and T. Gill), Elsevier, New York.

93. Kovats, S., Main, E.K., Librach, C. *et al.* (1990) A Class I antigen, HLA-G, expressed in human trophoblasts. *Science*, **248**, 220–3.

94. Ellis, S.A. and McMichael, A.J. (1990) Human trophoblast and the choriocarcinoma cell line BeWo express a truncated HLA Class I molecule. *J. Immunol.*, **144**, 731.

95. Feinman, M.A., Kliman, J.H. and Main, E.K. (1987) HLA antigen expression and induction by gamma-interferon in cultured human trophoblast. *Am. J. Obstet. Gynecol.*, **157**, 1429–34.

96. Anderson, D.J. and Berkowitz, R.S. (1985) Gamma interferon enhances expression of class I MHC antigens in the early HLA(+) human choriocarcinoma cell live BeWo but does not induce MHC expression in the HLA(−) choriocarcinoma cell live Jar. *J. Immunol.*, **135**, 2498.

97. Hill, J.A., Melling, G.C. and Johnson, P.M. (1995) Immunohistochemical studies of human uteroplacental tissues from first-trimester spontaneous abortion. *Am. J. Obstet. Gynecol.*, **173**, 90–6.

98. Hunt, J.S. and Hsi, B.L. (1990) Evasive strategies of trophoblast cells: selective expression of membrane antigens. *Am. J. Reprod. Immunol.*, **23**, 57–63.

99. Branch, D.W., Rote, N.S., Dostal, D. *et al.* (1987)

Association of lupus anticoagulant with antibody against antiphosphotidyl serine. *Clin. Immunol. Immunopathol.*, **42**, 63.

100. Alving, B.M., Baldwin, P.E., Richards, R.L. *et al.* (1985) The dilute phospholipid APTT: a sensitive assay for verification of lupus anticoagulants. *Thromb. Haemost.*, **54**, 709.

101. Rosner, F. and Grunwald, H.W. (1988) Thrombocytosis and spontaneous abortion. *Am. J. Hematol.*, **27**, 233.

102. Cowchuck, S., Dehoratius, R.D., Wapner, R.J. *et al.* (1984) Subclinical autoimmune disease and unexplained abortion. *Am. J. Obstet. Gynecol.*, **150**, 367.

103. Garcia de la Torre, I., Hernandez-Vasquez, L., Angulo-Vasquez, J. *et al.* (1984) Prevalence of antinuclear antibodies in patients with habitual abortion in normal and toxemic patients. *Rheumatol. Int.*, **4**, 87.

104. Regan, L., Brande, P.R. and Hill, D.P. (1981) A prospective study of the incidence, time of, appearance of, significance of anti-paternal lymphocytotoxic antibodies in human pregnancy. *Hum. Reprod.*, **6**, 294–8.

105. McConnachie, P.R. and McIntyre, J.A. (1984) Maternal antipaternal immunity in couples predisposed to repeated pregnancy losses. *Am. J. Reprod. Immunol.*, **5**, 145–50.

106. Regan, L. and Braude, P.R. (1987) Is antipaternal cytotoxic antibody a valid marker in the management of recurrent abortion? *Lancet*, **ii**, 1280–2.

107. Huang, J.L., Ho, H.N., Yang, U.S. *et al.* (1992) The role of blocking factors and antipaternal lymphocytotoxic antibodies in the success of pregnancy in patients with recurrent spontaneous abortion. *Fertil. Steril.*, **58**, 691–6.

108. Coulam, C.B. (1992) Immunological tests in the evaluating reproductive disorders: a critical review. *Am. J. Obstet. Gynecol.*, **167**, 1844–51.

109. Eroglu, G., Betz, G. and Torregano, C. (1992) Impact of histocompatibility antigens on pregnancy outcome. *Am. J. Obstet. Gynecol.*, **166**, 1364–9.

110. Cowchuck, F.S. and Smith, J.B. (1992) Predictors for live birth after unexplained spontaneous abortion: correlations between immunologic test results, obstetric histories, and outcome of next pregnancy without treatment. *Am. J. Obstet. Gynecol.*, **167**, 1208–12.

111. Cowchuck, F.S., Smith, J.B., David, S. *et al.* (1990) Paternal mononuclear cell immunization theory for repeated miscarriage: predictive variables for pregnancy success. *Am. J. Reprod. Immunol.*, **22**, 12.

112. Taylor, C. and Faulk, W.P. (1981) Prevention of recurrent abortion with leukocyte transfusions. *Lancet*, **ii**, 68–70.

113. Beer, A.E., Semprini, A.E., Ziaoyu, Z. and Quebbeman, J.F. (1985) Pregnancy outcome in human couples with recurrent spontaneous abortions: HLA antigen profiles; HLA antigen sharing; female serum MLR blocking factors; and paternal leukocyte immunization. *Exp. Clin. Immunogenet.*, **2**, 137–83.

114. Johnson, P.M., Ramsden, G.H., Chia, K.V. *et al.* (1991) A combined randomized double-blind and open study of trophoblast membrane infusion (TMI) in unexplained recurrent miscarriage, in *Cellular and Molecular Biology of the Maternal–fetal Relationship* (eds G. Chaouat and J. Mowbray), INSERM John Libbey Eurotext, **212**, 272–84.

115. Coulam, C.D. (1988) Treatment of recurrent spontaneous abortion. *Am. J. Reprod. Immunol. Microbiol.*, **17**, 149.

116. Christiansen, O.B., Mathiesen, O., Husth, M. *et al.* (1994) Placebo-controlled trial of active immunization with third party leukocytes in recurrent miscarriage. *Acta Obstet. Gynecol. Scand.*, **73**, 261–8.

117. Mowbray, J.F., Gibbings, C., Liddell, H. *et al.* (1985) Controlled trial of treatment of recurrent spontaneous abortion by immunostimulation with paternal cells. *Lancet*, **i**, 941–3.

118. Ho, H.N., Gill, T.J., Itsieh, H.J. *et al.* (1991) Immunotherapy for recurrent spontaneous abortions in a Chinese population. *Am. J. Reprod. Immunol.*, **25**, 10–15.

119. Cauchi, M.N., Lim, D., Young, D.E. *et al.* (1991) The treatment of recurrent aborters by immunization with paternal cells: controlled trial. *Am. J. Reprod. Immunol.*, **25**, 16–17.

120. Fraser, E.J., Grimes, D.A. and Schulz, K.F. (1993) Immunizations as therapy for recurrent spontaneous abortion: a review and meta-analysis. *Obstet. Gynecol.*, **82**, 854–9.

121. The Recurrent Miscarriage Immunotherapy Trialist Group (1994) World wide collaborative observational study and meta-analysis on allogenic leukocyte immunotherapy for recurrent spontaneous abortion. *Am. J. Reprod. Immunol.*, **32**, 55–72.

122. Relman, A.S. (1978) On controversy in medicine. *Pharos*, January, 18–22.

123. Report of the ASRI ad hoc Ethics Committee

appointed by Dr Joan Hunt, President of the ASRI 1994–1995.

124. Lubbe, W.F., Butler, W.S., Palmer, S.J. and Higgins, G.C. (1985) Fetal survival after prednisone suppression of maternal lupus anticoagulant. *Lancet*, **i**, 1361.

125. Lockshin, M.D., Druzin, M.L. and Qamar, T. (1989) Prednisone does not prevent recurrent fetal death in women with antiphospholipid antibody. *Am. J. Obstet. Gynecol.*, **160**, 439–43.

126. Cowchuck, F.S., Reece, E.A., Baladen, D. *et al.* (1992) Repeated fetal losses associated with anti phospholipid antibodies. A collaborative randomized trial comparing prednisone to low-dose heparin treatment. *Am. J. Obstet. Gynecol.*, **166**, 1318–27.

127. Csapo, A.L., Pulkkinen, M.O. and Wiest, W.G. (1973) Effects of luteectiomy and progesterone replacement in early pregnant patients. *Am. J. Obstet. Gynecol.*, **115**, 759.

128. Siiteri, P.K., Febres, F., Clemens, L.E. *et al.* (1977) Progesterone and maintenance of pregnancy. Is progesterone nature's immunosuppressant? *Ann. NY Acad. Sci.*, **286**, 334.

129. Clemens, L.E., Siiteri, P.K. and Stites, D.P. (1979) Mechanisms of immunosuppression of progesterone on maternal lymphocyte activation during pregnancy. *J. Immunol.*, **122**, 1978–85.

130. Wang, H.S., Kunzaki, H., Tokushige, M. *et al.* (1988) Effect of ovarian steroids on the secretion of immunosuppressive factors from human endometrium. *Am. J. Obstet. Gynecol.*, **158**, 629–57.

131. Feinberg, B.B., Tan, N.S., Gonik, B. *et al.* (1991) Increased progesterone concentrations are necessary to suppress interleukin-2-activated human mononuclear cell cytotoxity. *Am. J. Obstet. Gynecol.*, **165**, 1872–6.

132. Jones, G.E.S. (1949) Some new aspects of the management of infertility. *JAMA*, **141**, 1123.

133. Randomized clinical trials of progestational agents in pregnancy. *Br. J. Obstet. Gynecol.*, **96**, 265.

134. Daya, S., Ward, S. and Burrows, E. (1988) Progesterone profiles in luteal phase defect cycles and outcome of progesterone treatment in patients with recurrent spontaneous abortion. *Am. J. Obstet. Gynecol.*, **158**, 225–32.

135. Miles, R.A., Paulson, R.J., Lobo, R.A. *et al.* (1994) Pharmacokinetics and endometrial tissue progesterone after administration by intramuscular and vaginal routes: A comparative study. *Fertil. Steril.*, **62**, 485–90.

136. Scott, J.R., Branch, D.W., Kochenour, W.K. and Ward, K. (1988) Intravenous immunoglobulin treatment of pregnant patients with recurrent pregnancy loss caused by antiphospholipid antibodies and Rh immunization. *Am. J. Obstet. Gynecol.*, **159**, 1055.

137. Dwyer, J.M. (1992) Manipulating the immune system with immune globulin. *N. Engl. J. Med.*, **326**, 107–16.

138. Mueller-Eckhardt, G., Heine, O. and Poltrin, B. IVIG to prevent recurrent spontaneous abortion. *Lancet*, **i**, 424.

139. Maruyama, T., Makine, T., Iwasaki, K.I. *et al.* (1994) The influence of intravenous immunoglobulin treatment of maternal immunity in women with unexplained recurrent miscarriage. *Am. J. Reprod. Immunol.*, **31**, 7–18.

139a. Daya, S., Gunby, J., Clark D.A., (1998) Intravenous immoglobulin therapy for recurrent spontaneous abortion: a meta-analysis. *Am. J. Reprod. Immunol.*, **39**, 69–76.

140. Stein, Z.A. (1985) A women's age: child bearing and child rearing. *Am. J. Epidemiol.*, **121**, 327–40.

141. Regan, L., Braude, P.R. and Trembath, P.L. (1989) Influence of post reproductive performance on risk of spontaneous abortion. *Br. Med. J.*, **299**, 541–5.

142. Katz, I., Fisch, B., Amit, S. *et al.* (1992) Cutaneous graft-versus host-like reaction after paternal lymphocyte immunization for prevention of recurrent abortion. *Fertil. Steril.*, **57**, 927–9.

143. Johnson, P.M. and Ramsden, G.H. (1992) Recurrent miscarriage. *Baillieres Clin. Immunol. Allerg.*, **2**, 607–24.

144. Warburton, D. and Fraser, F.C. (1961) On the probability that a woman who has had a spontaneous abortion will abort in subsequent pregnancies. *Br. J. Obstet. Gynecol.*, **68**, 784–7.

145. Poland, B.J., Miller, J.P., Jones, D.C. *et al.* (1977) Reproductive counseling in patients who had a spontaneous abortion. *Am. J. Obstet. Gynecol.*, **127**, 685–91.

146. Vlaadneren, W. and Treffers, P.E. (1987) Prognosis of subsequent pregnancies after recurrent spontaneous abortion in first trimester. *Br. Med. J.*, **295**, 92–3.

147. Lubbe, W.F. and Liggins, G.C. (1988) Role of lupus anticoagulant and autoimmunity in

recurrent pregnancy loss. *Semin. Reprod. Endocrinol.*, **6**, 161–90.

148. Branch, D.W., Silver, R.M., Blackwell, J.L. *et al.* Outcome of treated pregnancies in women with antiphospholipid syndrome: an update of the Utah experience. *Obstet. Gynecol.*, **80**, 614–20.

149. Caruso, A., DeCarolis, S., Ferrazzani, S. *et al.* (1993) Pregnancy outcome in relation to uterine artery flow velocity wave forms and clinical characteristics in women with antiphospholipid syndrome. *Obstet. Gynecol.*, **82**, 970–7.

150. Frates, M., Doubilet, P., Brown, D. *et al.* (1996) Role of Doppler ultrasonography in the prediction of pregnancy outcome in women with recurrent spontaneous abortion. *J. Ultrasound Med.*, **15**, 557–62.

IMMUNOTHERAPY FOR RECURRENT MISCARRIAGE

10

J.R. Scott

Billingham[1] pointed out that pregnancy represents the only natural and completely successful grafting of tissue from one person to another. He raised the intriguing question about why all semiallogeneic conceptuses are not rejected. Therefore, it is not surprising that immunologic rejection has long been suspected as the cause of some cases of human spontaneous abortions. In fact, immunologic abnormalities have gradually become accepted by many physicians and patients as a common reason for early recurrent pregnancy losses. Nevertheless, despite the tremendous amount of research directed at this problem, definite proof for an alloimmune cause of recurrent miscarriage remains elusive.

THE HUMAN IMMUNE SYSTEM

In a classical immune response, antigen presenting cells of the non-specific (innate) system recognize, process, and remove non-self antigens. The specific (adaptive) system is also assisted by the innate system in processing and presenting antigens to T and B lymphocytes. T lymphocytes divide into specific subsets, and B lymphocytes differentiate into plasma cells which produce antibodies[2] (Figure 10.1). Each lymphocyte has surface adhesion molecules which recognize corresponding surface receptors. These surface markers have been designated clusters of differentiation (CD). Antigens associated with

cell surface markers are derived from the major histocompatibility complex (MHC) located on the short arm of chromosome 6. Class I MHC antigens consist of HLA-A, B and C which are involved in the activation of CD8+ T cells. Class II consists of DR, DP and DQ alleles, markers responsible for stimulating the CD4+ T cells. Communication between cells of the immune system is dependent on cytokines, a diverse group of soluble proteins which act as growth factors, direct cellular traffic, and orchestrate allograft rejection (Figure 10.2).

THE CONCEPTUS AS A SEMIALLOGRAFT

It is readily apparent that the successfully implanted fertilized ovum does not behave like usual transplanted tissue or organs. Although the fetus inherits a paternal set of the six major HLA antigens as well as the maternal HLA haplotype, no HLA antigens are expressed on the blastocyst or fetally derived placental syncytiotrophoblast[3]. Only HLA-G, an HLA variant, is present on cytotrophoblast[4]. Thus, the relatively inert tissue properties of trophoblast probably play an important protective role for the conceptus.

Active modulation of the maternal immune system may also participate in protecting the developing embryo. Whether immunologic tolerance or reactivity develops toward foreign tissue is dependent on many factors. These include the physical form of the presented

Clinical Management of Early Pregnancy. Edited by Walter Prendiville and James R. Scott.
Published in 1999 by Arnold, ISBN 0 340 74100 7

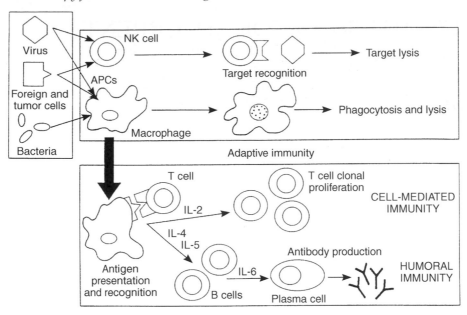

Figure 10.1. Interaction of innate and adoptive immune systems. (Reproduced with permission from Scott, J.R. and Branch, D.W. (1994) Potential alloimmune factors and immunotherapy in recurrent miscarriage. *Clin. Obstet. Gynecol.*, **37**, 761–7.)

antigen, the cell type that acts as antigen presenter, and the phase of the cell cycle of the T cells to which the antigen is presented. Circulating immunosuppressive factors proposed as necessary to prevent immunologic rejection of the conceptus include anti-idiotypic antibodies. Local factors which may be important include decidual cells, suppressor cells, soluble mediators, and certain cytokines[5]. However, none of these mechanisms has been definitively proven as responsible for protecting the fetal–placental unit.

ALLOIMMUNE-MEDIATED RECURRENT PREGNANCY LOSS

Abnormalities of any potential mechanism of fetal–maternal protection could theoretically be responsible for alloimmune rejection or spontaneous abortion.

HLA SHARING

Initial animal studies suggested that parental HLA heterozygosity was related to successful reproduction[6,7]. It was proposed that immunogenetic compatibility prohibited the proper activation of immunologic processes essential for pregnancy maintenance. However, recent studies fail to confirm the benefit of genetic heterogeneity in human pregnancy[8]. Testing couples with recurrent pregnancy loss (RPL) for HLA sharing is expensive and does not change the management[9].

MATERNAL ANTIFETAL ANTIBODY EXPRESSION

The mother can become sensitized against fetal MHC antigens by (1) transplacental transfer of

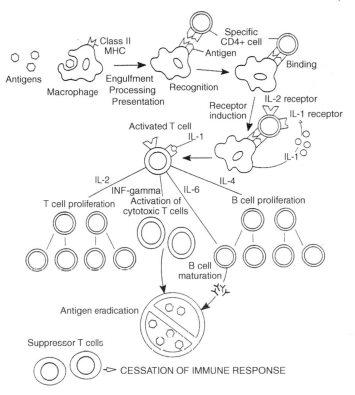

Figure 10.2. Components of the immune response. (Reproduced with permission from Scott, J.R. and Branch, D.W. (1994) Potential alloimmune factors and immunotherapy in recurrent miscarriage. *Clin. Obstet. Gynecol.*, **37**, 761–7.)

fetal cells into the maternal circulation, and (2) perhaps abnormal induction of class I MHC expression on trophoblast by interferon-gamma or other mechanisms[10]. These alloantibodies are commonly found in multiparous women and have also been proposed as necessary for normal pregnancy. However, in primigravidas these antibodies are absent early in gestation and even throughout pregnancies which progress normally. Moreover, both mice and humans incapable of generating any antibody responses still reproduce normally[11].

CIRCULATING IMMUNOSUPPRESSIVE FACTORS

Blocking factors are presumed to be anti-idiotypic antibodies, long alleged to be essential for successful pregnancies. It has been suggested that these circulating factors cover or mask fetal–trophoblast antigens or maternal lymphocyte receptors to interfere with the expected maternal immune response against the foreign conceptus. Detection of blocking antibodies relies on indirect immunologic tests, most commonly the one-way mixed lymphocyte reaction. There are a variety of technical problems with interpretation of these assays[12,13], and mixed lymphocyte culture has now proven to be an unreliable marker of either miscarriage risk or treatment success[9,12]. The validity of other circulating factors such as embryotoxic factor and TJ6 cytokine expression on CD56+ lymphocytes as causes of recurrent miscarriage have also not been adequately established[14,15]. None of these tests are proven to be clinically useful in the routine evaluation of RPL[9].

SUPPRESSOR CELLS AND IMMUNE MEDIATORS

A variety of immune cells and soluble mediators are present in the decidua, and women who have aborted reportedly have insufficient suppressor cells[16]. Theoretically, certain cytokines can be directly or indirectly cytotoxic to the conceptus. Conversely, maternal cell recognition of the fetal allograft may release cytokines that serve as growth factors for trophoblast and placental development required for embryonic survival (immunotrophism)[17]. Contemporary studies are focusing on local decidual/trophoblastic cytokines and other bioactive factors such as hormones, enzymes, growth factors, and endometrial proteins[18,19]. No practical clinical tests are yet available for these factors.

DIAGNOSIS

A fundamental understanding of issues related to the timing and causes of recurrent pregnancy loss is necessary to investigate ways that alloimmune mechanisms might be involved. Up to 5% of all couples trying to conceive have two consecutive miscarriages, and 1–2% experience three consecutive losses. Approximately 50% of women with RPL have no genetic, anatomic, endocrine, infectious or autoimmune causes. It is for this large group with no known reason for RPL that alloimmune causes have been implicated. Nevertheless, this diagnosis is ultimately one of exclusion since there are no definitive clinical or laboratory tests[9,20]. Because of the

uncertain etiology, I still prefer to categorize this subgroup as 'unexplained'.

IMMUNOLOGIC TREATMENT

LEUKOCYTE IMMUNIZATION

Original attempts to improve maternal immunotolerance were based on evidence that (1) pretransplant blood transfusions decreased rejection of organ allografts[21] and (2) the rate of resorptions or abortions in animal models was reduced by prior immunization with spleen cells from a paternally related strain[22]. Not all subsequent data favor an alloimmune pathogenesis of recurrent miscarriage. The beneficial effect of pretransplant blood transfusions to abrogate rejection has now been questioned. Moreover, extrapolation from animal models to the human situation is often irrelevant because of interspecies differences. For example, the immunologic implications of living fetuses and resorptions in the same uterine horn in rodents are uncertain. Early proponents of leukocyte immunization believed that normal pregnancy required maternal allogeneic recognition in order to stimulate the formation of blocking antibodies necessary for pregnancy maintenance. Since HLA heterogeneity does not predict pregnancy outcome, it now seems more likely that any benefit from immunotherapy involves local immunomodulation. These important changes in the premise and rationale for immunotherapy warrant re-evaluation of the biologic plausibility of this treatment.

A number of medical centers throughout the world now offer leukocyte immunization to prevent RPL. Immunization of the female partner with the male partner's leukocytes has been the most widely used regimen, but third party leukocytes, seminal plasma, and trophoblast preparations have also been utilized. There has been no consensus regarding the dose, route or timing of immunizations, and no reliable way to prospectively identify which patient would benefit from treatment has emerged.

Immunization technique

Despite attempts to standardize paternal cell immunization, regimens still vary[23]. The male partner, after testing negative for hepatitis, syphilis and human immunodeficiency virus, usually donates one unit of blood. The blood is centrifuged through a density gradient, and a highly enriched lymphocyte/monocyte population is extracted. These cells are washed, and 200–400 million mononuclear cells are resuspended in lactated Ringer's solution. A portion of the concentrated cell preparation is typically infused intravenously, and the remainder is injected into intradermal and subcutaneous sites.

Potential complications

Risks of blood-component immunotherapy include transfusion-related risks such as maternal sensitization and the possibility of viral transmission. Complications are rare, but reactions at the injection site, fever, myalgias, platelet and erythrocyte alloimmunization, and a cutaneous graft-versus-host-like reaction have occurred[24–26]. No increase above background congenital anomalies or other problems have been noted in the offspring to date[27].

Results

The efficacy of immunotherapy remains controversial. In initial uncontrolled series, the live birth rate in recurrent miscarriage patients following maternal immunization with paternal leukocytes ranged from 50% to 83%[28]. The results of more recent properly designed studies have been conflicting[29–33]. There have been two independent meta-analyses under the auspices of the American Society for Reproductive Immunology using results from individual patient data sheets in both published and unpublished prospective randomized trials[34]. One team of analysts found that 68% of women who received paternal leukocytes delivered a live infant in the next pregnancy compared to a 61% livebirth rate in untreated controls[35]. Thus, the percentage livebirth ratio (risk ratio) for recurrent miscarriage patients immunized with paternal leukocytes compared to control women was 1.164 (95% confidence interval = 1.014–1.335). The risk for another early pregnancy loss increased with maternal age and the number of previous miscarriages in both control and treated groups, and the effect of immunization was greater when adjusted for these variables. Improvement over control patients was not statistically significant when unadjusted. The other meta-analysis conducted from the same database confirmed the small improvement with leukocyte immunization[36].

Nevertheless, whether the difference in outcome between the treated and control groups is statistically significant depends largely on how the analysis is done[37]. Updated data on leukocyte immunization which includes our own patients are shown on Table 10.1 and Figure 10.3. Even the most optimistic interpretation indicates that paternal cell immunization is of marginal clinical benefit. Based on information available at this time, 11–13 patients would require this treatment to achieve one more livebirth. Which recurrent aborter should receive paternal cell immunization remains uncertain, and the treatment is expensive. Other immunization regimens, such as third-party donor cells[38], or trophoblast membrane infusion[39] have no apparent advantage over paternal cells (Table 10.1).

INTRAVENOUS IMMUNOGLOBULIN (IVIG)

Other investigators have treated women with alleged alloimmune recurrent pregnancy loss with IVIG[40–42]. Since immunoglobulins may

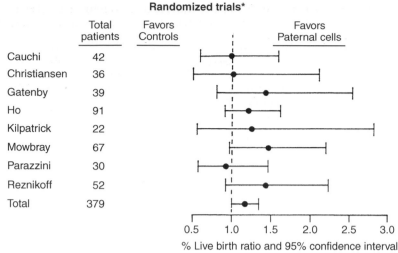

Figure 10.3. Randomized trials adjusted for age number of prior spontaneous abortions. Odds ratios and 95% confidence intervals of successful pregnancy outcome with paternal leukocyte immunization. (Reproduced with permission from Scott, J.R. and Branch, D.W. (1994) Potential alloimmune factors and immunotherapy in recurrent miscarriage. *Clin. Obstet. Gynecol.*, **37**, 761–7.)

contain both idiotype and anti-idiotype antibodies against trophoblast antigens, IVIG theoretically benefits women with RPL who do not produce sufficient 'blocking' antibodies. Other unknown immunologic mechanisms may also be involved. The five IVIG preparations commercially available differ slightly in their immunoglobulin levels and preparation procedures. A unified protocol has not been developed, and the cost may be substantially higher than leukocyte immunization. There have been four prospective randomized trials published to date[40–43]. In two studies, IVIG 0.5 mg/kg/month was started before conception and continued through 28–32 weeks' gestation[41,43]. The third regimen consisted of 600 ml (30 g) IVIG at 5 weeks' gestation followed by 400 ml (20 g) every three weeks to 25 weeks[40]. The fourth regimen was more complicated[42]. In one trial IVIG treatment resulted in improvement in the pregnancy success rate[41], but there was no statistically significant difference between treated and control groups in the others[40,42,43] (Table 10.1).

CONCLUSION

It is difficult to determine whether alloimmune factors are responsible for some cases of recurrent miscarriage. No diagnostic tests have been found to be clinically useful. When known non-immunologic causes are ruled out, approximately 60% of couples will achieve a successful pregnancy with no treatment. It appears that paternal cell immunization may increase the livebirth rate by 8–10%, but the results of large prospective, randomized studies presently ongoing are necessary to confirm this therapeutic effect. Better understanding of the immunology of pregnancy, and a reliable way to identify those women who do not need immunotherapy are urgently needed. Leukocyte immunization is associated with side effects, though they are rare. The treatment does not seem to produce adverse effects

Table 10.1 Comparison of livebirth rate between investigators by treatment for recurrent miscarriage in prospective randomized published and unpublished trials [34]

	Paternal cells		Controls	
Mowbray [29]	25/37	(67.6%)	14/30	(46.7%)
Ho [30]	33/42	(78.6%)	32/49	(65.3%)
Cauchi [31]	13/20	(65.0%)	16/22	(72.7%)
Gatenby [32]	12/20	(60.0%)	13/19	(68.4%)
Christiansen	4/8	(50.0%)	10/28	(57.1%)
Kilpatrick	8/12	(66.7%)	6/10	(60.0%)
Reznikoff	17/26	(65.4%)	14/26	(53.9%)
Parazzini	10/16	(62.5%)	11/14	(78.6%)
Stray-Pedersen	24/32	(75.0%)	22/30	(73.3%)
Scott	8/13	(61.5%)	5/13	(38.5%)
Total	154/226	(68.1%)	150/241	(62.2%)
	Donor cells		Controls	
Gatenby [32]	8/11	(72.7%)	12/20	(60.0%)
Christiansen [38]	27/40	(67.5%)	16/28	(57.1%)
Scott	7/18	(38.9%)	5/12	(41.7%)
Total	42/69	(60.9%)	33/60	(55.0%)
	Trophoblast membranes		Controls	
Johnson [39]	8/17	(47.1%)	14/20	(70.0%)
	IVIG		Controls	
Mueller-Eckhardt [40]	20/27	(74.0%)	21/30	(70.0%)
Coulam [41]*	18/29	(62.1%)	11/32	(34.4%)
Christiansen [42]	9/17	(52.9%)	5/17	(29.4%)
Stephenson [43]*	12/21	(57.0%)	11/22	(50.00%)
Total	59/94	(62.8%)	48/101	(47.5%)

*Patients with as few as two previous miscarriages were entered into these trials.

in the offspring, but there are no long-term published reports on these children.

Currently, the author recommends that physicians adopt a cautious approach to the diagnosis and management of potential alloimmune RPL. Leukocyte immunization is best reserved for patients who have no other options and who understand the cost, risks and benefits. Those who desire to pursue immunotherapy after appropriate counseling should be referred to a research center with an interest in this area.

REFERENCES

1. Billingham, R.E. (1964) Transplantation immunity and the maternal–fetal relation. *N. Engl. J. Med.*, **270**, 667–72, 720–5.
2. Dudley, D.J. (1992) The immune system in health and disease. *Balliere's Clin. Obstet. Gynaecol.*, **6**, 393–416.
3. Hunt, J.S. and Hsi, B.-L. (1990) Evasive strategies of trophoblast cells: selective expression of membrane antigens. *Am. J. Reprod. Immunol.*, **23**, 57–63.
4. Kovats, S., Main, E.K., Librach, C. *et al.* (1990) A Class I antigen, HLA-G, expressed in human trophoblasts. *Science*, **248**, 220–3.

5. Hill, J.A. and Anderson, D.J. (1990) Evidence for the existence and significance of immune cells and their soluble products in reproductive tissues. *Immunol. Allergy Clin. North. Am.*, **10**, 1.

6. Hull, P. (1964) Partial incompatibility not affecting litter size in the mouse. *Genetics*, **50**, 563.

7. Clarke, B. and Kirby, D.R.S. (1966) Maintenance of histocompatibility polymorphisms. *Nature (London)*, **211**, 999.

8. Balasch, J., Coll, O., Martorell, J. *et al.* (1989) Further data against HLA sharing in couples with recurrent spontaneous abortion. *Gynecol. Endocrinol.*, **3**, 63–9.

9. Coulam, C.B. (1992) Immunologic tests in the evaluation of reproductive disorders: a critical review. *Am. J. Obstet. Gynecol.*, **167**, 1844–51.

10. Feinman, M.A., Kliman, J.H. and Main, E.K. (1987) HLA antigen expression and induction by gamma-interferon in cultured human trophoblast. *Am. J. Obstet. Gynecol.*, **157**, 1429–34.

11. Rodger, J.C. (1985) Lack of a requirement for a maternal humoral immune response to establish or maintain successful allogeneic pregnancy. *Transplantation*, **40**, 372–5.

12. Neppert, J., Mueller-Eckhardt, G., Neumeyer, H. *et al.* (1989) Pregnancy-maintaining antibodies: workshop report (Giessen, 1988). *J. Reprod. Immunol.*, **15**, 159–67.

13. Park, M.I., Edwin, S.S., Scott, J.R. and Branch, D.W. (1990) Interpretation of blocking activity in maternal serum depends on the equation used for calculation of mixed lymphocyte culture results. *Clin. Exp. Immunol.*, **82**, 363–8.

14. Hill, J.A., Polgar, K., Harlow, B.L. and Anderson, D.J. (1992) Evidence of embryo- and tropho-blast-toxic cellular immune response(s) in women with recurrent spontaneous abortion. *Am. J. Obstet. Gynecol.*, **166**, 1044–52.

15. Coulam, C.B. and Beaman, K.D. (1995) Reciprocal alteration in circulating TJ6+CD19+ and TJ6+CD56+ leukocytes in early pregnancy predicts success or miscarriage. *Am. J. Reprod. Immunol.*, **34**, 219–24.

16. Daya, S., Clark, D.A., Devlin, C. and Jarrell, J. (1985) Preliminary characterization of two types of suppressor cells in the human uterus. *Fertil. Steril.*, **44**, 778–85.

17. Athanassakis, I., Bleackley, R.C., Paetkau, V. *et al.* (1987) The immunostimulator effect of T cells and T cell lymphokines on murine fetally derived placental cells. *J. Immunol.*, **138**, 37–44.

18. Johnson, P.M. (1992) Pregnancy immunology. *Fetal Matern. Med. Rev.*, **4**, 1–14.

19. Giudice, L.C. (1994) Growth factors and growth modulators in human uterine endometrium: their potential relevance to reproductive medicine. *Fertil. Steril.*, **61**, 1–17.

20. Cowchock, S.F. and Smith, J.B. (1992) Predictors of live birth after unexplained spontaneous abortions: correlations between immunologic test results, obstetric histories, and outcome of next pregnancy without treatment. *Am. J. Obstet. Gynecol.*, **167**, 1208–12.

21. Sollinger, H.W., Burlingham, W.J., Sparks, E.M.F. *et al.* (1984) Donor-specific transfusions in unrelated and related HLA mismatched donor recipient combinations. *Transplantation*, **38**, 612–14.

22. Chaouat, G., Kiger, N. and Wegmann, T.G. (1983) Vaccination against spontaneous abortion in mice. *J. Reprod. Immunol.*, **5**, 389–92.

23. Coulam, C.B. (1991) Workshop A: unification of immunotherapy protocols. The report from the tenth anniversary meeting of the American Society for the Immunology of Reproduction. *Am. J. Reprod. Immunol.*, **25**, 1–6.

24. Pearlman, S.A., Meek, R.S., Cowchock, F.S. *et al.* (1992) Neonatal alloimmune thrombocytopenia after maternal immunization with paternal mononuclear cells: successful treatment with intravenous gamma globulin. *Am. J. Perinatol.*, **9**, 448–51.

25. Katz, I., Fisch, B., Amit, S. *et al.* (1992) Cutaneous graft-versus-host-like reaction after paternal lymphocyte immunization for prevention of recurrent abortion. *Fertil. Steril.*, **57**, 927–9.

26. Takakuwa, K., Goto, S., Hasegawa, I. *et al.* (1989) Is immunotherapy for habitual aborters an immunologically hazardous procedure for infants? *Am.. J. Reprod. Immunol.*, **19**, 53–6.

27. Clark, D.A. and Daya, S. (1991) Trials and tribulation in the treatment of recurrent spontaneous abortion. *Am. J. Reprod. Immunol.*, **25**, 18–24.

28. Branch, D.W. and Scott, J.R. (1992) Immunologic aspects of pregnancy loss: Alloimmune and autoimmune considerations, in *Medicine of the Fetus and Mother* (eds E.A. Reece, J.C. Hobbins, M.J. Mahoney and R.H. Petrie), J.B. Lippincott, Philadelphia, pp. 217–33.

29. Mowbray, S.F., Gibbons, C., Liddell, H. *et al.* (1985) Controlled trial of treatment of recurrent spontaneous abortion by immunization with paternal cells. *Lancet*, **i**, 941–3.

30. Ho, H.N., Gill, T.H., Hsieh, H.J. *et al.* (1991) Immunotherapy for recurrent spontaneous

abortions in a Chinese population. *Am. J. Reprod. Immunol.*, **25**, 10–15.

31. Cauchi, M.N., Lim, D., Young, D.E. *et al.* (1991) Treatment of recurrent aborters by immunization with paternal cells – controlled trial. *Am. J. Reprod. Immunol.*, **25**, 16–17.

32. Gatenby, P.A., Cameron, K., Simes, R.J. *et al.* (1993) Treatment of recurrent spontaneous abortion by immunization with paternal lymphocytes: results of a controlled trial. *Am. J. Reprod. Immunol.*, **29**, 88–94.

33. Fraser, E.J., Grimes, D.A. and Schulz, K.F. (1993) Immunization as therapy for recurrent spontaneous abortion: a review and meta-analysis. *Obstet. Gynecol.*, **82**, 854–9.

34. Coulam, G., Clark, D.A., Collins, J. *et al.* (1994) Worldwide prospective collaborative observational study and meta-analysis on immunotherapy for recurrent spontaneous abortion. *Am. J. Reprod. Immunol.*, **32**, 55–72.

35. Scott, J.R. (1994) Immunotherapy for recurrent spontaneous abortion: analysis 2. *Am. J. Reprod. Immunol.*, **32**, 279–80.

36. Collins, J. and Roberts, R. (1994) Immunotherapy for recurrent spontaneous abortion: analysis 1. *Am. J. Reprod. Immunol.*, **32**, 275–8.

37. Jeng, G., Scott, J.R. and Burmeister, L. (1995) A comparison of meta-analytic results using literature versus individual patient data: paternal cell immunization for recurrent miscarriage. *JAMA*, **274**, 830–6.

38. Christiansen, O.B., Mathiesen, O., Husth, M. *et al.* (1994) Placebo-controlled trial of active immunization with third party leukocytes in recurrent miscarriage. *Acta Obstet. Gynecol. Scand.*, **73**, 261–8.

39. Johnson, P.M., Ramsden, G.H., Chia, K.V. *et al.* (1991) A combined randomized double-blind and open study of trophoblast membrane infusion (TMI) in unexplained recurrent miscarriage, in *Cellular and Molecular Biology of the Materno–Fetal Relationship* (eds G. Chaouat and J. Mowbray), Colleque INSERM/John Libbey Eurotext Ltd., **212**, 277–84.

40. Mueller-Eckhardt, G., Mohr-Pennert, A., Heine, O. *et al.* (1994) Controlled trial on intravenous immunoglobulin treatment for prevention of recurrent spontaneous abortion. *Br. J. Obstet. Gynaecol.*, **101**, 1072–7.

41. Coulam, C.B., Krysa, L., Stern, J.J. and Bustillo, M. (1995) Intravenous immunoglobulin for treatment of recurrent pregnancy loss. *Am. J. Reprod. Immunol.*, **34**, 333–7.

42. Christiansen, O.B., Mathiesen, O., Husth, M. *et al.* (1995) Placebo-controlled trial of treatment of unexplained secondary recurrent spontaneous abortions and recurrent late spontaneous abortions with IV immunoglobulin. *Hum. Reprod.*, **10**, 2690–5.

43. Stephenson, M.D., Dreher, K., Houlihan, E., Wu, V. (1998) Prevention of unexplained recurrent spontaneous abortion using intravenous immunoglobulin: a prospective, randomized, double-blinded, placebo-controlled trial. *Am. J. Reprod. Immunol.*, **39**, 82–8.

References   162

W. Prendiville

INTRODUCTION

Progesterone as its name implies is supportive of pregnancy. Does administration of this or other hormones during pregnancy prevent miscarriage? This chapter attempts to answer this question by assessing the available evidence, with particular reference to controlled trials.

Progesterone is necessary for the implantation and maintenance of early pregnancy. In the 1930s several publications described the pregnancy maintaining hormone produced by the corpus luteum. In 1935 a number of workers published a paper calling this hormone progesterone[1]. Among others Csapo et al.[2] confirmed the crucial role played by progesterone in maintaining early pregnancy. In this study, seven of eleven patients exhibited a decrease in serum progesterone and miscarried within 7 days of surgery, following luteectomy in the early part of the first trimester. This contrasted starkly with seven other patients subjected to the same surgery but subsequently treated with progesterone in whom pregnancy continued.

Although the precise role of progesterone is still debatable, further support for its therapeutic possibilities comes from the hormonal profile of women who experience recurrent miscarriage without any obvious non-hormonal etiology. Also, luteal phase defect has been shown to occur more frequently among women with recurrent miscarriage[3].

Because of this evidence it is not unreasonable to suppose that treatment in very early pregnancy might have an effect on the risk of pregnancy failure – be it miscarriage or even stillbirth. It is not surprising that progestogens have indeed been prescribed by a very large number of clinicians with just such aims in mind and a large number of trials, controlled and otherwise, have been undertaken to discover whether or not the supposed benefits were real.

Estrogen, progesterone and human chorionic gonadotrophin (hCG) are all needed to maintain the appropriate environment for a successful pregnancy[4].

Although this may be true, it does not necessarily follow that the therapeutic administration of hormones will prevent or rescue a miscarrying pregnancy. Sadly, it was just this argument which led workers to propose that the synthetic estrogen diethylstilbestrol (DES) was the therapeutic agent of choice in these circumstances[5].

ESTROGENS

The story of the administration of estrogens to women in order to prevent miscarriage is a tragic one. The lesson it provides is useful to every clinician and his/her patients.

Diethylstilbestrol (DES) was popular among a large number of obstetricians in the USA and to a lesser extent in the UK during the 1950s,

Clinical Management of Early Pregnancy. Edited by Walter Prendiville and James R. Scott.
Published in 1999 by Arnold, ISBN 0 340 74100 7

1960s and 1970s. Of the clinical trials performed to assess the potential value of DES a clear difference was highlighted by Goldstein *et al.*[4]. The broadly similar conclusion – that dimethylstilbestrol was an effective drug when used to reduce the risk of miscarriage – was reached in uncontrolled trials[5–10]. These trials did not use a control population with which to compare outcome and there was no attempt at blinding the investigators or patients.

In contrast, at about the same time, a number of controlled trials were implemented in which there were attempts to blind and to randomly or systematically allocate patients. These trials have been analyzed together by way of meta-analysis and the results of this analysis are presented in Table 11.1.

A number of meta-analyses have been performed on the available data from these controlled trials and no benefit is revealed from the use of DES on the risk of miscarriage, prematurity, stillbirth or neonatal death.

Table 11.1 reveals very clearly that in no single trial did DES appear to confer any benefit on these women in terms of the risk of miscarriage. The odds ratios between these trials is compatible with the drug having no effect and when analysed together as a typical odds ratio, the effect is more suggestive of an adverse effect. Furthermore, in each of the trials except Dieckman *et al.*[11] the confidence limits cross unity suggesting that the use of DES could have either a negative or positive effect. In Dieckman *et al.*'s trial, the odds ratio suggested that DES actually increased the chance of miscarriage for the women who took the drug.

Despite the results of these controlled trials, DES was prescribed for another 30 years until Herbst and Scully[12] revealed the link between DES and vaginal adenocarcinoma. Further work by Herbst *et al.*[13] and Greenwald *et al.*[14] confirmed the correlation between maternal stilbestrol and tumor development of female children born to these mothers.

A number of other serious side effects have since been shown to occur more frequently in the offspring of mothers who took DES during the first trimester of pregnancy. These include vaginal adenosis, circumferential cervical and vaginal ridges[15], irregular menses and reduced fecundity[16] as well as increased risks in the chance of premature birth, perinatal death, spontaneous miscarriage and ectopic pregnancy[17]. Bibbo *et al.*'s[15] study also showed an increased risk in the male offspring of the mothers who took DES of epididymal cysts, hypotrophic testes, as well as reduced sperm motility.

Finally, Swyer and Law's long-term follow-up study[18] which began in 1954 revealed an increased risk of psychiatric problems among those exposed to intrauterine DES. The subject is well reviewed by Goldstein *et al.*[4] who conclude their review by pointing out that despite the existence of a vast body of literature describing the failures of diethylstilbestrol, one non-randomized study, using historical controls, asserted that 'diethylstilbestrol was efficacious in improving pregnancy outcome when initiated in the early stages of high-risk pregnancies'[19].

HUMAN CHORIONIC GONADOTROPHIN

Human chorionic gonadodotrophin (hCG) continues to be prescribed in order to prevent miscarriage in women with a history of recurrent miscarriage. It is not currently used to prevent miscarriage in women presenting with threatened miscarriage.

The author has recently had the opportunity to review the available evidence from the known controlled trials of hCG used in this circumstance for the *Cochrane Database of Systematic Review* and the following section is reproduced by kind permission of the Cochrane Database of Systematic Reviews[20].

BACKGROUND

hCG is known to play a vital part in the establishment of pregnancy, although its precise

Table 11.1 Effect of diethylstilbestrol in pregnancy on miscarriage

Study	Experimental		Control		Odds ratio (95% CI)	Graph of odds ratios and confidence intervals
	n	(%)	n	(%)		0.01 0.1 0.5 1 2 10 100
Dieckmann et al. (1953)	34/840	(4.05)	17/806	(2.11)	1.19 (1.09–3.33)	
Medical Research Council (1955)	6/76	(7.89)	6/71	(8.45)	0.93 (0.29–3.02)	
Berle and Behnke (1977)	55/134	(41.04)	52/131	(39.69)	1.06 (0.65–1.73)	
Robinson and Shettles (1952)	6/51	(11.76)	10/42	(23.81)	0.43 (0.15–1.27)	
Ferguson (1953)	6/190	(3.16)	5/203	(2.46)	1.29 (0.39–4.27)	
Crowder et al. (1950)	31/63	(49.21)	16/37	(43.24)	1.27 (0.56–2.85)	
Typical odds ratio (95% confidence interval)					1.20 (0.89–1.62)	

Reproduced from Goldstein et al. [4] with permission of Oxford University Press.

role is still uncertain. Early uncontrolled series of patients treated with hCG in order to prevent miscarriage suggested that hCG was likely to offer hope to women with a history of repeated unexplained miscarriage. An association between recurrent spontaneous miscarriage (RSM) and follicular phase hormonal aberration has been postulated by several authors[21–23]. Also recent research supports a specific association between recurrent spontaneous miscarriage and polycystic ovaries[23–25], although some authors feel that more recent work has cast doubt on the importance of this work[26]. Quenby and Farquharson[27] found that oligomenorrhea was 10 times more important than any other identifiable risk factor in predicting a failed pregnancy in women with RSM. They did not, however, find any abnormality of luteinizing hormone in women with recurrent pregnancy loss and oligomenorrhea.

The objectives of this review were to assess the effect of hCG administration during early pregnancy on the risk of miscarriage in women with a history of recurrent spontaneous miscarriage, and further to investigate the effect of hCG on the risk of miscarriage in women with recurrent miscarriage who also had oligomenorrhea[20]. All trials which attempted to assess the effect of hCG on the risk of miscarriage when given to women with a history of recurrent miscarriage were considered for inclusion in this review.

The participants were women with a diagnosis of recurrent spontaneous miscarriage (alia recurrent miscarriage; recurrent abortion). In all the studies considered for inclusion the minimum number of previous miscarriages was two. The primary outcome measure was miscarriage. Some authors compared later pregnancy outcome.

Published and unpublished randomized and quasi-randomized comparisons of alternative forms of care given in pregnancy and childbirth were identified by a combination of systematic electronic search, systematic handsearch of selected journals, and informal discovery by a variety of methods including ad hoc reading, discussion, correspondence, conference abstracts and proceedings and reference lists of relevant papers.

One trial was excluded from the analysis: Pearce and Hamid (1994). This study was reported in the *British Journal of Obstetrics and Gynaecology* in August 1994. Since its publication evidence has come to light which casts serious doubt on the verity of the report. The *British Journal of Obstetrics and Gynaecology* has since withdrawn publication status from this paper (January 1995). Current evidence suggests that the trial did not actually take place (Chamberlain personal communication).

Trials included in this meta-analysis were Svigos (1982)[28], Harrison (1985)[29], Harrison (1992)[30] and Quenby and Farquharson (1994)[26]. No unpublished trials have been included in this review.

The methodological quality of these trials is variable. The method of randomization is not detailed in any of the first three trials. There were exclusions after randomization in Svigos' study. All four trials used a placebo preparation.

RESULTS

The data suggest that hCG may have a beneficial effect on the risk of miscarriage for all women with a history of recurrent miscarriage. This evidence should be interpreted with great caution. However, the apparent effect is greatly influenced by the two earliest studies (Svigos 1982[28] and Harrison 1985[29]), both of which had important methodological weaknesses.

The effect of hCG on the risk of miscarriage in specific populations of women who suffer recurrent spontaneous miscarriage appears to be substantial. The study by Quenby and Farquharson (1994)[26] provides evidence that women with a history of recurrent spontaneous miscarriage who have oligomenorrheic cycles have a reduced risk of miscarriage if treated with hCG. However, this evidence derives from comparison of very small numbers of patients with this particular clinical profile (11 of 13 pregnancies successful with hCG vs 4 of 10 pregnancies successful with placebo preparation).

In the two earlier and methodologically weaker studies (Svigos, 1982[28] and Harrison, 1984[29]) the protection from miscarriage derived from hCG is apparently greater than in the two later and methodologically stronger studies (Harrison, 1992[30] and Quenby and Farquharson, 1994[26]). Also in the two earlier studies the confidence limits do not approach unity whereas in the two latter studies the confidence limits both cross zero.

IMPLICATIONS FOR PRACTICE

There is insufficient evidence concerning the effectiveness of hCG when used to prevent miscarriage during pregnancy for women with a history of unexplained recurrent spontaneous miscarriage. There is evidence, however, that hCG may have a beneficial effect in this population of women who also have oligomenorrhea. However, the numbers involved in the one study which revealed this effect were small (total 21 patients).

PROGESTOGENS

No one disputes the crucial role that progesterone plays in the maintenance of pregnancy. Whether this is by the inhibition of oxytocin induced myometrial activity[31,32] or through inhibition of prostaglandin excitation[33,34] is less clear. Undoubtedly progesterone levels fall in association with a failing or failed pregnancy whether this is intrauterine or extra-uterine[35].

Progestogens have been prescribed for over 30 years by clinicians all over the world in the belief that they reduce the risk of pregnancy failures – in particular first trimester miscarriage. A large number of studies have been undertaken, many of which were uncontrolled. Perhaps because of this, opinions

concerning the efficacy of progestogen therapy have remained divided. In an attempt to derive an accurate assessment of the value of progestogens, a number of meta-analytical reviews have been undertaken.

In 1989 Goldstein *et al.*[36] published a meta-analysis of randomized controlled trials of progestational agents in pregnancy. In order to reduce the number of confounding variables the authors confined their review to papers fulfilling the following criteria.

1. All study patients must be considered to be in high risk pregnancies.
2. The study report must state that patients were randomly or quasi-randomly allocated to the treatment or control study group.
3. The study group patients received progesterone or progestogen.
4. The paper must provide data on outcome of pregnancy including livebirths and miscarriage or stillbirth or neonatal death.

After an exhaustive search of the literature Goldstein *et al.*[36] found 31 randomized controlled trials (RCTs), 33 non-RCTs, 36 reviews/editorials, 60 follow-up studies and 16 other miscellaneous papers. The actual meta-analysis was undertaken on 15 RCTs and subanalyses were performed on smaller numbers of studies according to eligibility. Tables 11.2 and 11.3 reveal the characteristics and results of the various comparisons which were undertaken.

Examination of Table 11.3 reveals that the odds ratios for miscarriage vs liveborn babies is 0.97 (95% CI 0.65–1.44) suggesting that there is no benefit to the use of progestogens in this circumstance but not excluding the possibility of either benefit or detriment. As the authors point out in their discussion, this reflects precisely the spectrum of opinion in medical textbooks with some authors advocating the use of progestogens, some considering its use inappropriate and yet others remaining equivocal in their advice.

In the same publication another meta-analytical review of the use of progestogens

Table 11.2 Studies included in the meta-analysis, listed in decreasing order of quality score. In all instances the control patients received no hormonal therapy

Study	Randomization blinded	Placebo	Regimen	Dosage	Gestation at start of therapy (weeks)
Johnson et al. (1975)	Yes	Yes	17-OH-PC[a]	250 mg/week	16.7 ± 4.4
Papiernik-Berkhauer (1970)	Unknown	Yes	OHPC[b]	Unknown	Unknown
Hartikainen-Sorri et al. (1980)	Unknown	Yes	17-OH-PC	250 mg/week	29.2 ± 1.9
Sondergaard et al. (1985)	Unknown	Yes	Progest[c]	200 mg/day	<11
Yemini et al. (1985)	No	Yes	17-OH-PC	250 mg/week	12.2 ± 3.3
Klopper and MacNaughton (1965)	Yes	Yes	EL[d]	100 mg/day	<10
Hauth et al. (1983)	Unknown	Yes	17-OH-PC	100 mg/week	16–20
Fuchs and Stakemann (1966)	No	Yes	Progest	Schedule	21–36
Le Vine (1964)	No	Yes	17-OH-PC	500 mg/week	<17
Dalton (1962)	No	No	Progest	Schedule	16–28
Goldzieher (1964)	Yes	Yes	MAP[e]	10 mg/day	<18
Brenner and Hendricks (1962)	Unknown	Yes	MAP	80 mg/day	36–38
Moller and Fuchs (1965)	No	Yes	MAP	Schedule	8–21+
Swyer and Daley (1953)	No + unknown	No	Progest	150-mg implant	<11
Tognoni et al. (1980)	Unknown	Yes	OHPC/AE[f]	OHPC–25 mg/day AE–10 mg/day	<15

[a]17-OH-PC = 17-alpha-hydroxyprogesterone caproate.
[b]OHPC = hydroxyprogesterone caproate.
[c]Progest = Progesterone.
[d]EL = Enol Luteovis (Vister), a cyclopentyl enol ether of progesterone.
[e]MAP = 6-alpha-17-alpha-acetoprogesterone (medroxyprogesterone acetate).
[f]AE = Allyloestrenol (a progestogen of the 19-nortestosterone series without androgenic properties).

Table 11.3 Pooled odd ratios of 15 randomized control trials using a progestogen for the maintenance of pregnancy

Analysis	No. of studies[a]	χ^{2d}	Odds ratio	(95% CI on odds ratio)
Neg[b] vs Live[c]	15	0.86	0.88	(0.66–1.15)
MIS vs Live	14	0.0027	0.97	(0.65–1.44)
SB vs Live	13	1.47	0.50	(0.2–1.28)
NND vs Live	7	1.41	2.37	(0.75–7.4)
MIS vs Term	8	0.76	0.75	(0.42–1.31)
SB vs Term	8	1.34	0.44	(0.15–1.34)
NND vs Term	6	0.51	1.89	(0.56–6.35)
PD vs Term	10	3.05	0.71	(0.49–1.02)

[a]Studies were included only in those analyses for which they provided data, either directly or indirectly.
[b]Negative, the sum of all miscarriages, stillbirths and neonatal deaths.
[c]Live, the sum of all preterm and term deliveries.
[d]$P > 0.05$.

was published by Daya[37]. In this review Daya confined his examination to studies where progestogens were used in controlled trials for women with recurrent miscarriage. The results of Daya's meta-analysis of three studies (Swyer and Daley, 1953[38], Goldzeiher, 1964[39] and LeVine, 1964[40]) are shown in Table 11.4.

Daya's criteria for inclusion were as follows.

1. Patients were allocated to treatment or control groups on a random or quasi-random basis.
2. Treatment with progesterone (or progestogen) was started in the first trimester.
3. The control group received placebo.
4. Women recruited to the studies had three or more previous consecutive miscarriages.

A third meta analytical review was published one year later by Keirse[41]. He argued that there are large differences among the many agents considered to be progestational. He, therefore, conducted another more restricted meta-analysis using data from all placebo-controlled studies which involved the prophylactic use of a single progestogen agent, i.e. 17 α-hydroxyprogesterone caproate. Only four of the seven eligible studies provided data concerning miscarriage: (Shearman, 1968[42], Yemini *et al.*, 1985[43], LeVine *et al.*, 1964[40] and Johnson *et al.*, 1975[44]).

Table 11.5 reveals the odds ratios of the individual trials and the summary or 'typical' odds ratio of 1.30 (95% CI 0.61–12.74).

This review concluded that 'there is currently no evidence from controlled trials to justify the clinical use of any progestational agent to prevent miscarriage'.

In order to keep abreast of the continued publication of randomized controlled trials in pregnancy and childbirth, Chalmers *et al.* have produced several electronic databases and reviews of RCTs. The first of these was the Oxford Database of Perinatal Trials[45] which has become the Cochrane Pregnancy and Childbirth Database[46]. Currently the reviews in these two publications are being updated to accommodate the format of the Cochrane Database of Systematic Reviews (CDSR)[47]. This latter database encompasses reviews from all branches of medicine and allied health professions and has already had its first disk issue. The task of creating such reviews and databases is a daunting one and the interested reader is referred to Chalmers *et al.*[48,49] and Chalmers and Soll[50].

The following review summaries have been abstracted from the Cochrane Pregnancy and Childbirth Database (1995) which were originally prepared by Keirse and updated by Prendiville[51].

Table 11.4 Effect of progesterone treatment on continuing pregnancy rate

No. Trial	Progestogen	Continuing pregnancy rate		Treatment effect[a] (%)	(95% CI on treatment effect)	P[b]	Odds ratio	(95% CI on odds ratio)
		Treatment	Control					
1 Sywer and Daley [38]	MPA	21/27 (77.8%)	11/20 (55.0%)	22.8	(8.1–49.3)	0.10	2.86	(0.69–12.37)
2 Goldzieher [39]	17-OHP-C	6/8 (75.0%)	6/10 (60.0%)	15.0	(−36.4–51.3)	0.51	2.00	(0.18–25.01)
3 Le Vine [40]	PP	12/15 (80.0%)	7/15 (46.7%)	33.3	(−7.7–61.4)	0.06	4.57	(0.72–32.52)
Overall odds ratio[c]							3.09	(1.28–7.42)

[a]Treatment effect is the difference in proportions of successful pregnancy between treatment and control groups. MPA, Medroxyprogesterone acetate; 17-OHP-C, 17-hydroxyprogesterone caproate; PP, progesterone pellet implants.
[b]χ^2 test on 1 d.f.
[c]Overall test of association using Mantel–Haenszel χ^2 test on 1 d.f. = 6.20 ($P < 0.01$).
Reproduced from Daya [37] with kind permission of the *British Journal of Obstetrics and Gynaecology*.

Table 11.5 Effects of 17 alpha-hydroxyprogesterone caproate administration in pregnancy on various pregnancy outcomes

Pregnancy outcome and study	17alpha-hydroxy progesterone	Placebo	Odds ratio (95% CI)
Miscarriage			
Searman (1968)	5/27	5/23	0–82 (0.21–3.25)
Yemini *et al.* (1985)	8/39	3/40	2.92 (0.82–10.36)
Le Vine (1964)	3/15	7/15	0.31 (0.07–1.39)
Johnson *et al.* (1975)	3/23	0/27	9.64 (0.95–97.98)
Typical odds ratio			1.30 (0.61–2.74)

From Keirse *et al.* [51] Reproduced with kind permission of Oxford University Press.

1. Progestogens in pregnancy[52]: This review attempted to assess the effects of progestogen administration (various agents) in pregnancy on the adverse pregnancy outcomes or miscarriage, stillbirth, neonatal death and prematurity. In the 25 studies included in this review 1700 women were recruited and systematically assigned to a progestational agent or placebo. Despite this, no clear answer is evident. Table 11.6 details the results of the overview which compared the effect of progestogens on miscarriage in 14 trials where data were available. The typical odds ratio of 1.07 and the confidence limits (0.78–1.47) suggest no benefit but are compatible with either a beneficial or detrimental effect.

2. Progestogens to prevent miscarriage and preterm birth[52,53]: This review differs from the preceding one in that it included only those trials which reported on the prophylactic use of progestogens (i.e. in

Table 11.6 Progestogens in pregnancy: outcome, miscarriage

Study identifier	Treatment Obs/Total	Control Obs/Total	Weight %	Log odds ratio (99% CI)	
Berle+ 1977	55/134	52/131	24.2		1.06 (0.56–2.01)
Berle+ 1980	58/154	46/146	25.8		1.31 (0.70–2.45)
Gerhard+ 1987	3/26	5/26	2.6		0.56 (0.08–3.98)
Goldzieher [39]	5/23	5/31	3.0		1.44 (0.24–8.78)
Johnson+ [44]	0/18	4/25	1.3		0.16 (0.01–2.36)
Klopper+ 1965	8/18	5/15	3.0		1.57 (0.26–9.64)
Le Vine 1964	3/15	7/14	2.5		0.28 (0.04–2.01)
Medical R. 1955	6/76	6/71	4.2		0.93 (0.20–4.37)
Shearman [42]	5/27	5/23	3.0		0.82 (0.13–5.01)
Sonderga.+ 1985	17/23	17/19	2.4		0.37 (0.05–2.78)
Souka 1980	17/25	14/25	4.5		1.65 (0.37–7.28)
Swyer [38]	11/60	13/53	7.2		0.69 (0.21–2.26)
Tognoni [56]	26/71	21/68	11.8		1.29 (0.51–3.24)
Yemini [43]	8/39	3/40	3.6		2.92 (0.55–15.42)
Totals	222/709	203/687			1/07 (0.78–1.47)

Between trial test for heterogeneity: Chi square (df = 13) = 14.49.
From *The Cochrane Pregnancy and Childbirth Database (1995, Issue 1).*

asymptomatic women). Again, no demonstrable benefit is revealed by these studies in terms of the risk of miscarriage. Table 11.7 reveals an odds ratio of 1.06 with confidence intervals of 0.53–2.13. This suggests that progestogens could either have a beneficial or detrimental effect but that neither is revealed by these studies when analysed meta-analytically.

3. Progestogen/estrogen prophylaxis in early normal pregnancy[54]: Only one randomized controlled trial has been found which compared a combination preparation of estradiol and 17 α-hydroxyprogesterone acetate[55]. This was administered on days 13 and 15 postembryo transfer in 120 normal pregnancies after *in vitro* fertilization. Patients were allocated to placebo or drug group by date of birth rather than randomly. Tables 11.8 and 11.9 suggest that this combination therapy reduces the risk of miscarriage in preclinical or 'biochemical' pregnancies but not in pregnancies between 7 and 12 weeks' gestation. This study should be repeated elsewhere using truly random allocation and with follow-up data concerning the risk of preterm delivery, stillbirths and neonatal deaths.

DISCUSSION

The difficulty in arriving at even a consensus view concerning the usefulness of progestogens to prevent miscarriage does not result from a paucity of experimentation. There have been numerous controlled and uncontrolled trials of progestogens in early pregnancy to prevent miscarriage. Several variables have confounded a summary analysis:

- Progestogens encompass a wide range of synthetic progesterone-like hormones.
- Progestogens have been studied in a large number of trials but using different entry criteria, different doses and different routes of administration.
- Most of the published (and unpublished) work was undertaken before it was possible to confirm a viable pregnancy using ultrasonography and endocrinological assay. As a result of this it is possible that progestogens do actually confer some protection from miscarriage but that this protection has not been revealed by these studies and reviews. This may be in part because several women with non-viable fetuses were recruited to these studies.

As referred to earlier the reason clinicians prescribe progestogens in pregnancy is because progesterone is necessary to support pregnancy. It may reasonably be supposed that a luteal phase (or later) deficiency in the production of progesterone may lead to a miscarriage. If, however, such progesterone deficiency is a result rather than a cause of miscarriage then it is plain that progesterone or

Table 11.7 Progestogens to prevent miscarriage and preterm birth: outcome, miscarriage

Study identifier	Treatment Obs/Total	Control Obs/Total	Weight %	Log odds ratio (99% CI)
Goldzieher [39]	5/23	5/31	14.8	1.44 (0.24–8.78)
Johnson+ [44]	3/23	0/27	5.2	9.64 (0.46–202.98)
Le Vine [40]	3/15	7/15	12.6	0.31 (0.04–2.23)
Shearman [42]	5/27	5/23	14.8	0.82 (0.13–5.01)
Swyer [38]	11/60	13/53	34.8	0.69 (0.21–2.26)
Yemini [43]	8/39	3/40	17.5	2.92 (0.55–15.42)
Totals	35/187	33/189		1.06 (0.53–2.13)

Between trial test for heterogeneity: Chi square (df = 5) = 9.69.
From *The Cochrane Pregnancy and Childbirth Database (1995, Issue 1).*

Table 11.8 Progestogen/estrogen prophylaxis in early normal pregnancy (preclinical pregnancies)

Study identifier	Treatment Obs/Total	Control Obs/Total	Log odds ratio (99% CI)	
Prietl+ 1992 [55]	1/54	17/64	— · —	0.15 (0.04–0.56)
Totals	1/54	17/64	—■—	0.15 (0.04–0.56)

From *The Cochrane Pregnancy and Childbirth Database* (1995).

Table 11.9 Progestogen/estrogen prophylaxis in early normal pregnancy (7–12 weeks' gestation)

Study identifier	Treatment Obs/Total	Control Obs/Total	Log odds ratio (99% CI)	
Prietl+ 1992 [55]	5/54	9/64	— · —	0.63 (0.15–2.75)
Totals	5/54	9/64	—■—	0.63 (0.15–2.75)

From *The Cochrane Pregnancy and Childbirth Database* (1995).

progestogen administration will not effect the *fait accompli* outcome.

CONCLUSION

Of all the drugs prescribed during pregnancy in order to prevent miscarriage progestogens are the most widely used. Their popularity varies between countries and between individual clinicians[56].

Everett *et al.*[57] reported that nearly 17% of general practitioners used progestogens in order to prevent miscarriage. Is such widespread use of progestogens justified? There is not good evidence to support their use in order to prevent miscarriage.

What useful advice can be derived from these reviews? Some clear statements can reasonably be made.

- The available evidence does not justify the continued use of progestogens, hCG or estrogens in clinical practice in early pregnancy outside the context of appropriately sized randomized controlled trials.
- The available evidence does not conclusively rule out benefit from the use of progestogens in early pregnancy.
- Most of the studies were too small to rule out or reveal a clinically important benefit.
- These studies were undertaken when ultrasonography was not sufficiently sensitive in very early pregnancy to be able to recognize a fetal heart. Thus any possible benefit of progestogens could have been missed.
- In none of these studies was an abnormally low serum progesterone demonstrated before recruitment to the study.

IMPLICATIONS FOR RESEARCH

There is an urgent need for a large randomized controlled trial of hCG in women who have oligomenorrhea and recurrent spontaneous miscarriage (RSM). In addition, because it is reasonable to hypothesize that this effect may extend to women with oligomenorrhea without RSM, there is a need for a randomized controlled trial of the use of hCG to prevent miscarriage in women with oligomenorrhea who have not yet suffered RSM.

REFERENCES

1. Allen, M.W., Butenandt, A., Corner, G.W. and Slotta, K.H. (1935) Zur Nomenklatur des Corpus luteumhormons. *Klin. Wochenschr.*, **14**, 1182.
2. Csapo, A.L., Pulkinen, M.O. and Weist, W.G. (1973) Effects of lutectomy and progesterone replacement therapy in early pregnancy patients. *Am. J. Obstet. Gynecol.*, **115**, 759–65.
3. Daya, S., Ward, S. and Burrows, E. (1988) Progesterone profiles in luteal phase defect cycles and outcome of progesterone treatment in patients with recurrent spontaneous abortion. *Am. J. Obstet. Gynecol.*, **158**, 225–32.
4. Goldstein, P.A., Sacks, H.S. and Chalmers, T. (1989) Hormone administration for the maintenance of pregnancy, in *Effective Care in Pregnancy and Childbirth* (eds I. Chalmers, M. Enkin and M. Keirse), Oxford University Press, Oxford, pp. 612–23.
5. Smith, O.W. and Smith, G.V.S. (1944) Pituitary stimulating property of stilbestrol as compared with that of esterone. *Proc. Soc. Exp. Biol. Med.*, **57**, 198–200.
6. Gitman, L. and Koplowitz, A. (1950) Use of diethylstilbestrol in complications of pregnancy. *N.Y. State J. Med.*, **50**, 2823–4.
7. Davis, M.E. and Fugo, N.W. (1950) Steroids in the treatment of early pregnancy complications. *JAMA*, **142**, 778–85.
8. Ross, J.W. (1953) Further report on the use of diethylstilbestrol in the treatment of threatened abortion. *J. Natl. Med. Assoc.*, **45**, 223.
9. Pena, E.F. (1954) Prevention of abortion. *Am. J. Surg.*, **87**, 95–6.
10. White, P., Koshy, P. and Duckers, J. (1953) The management of pregnancy complicating diabetes and of children of diabetic mothers. *Med. Clin. North Am.*, **37**, 1481–96.
11. Dieckmann, W.J., Davis, M.E., Rynkiewicz, L.M. and Pottinger, R.E. (1953) Does the administration of diethylstilbestrol during pregnancy have therapeutic value? *Am. J. Obstet. Gynecol.*, **66**, 1062–75.
12. Herbst, A.L. and Scully, R.E. (1970) Adenocarcinoma of the vagina in adolescence: a report of 7 cases including 6 clear-cell carcinomas (so called mesonephromas). *Cancer*, **25**, 745–57.
13. Herbst, A.L., Ulfelder, H. and Poskanzer, D.C. (1971) Adenocarcinoma of the vagina: association of maternal stilbestrol therapy with tumor appearance in young women. *N. Engl. J. Med.*, **284**, 878–81.
14. Greenwald, P., Barlow, J.J., Nasca, P.C. and Burnett, W.S. (1971) Vaginal cancer after maternal treatment with synthetic estrogens. *N. Engl. J. Med.*, **285**, 390–2.
15. Bibbo, M., Gill, W.B., Azizi, F. *et al.* (1977) Follow-up study of male and female offspring of DES-exposed mothers. *Obstet. Gynecol.*, **49**, 1–8.
16. Senekjian, E.K., Potjul, R.K., Frey, K. and Herbst, A.L. (1988) Infertility among daughters either exposed or not exposed to diethylstilbestrol. *Am. J. Obstet. Gynecol.*, **158**, 493–8.
17. Herbst, A.L., Hubby, M.M., Blough, R.R. and Azizi, F. (1980) A comparison of pregnancy experience in DES-exposed and DES-unexposed daughters. *J. Reprod. Med.*, **24**, 62–9.
18. Swyer, G.I.M. and Law, R.G. (1954) An evaluation of the prophylactic ante-natal use of stilbestrol: preliminary report. *J. Endocrinol.*, **10**, 6–7.
19. Horne, H.W. (1985) Evidence of improved pregnancy outcome with diethylstilbestrol (DES) treatment of women with previous pregnancy failures. A retrospective analysis. *Chron. Dis.*, **38**, 873–80.
20. Prendiville, W.G. (1995) hCG for recurrent miscarriage (revised 18 July 1995), in *Pregnancy and Childbirth Module* (eds M.W. Enkin *et al.*). The Cochrane Database of Systematic Reviews (database on disk and CDROM). The Cochrane Collaboration; Issue 2, Oxford: Update Software; 1995. Available from BMJ Publishing Group, London.
21. Johnson, P. and Pearce, J.M. (1990) Recurrent spontaneous abortion and polycystic ovarian disease: comparison of two regimes to induce ovulation. *Br. Med. J.*, **300**, 154–6.
22. Hamilton-Fairley, D., Kiddy, D., Watson Sagle, H. and Franks, S. (1991) Low dose-gonadotrophin therapy for induction of ovulation in 100 women with PCOS. *Hum. Rep.*, **6**, 1095–9.
23. Regan, L. (1991) Recurrent miscarriage. *Br. Med. J.*, **302**, 542–4.
24. Pearce, J.M. and Leigh, A.J. (1993) Luteinising hormone hyoersecretation. *Contemp. Rev. Obstet. Gynaecol.*, **5**, 142–51.
25. Sagle, M., Bishop, K., Ridley, N. *et al.* (1988) Recurrent early miscarriage and polycystit ovaries. *Br. Med. J.*, **297**, 1027–8.
26. Quenby, S. and Farquharson, R.G. (1994) hCG supplementation in recurring pregnancy loss: a controlled trial. *Fertil. Steril.*, **62**, 708–10.
27. Quenby, S. and Farquharson, R.G. (1993)

Predicting recurring miscarriage: what is important? *Obstet. Gynecol.*, **82**, 132–8.

28. Svigos, J. (1982) Preliminary experience with the use of human chorionic gonadotrophin therapy in women with repeated abortion. *Clin. Reprod. Fertil.*, **1**, 131–5.

29. Harrison, R.F. (1985) Treatment of habitual abortion with human chorionic gonadotrophin: results of open and placebo-controlled studies. *Eur. J. Obstet. Gynecol. Reprod. Biol.*, **20**, 159–68.

30. Harrison, R.F. (1992) Human chorionic gonadotrophin (hCG) in the management of recurrent abortion; results of a multi-centre placebo-controlled study. *Eur. J. Obstet. Gynecol. Reprod. Biol.*, **47**, 175–9.

31. Fuchs, F. and Fuchs, A.R. (1958) Induction and inhibition of labour in the rabbit. *Acta Endocrinol.*, **29**, 615–24.

32. Csapo, A.L., Pulkinen, M.O., Ruttner, B. *et al.* (1972) The significance of the human corpus luteum in pregnancy maintenance. *Am. J. Obstet. Gynecol.*, **112**, 1061–7.

33. Csapo, A.I., Henzl, M.R., Kaihola, H.L. *et al.* (1974) Suppression of uterine activity and abortion by inhibition of prostaglandinsynthesis. *Prostaglandins*, **7**, 39–47.

34. Csapo, A.I. (1976) Effects of progesterone, prostaglandin F and its analogue ICI 81008 on the excitability and threshold of the uterus. *Am. J. Obstet. Gynecol.*, **124**, 367–78.

35. Al-Sebal, M.A.H., Kingsland, C.R., Diver, M. *et al.* (1995) The role of a single progesterone measurement in the diagnosis of early pregnancy failure and the prognosis of fetal viability. *Br. J. Obstet. Gynaecol.*, **102**, 364–9.

36. Goldstein, P., Berrier, J., Rosen, S. *et al.* (1989) A meta-analysis of randomized control trials of progestational agents in pregnancy. *Br. J. Obstet. Gynaecol.*, **96**, 265–74.

37. Daya, S. (1989) Efficacy of progesterone support for pregnancy in women with recurrent miscarriage. A meta-analysis of controlled trials. *Br. J. Obstet. Gynaecol.*, **96**, 275–80.

38. Swyer, G.I.M. and Daley, D. (1953) Progesterone implantation in habitual abortion. *B. Med. J.*, **i**, 1073–7.

39. Goldzeiher, J.W. (1964) Double-blind trial of a progestin in habitual abortion. *JAMA*, **188**, 651–4.

40. LeVine, L. (1964) Habitual abortion. A controlled study of progestational therapy. *West. J. Surg. Obstet. Gynecol.*, **72**, 30–6.

41. Keirse, M.J.N.C. (1990) Progestogen administration in pregnancy may prevent preterm delivery. *Br. J. Obstet. Gynaecol.*, **97**, 149–54.

42. Shearman, R.P. (1968) Hormonal treatment of habitual abortion, in *Progress in Infertility* (eds S.J. Behrman and R.W. Kistner), J. & A. Churchill, London, pp. 767–77.

43. Yemini, M., Borenstein, R., Dreazen, E. *et al.* (1985) Prevention of premature labour by 17 alpha hydroxyprogesterone-caproate. *Am. J. Obstet. Gynecol.*, **151**, 5474–7.

44. Johnson, J.W.C., Austin, K.L., Jones, G.S. *et al.* (1975) Efficacy of 17 alpha hydroxyprogesterone caproate in the prevention of premature labour. *N. Engl. J. Med.*, **293**, 675–80.

45. Chalmers. I. (ed.) (1988) *The Oxford Database of Perinatal Trials*, Oxford University Press, Oxford.

46. *Cochrane Pregnancy and Childbirth Database* (1995) Update Software, Oxford OX2 7YX.

47. *Cochrane Database of Systematic Reviews* (1997) The Cochrane Library. Update Software, P.O. Box 696, Oxford OX2 7YX, UK.

48. Chalmers, I., Hetherington, J., Elbourne, D. *et al.* (1989) Materials and methods used in synthesising evidence to evaluate the effects of care during pregnancy and childbirth, in *Effective Care in Pregnancy and Childbirth* (eds I. Chalmers, M. Enkin and M.J.N.C. Keirse), Oxford University Press, Oxford, pp. 39-65.

49. Chalmers, I., Enkin, M. and Keirse, M.J.N.C. (1993) Establishing systems for creating and updating overviews of controlled trials of health care. *Milbank Q.*, **71**, 411–37.

50. Chalmers, I. and Soll, R. (1991) Progress and problems in establishing an International Registry of Perinatal Trials. *Controlled Clin. Trials*, **12**, 630.

51. Keirse, M.J.N.C. (1990) Progestogen in pregnancy may prevent pre-term delivery. *Br. J. Obstet. Gynaecol.*, **97**, 149–54.

52. Prendiville, W.J. (1993) Progestogens in pregnancy. *The Cochrane Pregnancy and Childbirth Database*, Issue I, 1995.

53. Prendiville, W.J. (1993) Progestogens to prevent miscarriage and pre-term birth, in *Oxford Database of Perinatal Trials* (ed. I. Chalmers), version 1.3, disc issue 7, record 4398.

54. Prendiville, W.J. (1995) Progestogen/estrogen prophylaxes in early normal pregnancy. *Cochrane Pregnancy and Childbirth Database*, Issue I.

55. Prietl, G., Diedrich, K., Van der Ven, H.H.,

Luckhaus, J. and Krebs, D. (1992) The effect of 17 alpha-hydroxyprogesterone caproate/estradiol valerate on the development and outcome of early pregnancies following in vitro fertilisation and embryo transfer: a prospective and randomised controlled trial. *Hum. Reprod.*, **7**, 1–5.

56. Tognoni, G., Ferrario, L., Inzalco, M. and Grosignani, P.G. (1980) Progestogens in threatened abortion. *Lancet*, **ii**, 1242–3.

57. Everett, C., Ashurst, H. and Chalmers, I. (1987) Reported management of threatened miscarriage by general practitioners in Wessex. *Br. Med. J.*, **295**, 583–6.

12

PSYCHOLOGICAL ASPECTS OF MISCARRIAGE IN EARLY PREGNANCY AND THEIR IMPLICATIONS FOR ANTENATAL CARE

H.M. McGee and S. Daly

INTRODUCTION

The focus on psychological issues associated with loss early in pregnancy has developed only very recently. A significant literature is available on psychological factors and induced abortion, much of it relating to early pregnancy. This is not addressed here because of the different psychological and social context of therapeutic abortion. Interested readers are referred to recent reviews[1–3]. Concern with spontaneous abortion (miscarriage) has evolved from an initial focus on the psychological aspects of stillbirth and perinatal events.

Miscarriage is a relatively common event with estimates of 10–20% of all pregnancies ending in miscarriage, mainly first trimester miscarriage[4]. However, early miscarriage has often been considered a non-event with regard to the significance of the loss. This in part may relate to the fact that miscarriage early in pregnancy is often a 'hidden grief'[5] since many people in the woman's social circle may not be aware of the pregnancy and also because of beliefs regarding the need for attachment to a 'palpable' object before the experience of separation and loss can be achieved. However, considerable distress has been documented in samples of first trimester miscarriages[6].

A range of studies have directly assessed psychological functioning in women following early miscarriage. Most of the available studies have been reviewed[7]. Details of larger studies which incorporate a concurrent (as distinct from a retrospective) research design are presented in Table 12.1.

Overall, depression is evident in one-fifth to one-half of the women in the various studies. Depression appears to diminish significantly over time from the miscarriage with evidence that anxiety fluctuates more and is more likely to be evident some time after the event than is depression. Psychological experiences other than depression and anxiety, e.g. guilt, have been studied less often. An early retrospective study found that 22% of 32 women experienced guilt for many months after the event[16]. Other studies have documented guilt levels of 18% ($n = 82$)[14] and 71% ($n = 32$)[6]; in the latter study 25% reported extreme guilt following miscarriage. These less well-documented emotions should nonetheless be considered in the clinical setting as they may have a significant bearing on the management of the individual patient. Furthermore, it may be that the focus should shift from a view of miscarriage as a once-off loss event (i.e. loss of the pregnancy and its attendant emotions) to a conceptualization of miscarriage as a first step

Clinical Management of Early Pregnancy. Edited by Walter Prendiville and James R. Scott.
Published in 1999 by Arnold, ISBN 0 340 74100 7

Table 12.1 Psychological consequences of early miscarriage: summary of larger studies using concurrent assessment of emotional functioning

Study	n	Interview time	Measure	Outcome
Friedman and Gath (1988) [8]	67	4 weeks	Present state examination Beck Depression Inventory	Psychiatric cases (48%) Significant depression (22%)
Garel et al. (1992) [9]	144 98	Immediate (T_1) 3 months (T_2)	DSM III criteria	Intense depression (43%) Major depression (51%)
Prettyman et al. (1993) [10]	65	1 week (T_1) 6 weeks (T_2) 12 weeks (T_3)	Hospital Anxiety and Depression Scale (HAD)	Depressed (22%) Anxious (41%) Depressed (8%) Anxious (18%) Depressed (8%) Anxious (32%)
Thapar and Thapar (1992) [11]	60	1 day (T_1) 6 weeks (T_2)	GHQ-28 Hospital Anxiety and Depression Scale	6 (median) Depressed (9%) Anxious (5%) 10 (median) Depressed (9%) Anxious (4%)
Cecil and Leslie (1993) [12]	48 26	Hospital (T_1) Varied (T_2)	State-Trait Anxiety Inventory (State results given)	Mean = 47.6 Mean = 39.0
Neugebauer et al. (1992) [13]	232	2 weeks (T_1) 6 weeks (T_2) 6 months (T_3)	Center for Epidemiological Studies – Depression (score >30)	Depression (36%) Depression (12%) Depression (10%)
Seibel and Graves (1980) [14]	93	Following dilatation and curettage	Multi-attribute Adjustment Checklist (MAACL)	Depressed (54%) Anxious (51%)
Hamilton (1989) [15]	42	Hospital (T_1)	Symptom list	Tearfulness (93%) Irritability (57%)

in a process in which a range of issues for the future need to be addressed. These issues include dealing with returning menstruation and with decisions about pregnancy in the future.

A NEW TECHNOLOGICAL AND SOCIAL CONTEXT

A range of social and technological changes in recent decades creates an environment which may influence the experience of miscarriage. Family size has decreased throughout the western world and many women now delay pregnancy to later in life. The occasion of pregnancy may thus be one that is now more often planned and contemplated in advance. With regard to technology, services such as early fetal scanning by ultrasonography now allow the woman to have visible evidence of her pregnancy some time before she can feel movement. These services may also make the pregnancy more accessible to men earlier in the process. Alongside this, there has developed a significant momentum to acknowledge pregnancy loss in general, including in early pregnancy, in a more public form than previously. Layne[17] describes campaigns for 'legitimizing' the loss of pregnancy in the US with issues ranging from bereavement leave from work to separation rites and artefacts. She describes this increasingly public acknowledgement of pregnancy loss as 'culture-in-the-making' and acknowledges the sociopolitical issues surrounding this from the feminist and anti-abortion stances.

Recent technologies have provided some possibilities for identifying problem pregnancies at an early stage. One US observer has noted that some women now wait until after amniocentesis before publicly announcing their pregnancy[18]. Prenatal screening has been shown to have its psychological costs even for those women who screen negative for a variety of problems and for whom the results would be expected to provide reassurance[19]. Early pregnancy loss and its psychological consequences are, in the future, likely to be expanded from its traditional conceptualization to include loss or failure surrounding *in vitro* fertilization (IVF) and to include the 'loss' of a healthy pregnancy induced by news of a genetic or other defect from prenatal screening technologies. This issue is returned to in a later section.

HEALTH CARE INITIATIVES FOR EARLY PREGNANCY LOSS

Early pregnancy loss or miscarriage is the commonest complication of pregnancy. Its management is therefore all the more important and a management strategy to encompass all aspects of care needs to be instituted in any unit in which pregnant women are treated. This should provide an adequate diagnostic service and a provision for surgical or medical treatment as well as information and follow-up. In a large maternity unit such as that of the Coombe Women's Hospital, over 750 women experiencing spontaneous early pregnancy

loss are seen each year[20]. The use of terms to describe pregnancy loss is important. Chalmers[21] has shown that certain ethnic groups find the term 'abortion' distressing. It is not always clear what reaction an individual woman may have to particular terms in this area. Thus staff need to be constantly aware of the individual woman's responses (verbal and non-verbal) to the words used to explain what has happened to her. The recognition that a miscarriage has occurred is usually made once either pain or bleeding begin. Recent developments mean that confirmation of miscarriage may happen in a manner removed from traditional expectations of symptoms such as pain and bleeding. Occasionally, for instance, the diagnosis is made after an ultrasound scan in which there was no prior history suggestive of a miscarriage. Irrespective of the presentation, the subsequent management can contribute to the morbidity associated with miscarriage[6]. The diagnosis of a failed intrauterine pregnancy may now be possible using a serum progesterone or beta human chorionic gonadotrophin (β hCG) assay[22]. This can be performed within the first six weeks of pregnancy and may have a role to play in women who are considered to be at high risk of pregnancy loss, for example, women with a poor obstetric history. It may also give reassurance to women who, although not at an increased risk of pregnancy loss believe themselves to be at risk of miscarriage (for example women whose first or most recent pregnancy resulted in a miscarriage). An ultrasonographic examination and in particular a vaginal ultrasonographic examination can detect fetal heart activity at 45–50 days after the first day of the last menstrual period[23]. The diagnostic accuracy may be improved using a color Doppler system[24] but these are not available in most units. It is likely that the majority of early pregnancy losses will still be suspected clinically and the diagnosis then confirmed with either transvaginal or transabdominal ultrasonography.

The management of early miscarriage is

usually an evacuation of the retained products of conception (ERPC). The possibility of using medical treatment has been described[25]. This would require giving an antiprogesterone agent and then stimulating uterine action with prostaglandin. The medical management of spontaneous early pregnancy loss may offer some advantages in terms of psychological morbidity. Jackman *et al.*[6] reported that among a group of 25 women who underwent an ERPC, the procedure was blamed for inducing 'negative' emotions in 22. However, Sharma[26] reviewed a group of women whose miscarriage was treated medically and reported considerable distress among this group and a preference for a surgical option if the need arose again. If, or before, medical treatment of failed intrauterine pregnancy becomes more widespread, then the question of the relative acceptability of these procedures needs careful evaluation.

In the past, the management of a miscarriage was reassurance and discharge if the miscarriage was complete, and an ERPC if the miscarriage was incomplete. The woman may have been admitted to an obstetric ward or may have been returned to the obstetric ward after surgery. A follow-up appointment would be given, usually for a general gynecological clinic. Over the past few years this form of management has been superseded by a more informative approach. Although the diagnosis and surgical management has changed little, there has been a recognition that the psychological aspects of care are those that dictate long-term morbidity. The role of the doctor as diagnostician and healer needs to be widened to encompass an ability to inform, communicate and counsel. This begins with explanation by staff, supplemented by information in a written format, before discharge from the hospital. Questions can be answered immediately about the possibility that some action of the mother may have induced a miscarriage. Many women will blame themselves for the loss: 'I lifted a heavy weight', 'I had a drink', 'We had intercourse just before I started to

bleed'. A brief explanation before discharge from hospital can ensure that the first weeks after the miscarriage are not fraught with guilt. Any aspiration to improve services offered to women who experience an early pregnancy loss must ensure adequate and appropriate follow-up. The provision of a specific miscarriage clinic may help[20]. The role of such a service is to provide an individualized management approach since each woman may have different requirements. Some women may feel that they are 'abnormal' because they are not experiencing any grief associated with their miscarriage, whereas others will be relating every action in the weeks before the miscarriage as being the cause for the loss and that they are therefore somehow to blame.

An explanation of the possible cause is always required. This may involve a discussion about the possibility of a chromosomal abnormality or early placental failure. Maternal age and general health are often questions raised by the woman or her partner. Although these are generally not applicable to the preceding loss, appropriate advice about risks for a future pregnancy is important and should be given honestly. The risk of recurrence should be outlined and the couple reassured that in general an isolated spontaneous early pregnancy loss does not increase the chance of a subsequent loss. The management of recurrent early pregnancy loss is not included in this review. However, it has been shown that psychological support alone has improved the outcome of subsequent pregnancies[27].

DURATION OF PREGNANCY

The bereavement of parents after a perinatal loss is well described[28,29]. Kirkley-Best[30] found that losses in late pregnancy were associated with a more intense grief reaction than losses in early pregnancy. This is not a universal finding. Peppers and Knapp[31] studied maternal grief reactions to miscarriage, stillbirth and neonatal death and found no quantifiable differences between the three groups. Leppert and Pahika[32] interviewed women shortly after a spontaneous early pregnancy loss and found that the grief was as intense as that occurring after stillbirth or neonatal death. It was not until 3–4 months after the loss that the grief began to resolve.

THE PARTNER'S ROLE IN MISCARRIAGE

The response to pregnancy loss has in general focused on the maternal response although several studies do evaluate the psychological response of both parents. This work has concentrated on perinatal or late pregnancy loss and although there may be differences between men and women after perinatal death there does appear to be significant morbidity in both partners. Toedter *et al.*[33] has reported higher overall levels of grief among women using the Perinatal Grief Scale. This was in the initial postpregnancy period only. Theut *et al.*[34] reported that mothers experiencing late pregnancy loss grieved more than fathers. In another study with longer follow-up, the levels of grief of both parents became similar[35].

The reasons why we perceive grief in an individual are either that we look for it or it is expressed spontaneously. Cook[36] has argued that the common belief that mothers feel more grief than fathers may reflect a sampling bias in that most studies have assessed the grief reaction of women only. Women are also seen to grieve more than men who may be less inclined to express their feelings[31]. A possible reason for this is that there is little or no opportunity for men to grieve and little support is offered. The reason may be that the need has not been identified. The Miscarriage Clinic in the Coombe Women's Hospital encourages partners to attend and based on anecdotal experiences a small study ($n = 25$) was undertaken to assess psychological functioning. Using the Hospital Anxiety and Depression Scale]37], significant morbidity in terms of high anxiety and depression levels among partners was evident. This population was biased in that they were a self-selecting population of men who chose to attend the clinic six weeks after their partner's miscarriage, but with the prevalence of morbid levels of anxiety at 36% and depression at 12%, the findings do suggest a previously unacknowledged group of men who might benefit from additional care[38].

RESEARCH ISSUES IN EARLY PREGNANCY LOSS

Research design for future studies in this area needs to be explicit and precise in the sampling procedures. Thus, time since event, management (e.g. surgical vs medical evacuation) and response rates need to be documented. The challenge of identifying miscarriages which are managed outside of the hospital setting is considerable. Studies such as the Avon Longitudinal Study of Pregnancy and Childhood[39] provide some method of considering this. Here a large cohort of pregnant women are being included in a longitudinal study. From these, a subgroup who miscarry ($n = 115$) have been identified. Premiscarriage psychological information is available on this group and their inclusion in the study is not dependent on their source of health care (if any) following the miscarriage.

Legitimate comparison or control groups are another challenge to the researcher studying miscarriage. Psychological response to pregnancy loss is likely to be best understood against a backdrop of the range of emotions experienced across completed pregnancies. Research in this area also needs to incorporate multivariate designs and to move towards theoretically driven studies which test for predictive capacity. Included in theoretically based studies there should be an expansion of psychological considerations from depression (as a marker of a 'loss' event) to a consideration of other emotions but also to evaluating the cognitive representations of women. For instance do women see miscarriage as within or beyond their control and what consequences does this have for psychological well-being?

Finally, studies need to incorporate well-validated research instruments into their design so that a level of quality and comparability across projects can be achieved. Many psychometrically adequate general measures exist, e.g. the Hospital Anxiety and Depression Scale[37]. A number of measures tailored for obstetric groups have also been developed, for instance the Edinburgh Postnatal Depression Scale[40], the Maternal Attachment Scale[41], the Pregnancy Anxiety Scale[42] and the Perinatal Grief Scale[33]. These may be particularly relevant to the issues considered in the study of women and miscarriage.

THE RESPONSE OF HEALTH PROFESSIONALS

An adequate and acceptable response to any tragedy depends on knowledge that addresses the possible causes of the problem, as well as an individualized explanation of what has happened. Medical training, in general, provides inadequate formal teaching on how to provide difficult news and advise and assist patients in dealing with the subsequent trauma. Finlay and Dallimore[43] asked 150 bereaved parents about the loss and the communication skills of those that had initially reported the loss to them. Police officers were rated as being more sympathetic than either doctors or nurses. This should not be a surprise as they receive formalized training in how to break bad news and deal with the questions that may follow. In undergraduate obstetrics and gynaecology teaching programs, little emphasis is given to spontaneous early pregnancy loss as many of the women who miscarry spend only a short time in hospital and the medical students are usually kept at a distance lest they might cause further upset. However, perhaps miscarriage needs to be given a higher priority in medical training. In fact miscarriage will be encountered much more commonly in general practice than for example invasive carcinoma of the cervix, which is rightly perceived as an important clinical condition about which every student would be expected to understand the most up to date management protocols. Siebel and Graves[14] provide a verbatim example of how to explain miscarriage and its management to patients in the immediate aftercare setting. This could provide a focus for discussion and teaching for students in their early medical years.

There are other problems associated with giving the bad news of miscarriage. Fallowfield[44] discusses the relative ease of imparting information on a subject where there are answers to the questions. An explanation of 'It's nature's way' is not enough for most couples after miscarriage and the anxiety of being unable to offer a solution makes the consultation all the more difficult for the doctor. This can result in a woman being discharged, often after an ERPC, with no real explanation. She may spend the next four to six weeks trying to find a cause for this loss and often ends up blaming herself or some event which she associates with the miscarriage.

The opportunity to discuss the events with the couple before discharge from hospital is important. Oakley *et al.*[45] report that women perceive the general practitioner to be second only to husbands as a source of help at the time of the miscarriage. The general practitioner appeared to listen more and discussed the possibility of a psychological reaction whereas hospital medical staff were seen as not fulfilling this role. Ongoing professional evaluation and audit is an appropriate method of assessing patient satisfaction and unmet needs in this context. Following a number of reports of dissatisfaction with general practitioner care of women after miscarriage[46], Roberts[47] reported an evaluation among general practitioners in one Scottish training practice of their management of miscarriage with a view to optimizing care.

WHAT SHOULD HEALTH PROFESSIONALS DO?

A number of recommendations can be made for good practice in the context of miscarriage. First, a proper consultation should take place at the time of the miscarriage or in the immediate postmiscarriage period. The consultation should be specifically structured for the management of 'bad' or 'sad' news. Cunningham *et al.*[48] provide such a structure. In brief, the consultation should be unhurried, honest, balanced and empathic. People need time to absorb the news, time that is not interrupted by a 'bleep' or a call to go elsewhere. The honesty of admitting that one does not know the reason for a given miscarriage is preferable to an uninformed opinion which may later be discredited. Such approaches have been shown not only to reduce anxiety in those receiving the news but also to increase patient satisfaction with the consultation. Patient satisfaction was evaluated six months after the consultation and differences between trained and untrained staff were clearly evident. In a small study of the views of women about viewing and disposal arrangements for a first trimester miscarriage, there was a variety of responses including most wishing for the hospital to make disposal arrangements[49]. There was, however, unanimous agreement that they should be consulted and informed of the proposed management by the medical team.

The location of the woman during her stay in hospital is important; a separate ward away from the obstetric unit may be of benefit. After miscarriage women may find it very distressing to be located with others who are about to deliver or who have just had a healthy baby.

However, isolation may lower self-esteem and inhibit expressions of grief. Therefore, contact with medical and nursing staff is important. Information given verbally is likely to be either completely or partially forgotten; written information is therefore essential. Roberts[47] highlights that there may be a difference between what doctors think they are telling patients and the message these patients are receiving. A doctor who tells a woman that her miscarriage was 'normal' is intending to give a comforting message. The woman may justifiably feel that this is not normal since at a pragmatic level only 15% of pregnancies result in miscarriage and at an emotional level, 'normal' implies healthy. The modern health care system incorporates many disciplines and these should be complementary. The problem may arise as to their separate roles. In an area such as miscarriage there is the chance that, although all health care professionals may believe it to be traumatic and require additional care, each group of professionals may expect that somebody else is providing that care. The woman or couple involved can then 'fall between stools'. Prettyman and Cordle[50] published a study on the attitudes of the primary health care team. A questionnaire was sent to equal numbers of general practitioners, health visitors, community midwifes and district nurses. The vast majority in all groups agreed that miscarriage was frequently associated with significant psychological sequelae and that women should be routinely offered the opportunity to discuss their feelings. The reality is that most women express high levels of dissatisfaction with the care and information provided[46]. Improvements will occur with a more formal approach. Forrest *et al.*[51] reported the results of introducing a counseling service in the management of perinatal bereavement and concluded that the duration of bereavement reaction after perinatal death was appreciably shortened by support and counseling. There is a need to evaluate such a service in the management of couples experiencing early pregnancy loss. The in-hospital management can be changed as already outlined. The subsequent follow-up is then either hospital or community based. In Prettyman and Cordle's[50] study most of the respondents felt that community midwifes or health visitors were the most appropriate professionals to offer psychological support to women after a miscarriage. However, in all groups the majority of individuals did not feel confident enough to give the counseling alone. Indeed only 21% of general practitioners reported being confident enough to provide counseling. These results imply that successful follow-up, counseling and care is likely to involve all members of the health care team. The initial management could occur in the hospital. Before discharge a nurse or doctor would explain the likely causes and give written information. A letter would be sent to the general practitioner informing him/her of the events. An appointment for a miscarriage clinic would be made for four weeks and the partner encouraged to attend. In the intervening weeks the general practitioner should be involved as well as the other members of the primary health care team. At the miscarriage clinic, explanation of the cause should be possible and a consultation as outlined by Turner *et al.*[20] can be undertaken. The value of listening alone cannot be overstated. If further counseling or treatment is required then this can be organized in conjunction with the general practitioner and primary health care team. Trigger events such as family occasions, or the birth of other family members can be distressing. A knowledge that such a reaction is normal may prevent guilt at being jealous of a sibling's new born baby. Hayton[52] has reported a high risk of a depressive reaction at the time of the expected birth of the lost baby. Once again the knowledge that this may occur will help in dealing with it. Although it can be difficult to predict women in need of extra care, Friedman and Gath[8] were able to identify two groups of factors which are significantly associated with psychiatric morbidity after spontaneous miscarriage. Personal factors such as single status, past psychiatric history, as well as obstetric factors such as previous spontaneous pregnancy loss and nulliparity may identify women at risk of long-term depressive illness.

FUTURE PERSPECTIVES

Within the maternity hospital of the future, there will continue to be a number of 'traditional' reproductive failure events, such as miscarriage, which have negative psychological consequences for patients and which require careful psychosocial as well as medical care. The advent of a range of modern technologies such as IVF and reproductive genetic testing also create new situations of reproductive failure for women and their partners. The psychological concomitants of these procedures are considerable[53–55], for instance 40% of women and 15% of men (of 200 couples undergoing IVF) considered infertility as the most upsetting experience of their lives[38]. It is to be recommended that hospitals adopt a generic approach to the psychosocial management of patients so that staff working in various services have a common, systematic approach to management in their designated area. Obstetrics in general has very high rates of litigation. Thus there is every reason to develop broad protocols for the management of psychosocial aspects of patient consultations in the maternity hospital, including for miscarriage services.

In conclusion, there is now a substantial body of evidence documenting the psychological difficulties of patients after miscarriage. There is also emerging a body of scientifically documented good practice which can provide pointers to clinicians about methods to develop their own services to the level of those currently pioneering the field.

REFERENCES

1. Adler, N.E., David, H.P., Major, B.N. *et al.* (1990) Psychological responses after abortion. *Science*, **248**, 41–4.
2. Dagg, P.K.B. (1991) The psychological sequelae of therapeutic abortion – denied and completed. *Am. J. Psychiatry*, **148**, 578–85.
3. Zolese, G. and Blacker, C.V.R. (1992) The psychological complications of therapeutic abortion. *Br. J. Psychiatry*, **10**, 742–9.

4. Aberman, E. (1988) The epidemiology of repeated abortion, in *Early Pregnancy Loss* (eds R.W. Beard and F. Sharp), Springer-Verlag, London.

5. Turner, M. (1989) Spontaneous miscarriage: 'this hidden grief'. *Ir. Med. J.*, **82**, 145.

6. Jackman, C., McGee, H.M. and Turner, M. (1991) The experience and psychological impact of early miscarriage. *Ir. J. Psychol.*, **12**, 108–20.

7. Gannon, K. (1994) Psychological factors in the aetiology and treatment of current miscarriage. A review and critique. *J. Infant Reprod. Psychol.*, **12**, 55–64.

8. Friedman, T. and Gath, D. (1989) The psychiatric consequences of spontaneous abortion. *Br. J. Psychiatry*, **155**, 810–13.

9. Garel, M., Blondel, B., Lelong, N. *et al.* (1992) Reactions depressives apres une fausse couche. *Contraception, Fertil. Sexual.*, **20**, 75–81.

10. Prettyman, R.J., Cordle, C.J. and Cook, G.D. (1993) A three-month follow-up of psychological morbidity after early miscarriage. *Br. J. Clin. Psychol.*, **66**, 363–72.

11. Thapar, A.K. and Thapar, A. (1992) Psychological sequelae of miscarriage: a controlled study using the general health questionnaire and the hospital anxiety and depression scale. *Br. J. Gen. Pract.*, **42**, 94–6.

12. Cecil, R. and Leslie, J.C. (1993) Early miscarriage: preliminary results from a study in Northern Ireland. *J. Reprod. Inf. Psychol.*, **11**, 89–95.

13. Neugebauer, R., Kline, J., O'Connor, P. *et al.* (1992) Determinants of depressive symptoms in the early weeks after miscarriage. *Am. J. Public Health*, **82**, 1332–9.

14. Siebel, M. and Graves, W.L. (1980) The psychological implications of spontaneous abortion. *J. Reprod. Med.*, **25**, 161–5.

15. Hamilton, S.M. (1989) Should follow-up be provided after miscarriage? *Br. J. Obstet. Gynaecol.*, **96**, 743–5.

16. Simon, N.M., Rothman, D., Goff, J.T. and Senturia, A. (1969) Psychological factors related to spontaneous and therapeutic abortion. *Am. J. Obstet. Gynaecol.*, **104**, 799–806.

17. Layne, L.L. (1990) Motherhood lost: cultural dimensions of miscarriage and stillbirth in America. *Women Health*, **16**, 69–98.

18. Rothman, B.K. (1986) *The Tentative Pregnancy: Prenatal Diagnosis and the Future of Motherhood*, Penguin, New York.

19. Marteau, T.M. (1989) Psychological costs of screening. *Br. Med. J.*, **291**, 97.

20. Turner, M.J., Flanelly, G.M., Wingfield, M. *et al.* (1991) The miscarriage clinic: an audit of the first year. *Br. J. Obstet. Gynaecol.*, **98**, 306–8.

21. Chalmers, B. (1992) Terminology used in early pregnancy loss. *Br. J. Obstet. Gynaecol.*, **99**, 357–8.

22. Carson, S.A. and Buster, J.E. (1993) Ectopic pregnancy. *N. Engl. J. Med.*, **329**, 1174–81.

23. Bateman, B.R., Nunley, W.C. Kolp, L.A. *et al.* (1990) Vaginal sonography findings and hCG dynamics of early intrauterine and tubal pregnancies. *Obstet. Gynecol.*, **75**, 421–7.

24. Emerson, D.S., Cartier, M.S., Altieri, L.A. *et al.* (1992) Diagnostic efficacy of endovaginal colour doppler flow imaging in an ectopic pregnancy screening program. *Radiology*, **183**, 413–20.

25. de Jonge, E.T., Makim, J.D., Manefeldt, Z. *et al.* (1995) Randomised clinical trial of medical evacuation and surgical curettage for incomplete miscarriage. *Br. Med. J.*, **311**, 662.

26. Sharma, J.B. (1993) Medical management of miscarriage. Psychological impact understated. (letter). *Br. Med. J.*, **306**, 1540.

27. Stray-Pederson, B. and Stray-Pederson, S. (1988) Recurrent abortion: the role of psychotherapy, in *Early Pregnancy Loss: Mechanisms and Treatment*. Proceedings of the eighteenth study group of the Royal College of Obstetricians and Gynaecologists, London, pp. 23–37.

28. Kennell, J.H., Slyter, H. and Klaus, M.H. (1970) The mourning response of parents to the death of a newborn infant. *N. Engl. J. Med.*, **283**, 344–9.

29. Lewis, E. (1979) Mourning by the family after a stillbirth or neonatal death. *Arch. Dis. Child.*, **54**, 303–6.

30. Kirkley-Best, E. (1981) Grief in response to prenatal loss: an argument for the earliest possible maternal attachment. *Dissert Abstr Int.*, **42**(B), 2560.

31. Peppers, L.G. and Knapp, R.J. (1980) Maternal reactions to involuntary fetal/infant death. *Psychiatry*, **43**, 155–9.

32. Leppert, P.C. and Pahika, B.S. (1984) Grieving characteristics after spontaneous abortion: a management approach. *Obstet. Gynecol.*, **64**, 119–22.

33. Toedter, L.J., Lasker, L.N. and Alhadeff, J.M. (1988) The perinatal grief scale: development and initial validation. *Am. J. Orthopsychiatry*, **53**, 435–99.

34. Theut, S.K., Pedersen, F.A., Zaslow, M.J. *et al.* (1989) Perinatal loss and parental bereavement. *Am. J. Psychiatry*, **146**, 635–9.

35. Goldbach, K.R., Dunn, D.S., Toedter, L.J. and

Lasker, J.N. (1991) The effects of gestational age and gender on grief after pregnancy loss. *Am. J. Orthopsychiatry*, **61**, 461–7.

36. Cook. J.A. (1988) Dads' double binds: rethinking fathers bereavement from a men's studies perspective. *J. Contemp. Ethnogr.*, **17**, 285–308.

37. Zigmond, A.S. and Snaith, R.P. (1983) The Hospital Anxiety and Depression Scale. *Acta Psychiatry Scand.*, **67**, 361–70.

38. Daly, S.F., Hickey, L. and O'Beirne, E. (1994) Does miscarriage affect the fathers? Proceedings of the annual conference of the Society for Reproductive and Infant Psychology. September, Dublin.

39. Harker, L. (1993) Emotional wellbeing following miscarriage. *J. Obstet. Gynecol.*, **13**, 262-5.

40. Murray, L. and Cox, J.L. (1990) Screening for depression during pregnancy with the Edinburgh Postnatal Depression Scale (EPDS). *J. Reprod. Inf. Psychol.*, **8**, 99–107.

41. Cranley, M.S. (1981) Development of a tool for the measurement of maternal attachment during pregnancy. *Nurs. Res.*, **30**, 281–4.

42. Levin, J.S. (1991) The factor structure of the Pregnancy Anxiety Scale. *J. Health Soc. Behav.*, **32**, 368–81.

43. Finlay, I. and Dallimore, D. (1991) Your baby is dead. *Br. Med. J.*, **302**, 1524–5.

44. Fallowfield, L. (1993) Giving bad and sad news. *Lancet*, **341**, 476–8.

45. Oakley, A., McPherson, A. and Roberts, H. (1990) *Miscarriage*. Penguin, London.

46. Friedman, T. (1989) Women's experiences of general practitioner management of miscarriage. *J. R. Coll. Gen. Pract.*, **39**, 456–8.

47. Roberts, H. (1991) Managing miscarriage: the management of the emotional sequelae of miscarriage in training practices in the west of Scotland. *Fam. Pract.*, **8**, 117–20.

48. Cunningham, C., Morgan, P. and McGucken, R. (1984) Down's syndrome: is dissatisfaction with disclosure of diagnosis inevitable? *Dev. Med. Child Neurol.*, **26**, 33–9.

49. Jackman, C., McGee, H.M. and Turner, M. (1993) Maternal views of the management of foetal remains following early miscarriage. *Ir. J. Psychol. Med.*, **10**, 93–4.

50. Prettyman, R.J. and Cordle, C. (1992) Psychological aspects of miscarriage: attitudes of the primary health care team. *Br. J. Gen. Pract.*, **42**, 97–9.

51. Forrest, G.C., Standish, E. and Baum, J.D. (1982) Support after perinatal death: a study of support and counselling after perinatal bereavement. *Br. Med. J.*, **285**, 1475–9.

52. Hayton, A. (1988) Miscarriage and delayed depression [letter]. *Lancet*, **i**, 834.

53. Edelmann, R.J. and Connolly, K.J. (1994) Reproductive failure and the reproductive technologies: a psychological perspective, in *Health Psychology: a Lifespan Perspective* (eds G.N. Penny, P. Bennett and M. Herbert), Harwood, Reading.

54. Black, R.B. (1993) Psychosocial issues in reproductive genetic testing and pregnancy loss. *Fetal Diagn. Ther.*, **8**(Suppl 1), 164–73.

55. Freeman, E.W., Boxer, A.B., Rickels, K. *et al.* (1985) Psychological evaluation and support in a program of *in vitro* fertilisation and embryo transfer. *Fertil. Steril.*, **43**, 48–53.

13

AVENUES OF INVESTIGATION IN THE STUDY OF RECURRENT ABORTION

D.W. Branch, D.J. Dudley and D. Dizon-Townson

Depending on one's biases and the patients selected for study, 50–85% of women with recurrent miscarriage have no discoverable reason for their pregnancy losses. Most women seeking consultation for this problem have repetitive first trimester losses. Excluding controversial 'causes', some authorities hold that no more than 15% of women with recurrent first trimester losses have a believable etiology such as a parental karyotype abnormality or a unicornuate uterus[1]. Several alleged causes of recurrent pregnancy loss, such as infection, luteal phase defect and alloimmune factors, are controversial if not dubious. Others, such as antiphospholipid antibodies, are clearly associated with second- or third-trimester fetal loss but distinctly uncommon in association with recurrent first trimester losses. Thus, we believe the field of recurrent pregnancy loss, especially that of recurrent first trimester abortion, offers unlimited opportunities for basic scientific and clinical investigations. Throughout this review, the term 'sporadic' will be used in reference to non-recurrent pregnancy loss.

MORPHOLOGY AND CHROMOSOMAL CHARACTERISTICS OF RECURRENT PREGNANCY LOSS (RPL)

A fundamental understanding of the morphological and chromosomal abnormalities of abortuses is a necessary first step in the identification of the mechanism(s) by which RPL occurs. Indeed, the allegation that many women with RPL have no explanation for their losses (or have an alleged hormonal, infectious or immune cause) rests in part on a dearth of objective information regarding the morphological details of recurrent abortions.

Embryologists divide pregnancy into the pre-embryonic postmenstrual (weeks 3–5), embryonic (weeks 6–10), and fetal (week 11 until delivery) periods. The embryonic period is characterized by embryonic tissue differentiation, organ formation and early placental development and vascularization. By the end of the 10th postmenstrual week of gestation, development of all major organ systems is complete and the fetal period begins. This stage is characterized by further fetal growth, limited tissue differentiation and further placental development and vascularization.

It is virtually certain that the causes of pregnancy loss during the pre-embryonic, embryonic, and fetal periods are largely different, yet little has been done to improve categorization of the 'causes' of RPL in these different developmental periods. Pre-embryonic pregnancy losses often, if not usually, go unrecognized. Whether or not recurrent pre-embryonic loss is an important clinical problem is uncertain. If so, such patients likely present with a chief complaint of infertility and are not regarded as having RPL.

Clinical Management of Early Pregnancy. Edited by Walter Prendiville and James R. Scott.
Published in 1999 by Arnold, ISBN 0 340 74100 7

EMBRYONIC PREGNANCY LOSS

Embryonic pregnancy loss has been most extensively studied in sporadic pregnancy losses which typically occurs between 5th and 12th postmenstrual weeks of gestation[2,3]. In most cases, the demise of the conceptus precedes clinical symptoms of miscarriage by several days-to-weeks, with most occurring before 8 weeks' gestation. Approximately one-third of sporadic first trimester abortions contain no identifiable embryo or fetus. The embryo is morphologically abnormal in another 25–30% of cases[4,5]. In addition, at least 40% of sporadic embryonic abortuses are chromosomally abnormal[5,6]. Thus, the majority of sporadic spontaneous abortions are embryonic losses associated with morphological abnormalities, chromosomal abnormalities, or both.

Far less is known about the morphological and chromosomal characteristics of recurrent embryonic losses. Sonographic studies indicate that up to 40% of recurrent abortions are anembryonic, and another 2–17% have no identifiable gestational sac[7–9]. Limited studies suggest that at least 65% of embryos or fetuses retrieved from women with recurrent pregnancy loss are morphologically abnormal[10]. At least three-quarters of these are chromosomally abnormal[5,10].

Unfortunately, the data regarding the morphological and chromosomal characteristics of recurrent losses do not include appropriate controls, and the definition of RPL varies from one study to another. The systematic, prospective study of early pregnancy and the morphological and chromosomal characteristics of abortuses is necessary for any future considerations of the etiology of RPL. Such studies also would yield a wealth of epidemiological information and allow for the creation of tissue and DNA banks for additional important studies.

FETAL DEATH

Death of the fetus (subsequent death of a fetus alive ≥ 10 weeks' gestation) is far less common than pre-embryonic or embryonic loss, occurring in less than 3.5% of all pregnancies[2]. Many pregnancy losses occurring in the late first trimester or early second trimester, when one might assume that a fetus is present, are actually anembryonic pregnancies or embryonic deaths that had not yet proceeded to clinical miscarriage. The only certain proofs of fetal death are (1) passage of a dead conceptus measuring 30 mm or more in length, (2) ultrasonographic documentation of a dead fetus, or (3) death of the conceptus after documented fetal cardiac activity at or beyond 10–11 weeks' gestation. Some second trimester 'pregnancy losses' involve the passage of a live fetus, or one alive at the time of the onset of labor. Such a history suggests a problem such as placental abruption or cervical incompetence as possible causes.

Approximately 30% of sporadic early-to-mid second trimester (14–24 weeks' gestation) fetal losses are chromosomally abnormal, but the rate is only 1–2% if the fetus is morphologically normal[6]. The rate of malformations in sporadic early second trimester fetal abortuses is less certain than for embryonic losses, but approaches 15%[4]. As with embryonic loss, the morphology and chromosomal characteristics of recurrent fetal death are uncertain.

PROPOSED STUDIES

It is obvious that a meticulous study of the morphological and chromosomal characteristics of RPL is urgently needed. Not only would the data be interesting in their own right, but the results would be telling with regard to correlation with tests for the traditionally suggested causes of RPL and the results of proposed treatments. Such a study could form the basis for uncovering the etiologies of RPL by providing baseline patient information, parental blood samples, and abortus tissues.

As with any medical study, the final design would be influenced by the amount of available resources, and there are several approaches. Non-pregnant individuals with RPL or with successful prior pregnancies (fertile controls) who intended to undertake another pregnancy should be recruited into longitudinal, prospective, observational study. Those with RPL would be selected because they had two, three or four prior consecutive losses, and no more than one or two prior successful pregnancies, but this variable could be accounted for in the data analysis. Appropriate controls would be women of similar age and gravidity with no prior pregnancy losses.

All women with RPL should have a 'standard' evaluation for known or suspected etiologies. As a minimum, the authors would include hysterosalpingography, luteal phase endometrial biopsy or two or more luteal phase progesterone determinations, antiphospholipid antibody determinations and parental karyotyping. More debatable evaluations might include cervical or endometrial cultures for Chlamydia or mycoplasmas. A well-funded study would also include controversial immunological tests, such as determination of maternal antipaternal leukocyte binding antibodies, and parental human leukocyte antigen determinations[11,12]. Ideally, all controls would also have these tests performed, though cost considerations would be influential in this regard. When parental bloods were collected, DNA and sera from each partner would be processed and stored. It may also be worthwhile to collect information regarding maternal medications and the use of recreational drugs, cigarettes, caffeine and alcohol. Once recruited and evaluated, it would be reasonable to advise all women to take a multivitamin containing 0.4 mg of folic acid per day[13].

All participants would be advised to obtain a pregnancy test as soon as they think they may be pregnant. If a pregnancy is confirmed, a transvaginal ultrasonogram would be performed at 5–6, 7–8 and 9–10 weeks' gestation and pertinent ultrasonographic characteristics of the pregnancy described. If a 'blighted ovum' or embryonic death is detected, reasonable efforts should be made to collect the gestational tissue early and asceptically so that the best possible morphological examination could be performed and culture of the tissue for karyotype is feasible. Morphological examination of the abortus specimen should be done by an experienced and interested pathologist according to the methods described by Fantel and Shepard[5] and in a blinded fashion. Every effort should be made to determine the time of embryonic or fetal demise; often this will be done using the crown–rump length determined by ultrasonography. Ideally, embryonic (or fetal) and placental tissue would be separately identified, and samples of each snap frozen for future studies. Other samples of each would be processed to yield DNA and tissues for histopathological examination.

Approximately 25% of women with RPL and 10% of controls will have abortions in the study pregnancy. Thus, meaningful numbers of abortuses will require fairly large numbers of RPL and control enrollees if the prospective, longitudinal study is to be accomplished. It may be possible to organize a retrospective, case-control type study, but we are not aware of any collection of abortion patients with the sequence of serial first trimester transvaginal ultrasonography, proper collection of abortus tissue and appropriate examinations of abortus tissues. Typical pathology laboratory processing of abortion material leaves inadequate material for determining the gestational age of demise and detailed morphological examination. It may be possible, however, to perform karyotypes on abortus material stored in paraffin blocks using new molecular genetic approaches.

This study protocol would provide sufficient observational data to interrelate the morphological and karyotypic features of recurrent abortions with the timing of the loss and the ultrasonographic features of the pregnancy.

Abortus findings would also be correlated with the parental findings obtained as a part of the evaluation for RPL. Finally, the differences in findings of abortuses from RPL patients and controls would greatly help to pinpoint etiologies of RPL.

The study of fetal death is hampered by its relative infrequency (only about 3% of pregnancies end in fetal death). However, fetal deaths after 18–20 weeks' gestation are often terminated using prostaglandin induction of labor. This method usually yields an intact fetus which may be examined in detail. In some areas, sufficient numbers of *post-mortem* studies on late fetal deaths (e.g. 18–28 weeks' gestation), as well as fetal tissue in paraffin storage, may be available for retrospective analysis.

ANTIPHOSPHOLIPID ANTIBODIES AND PREGNANCY LOSS

A relationship between antiphospholipid antibodies and pregnancy loss has been recognized for at least two decades, yet the underlying mechanism remains uncertain. Many authorities believe that the mechanism of pregnancy loss is similar to, if not identical to, the mechanism(s) of thrombosis associated with antiphospholipid antibodies. Numerous *in vitro* studies address proposed mechanisms of antiphospholipid-related thrombosis. These have been reviewed by Triplett[14] and Asherson and Hughes[15]. Alternatively, a non-thrombogenic effect of antiphospholipid antibodies may be involved, or the antibodies themselves may not be a causative factor.

Clinical investigations of antisphospholipid-related pregnancy loss have been confounded by poor characterization of the pregnancy losses in many case series. Relatively few authors have clearly reported the gestational age or status of the conceptus. In a 1987 review, Branch[16] concluded that a surprisingly high 30–40% of antiphospholipid-related pregnancy losses were second or early third trimester fetal deaths. A 1992 series of well-characterized antiphospholipid syndrome patients confirmed this: 79 of 195 (41%) previous pregnancies were fetal deaths[17]. Oshiro *et al.*[18] recently confirmed the high rate of fetal death in women with well-characterized antiphospholipid syndrome. In this study of 290 women without antiphospholipid antibodies and 77 women with antiphospholipid syndrome, nearly 50% of the pregnancy losses occurring in the antiphospholipid cases were fetal deaths. In contrast, less than 15% of pregnancy losses in the antiphospholipid-negative women were fetal deaths. These data have important implications for antiphospholipid-related pregnancy loss and underscore the necessity for clearly defining the type of pregnancy losses included in future studies. For example, if one wanted to identify women with antiphospholipid antibodies or enrich a study population with such patients, one would be best served by investigating women with second- or third-trimester fetal deaths. Also, initial studies of the mechanism of antiphospholipid-related pregnancy loss should focus on fetal death, not embryonic loss.

In cases of antiphospholipid-related fetal death that we have followed, the death of the fetus is typically preceded by ultrasonographic evidence of severe fetal growth impairment and the development of oligohydramnios. Both are most likely a consequence of what obstetricians call 'uteroplacental insufficiency' or 'placental insufficiency' due to inadequate uteroplacental blood flow. In turn, this is due to abnormalities in the formation of the spiral arteries feeding the intervillous space. The few reported cases in which detailed histopathological examination of the gestational tissues has been performed support this view. The seminal histopathological work in antiphospholipid-related fetal death was reported by De Wolf *et al.* in 1982[19]. Gross examination of the placenta showed infarction involving more than 50% of the placenta. The authors focused on the relative absence of normal physiological changes in the spiral arteries coursing through the decidua. These vessels were of small diameter, demonstrated intimal thickening, fibrinoid necrosis, acute atherosis and intraluminal thrombosis, findings typical of a spiral arterial vasculopathy.

Out *et al.*[20] published the largest and best designed histopathologic analysis to date and included placental histopathology from patients without antiphospholipid antibodies for comparison. All placental examinations were performed by the same pathologist who was blinded to the underlying disease and whether or not the patients had antiphospholipid antibodies. The placentas taken from fetal deaths in the 16 women with antiphospholipid antibodies were statistically more likely to have a decrease in vasculosyncytial membranes, an increase in fibrosis, an increase in hypovascular villi, and signs of 'thrombosis or infarction'. All of these findings are consistent with placental hypoxia. These findings also occurred in some placentas taken from non-antiphospholipid cases, and thus, none could be considered highly specific. In contrast to the findings of De Wolf *et al.*[19] atherosis was present in none of the eight cases in which maternal spiral arteries could be found.

PROPOSED STUDIES

Available clinical and histopathological information is consistent with a hypoxic cause for antiphospholipid-related fetal loss. In turn, this may be due to impairment of the maternal spiral arterial blood flow, though this would appear controversial. Further study of the histopathology and placental morphology of antiphospholipid-related pregnancy loss should be a priority in this area. A good design would be a case–control study of systematically collected and analyzed gestational tissues from women with pregnancy losses who are tested for antiphospholipid antibodies. The limited histological studies done thus far suggest that the decidual vasculature should be carefully scrutinized. To this end, investigators must make every attempt to examine decidual vasculature in the central placenta. A thorough study would include placental bed biopsies, but these are difficult to obtain after vaginal delivery of a dead fetus. At least two pathologists should be involved and should be blinded to the antiphospholipid status of the cases. A thorough examination of the fetus should be performed to exclude other causes of fetal death such as malformations.

Antiphospholipid syndrome is not a common disease, and this will make its study particularly difficult. The authors estimate that at least 100 women with unexplained fetal death will be required to obtain more than a handful with significant levels of antiphospholipid antibodies. Thus, a multicenter effort would almost certainly be required. Also, many women with obvious antiphospholipid syndrome will be excluded because they had been previously identified and treated with medications that probably improve the pregnancy outcome. Controls would include the cases without antiphospholipid antibodies and those with explanations for their losses (e.g. non-immune hydrops, abruption, pre-eclampsia) and pregnancies delivered of live fetuses of similar gestational age (e.g. idiopathic preterm labor)

Another approach to the study of the relationship between antiphospholipid antibodies and pregnancy loss is to measure antiphospholipid antibodies in early pregnancy in a cohort of women of unknown antiphospholipid antibody status and to observe the outcomes without intervention, collecting appropriate maternal history, current pregnancy data and gestational tissues. This sort of study would probably exclude those women with obvious antiphospholipid syndrome, since most would be treated. Because the prevalence of antiphospholipid antibodies is only about 5%[21,22], including women with low levels, several thousand women would have to be tested in order to gather enough positive cases for reasonable analysis. Participating women would have to be tested early in pregnancy, if not before pregnancy, in order to avoid excluding those with attributable late first trimester losses. Pregnancy outcomes, including placental pathology, would be prospectively collected with as much clinical detail as possible. Outcomes among those with antiphospholipid antibodies would be compared and contrasted to those without antiphospholipid antibodies. Again, the personnel collecting the information and analyzing the samples should be blinded to the antiphospholipid status of the subjects.

The matter of antiphospholipid antibody testing deserves special comment. The results from some laboratories are difficult to interpret or associated with unacceptable day-to-day variability. A large, blinded study confirmed this suspicion[23]. Future well-designed studies should include blind testing in at least two reliable laboratories, or at least confirmation of the results in a second laboratory. It would be wise to store aliquots of sera for confirmation of results at a later date, since women with suspicious clinical histories may initially test negative for antiphospholipid antibodies, only to be found to have significant levels upon repeat testing several months to years later[24]. Thus, repeat testing should be included in any study of the relationship between antiphospholipid antibodies and pregnancy loss. Finally, IgM anticardiolipin antibodies and low levels of IgG anticardiolipin antibodies are not associated with the same risks as lupus anticoagulant and moderate-to-high levels of IgG anticardiolipin antibodies[24]. Adequate study designs should account for the proper analysis of semiquantitative anticardiolipin results and the presence or absence of lupus anticoagulant.

If a decidual or placental vascular damage leading to hypoxemia is the immediate cause of fetal loss in antiphospholipid syndrome, how does it occur? According to one hypothesis[25] the damage to the spiral arterioles occurs during the physiological alterations of the spiral arteries in the first and second trimesters. Seemingly useful tools for investigation in this area are the *in vitro* models of cytotrophoblastic growth, invasion and differentiation currently available in several laboratories[26,27]. Monoclonal or affinity-purified antiphospholipid antibodies could be incorporated into these human trophoblast cultures. Quantifiable results defining trophoblast growth, depth of invasion and the elaboration of pertinent surface cell markers (e.g. cell adhesion molecules) could be measured. Other experiments could be performed to measure the influence of antiphospholipid antibodies on the expression of procoagulant factors in the cells, matrix or culture fractions.

Murine models of antiphospholipid syndrome have been described[28,29] and provide one of the most convincing arguments that antiphospholipid antibodies *per se* cause pregnancy loss. Detailed murine placental examinations have been done in only a few experiments[28,30], and there is clearly a need for adequate and systematic histopathological examination of the pertinent tissues in these models. Also, the ability immunologically to manipulate mouse models is far greater than in the human, providing opportunities to better focus on the key initial events in antiphospholipid-related fetal loss. It must be said, however, that murine placentation is sufficiently different from human placentation that cautious interpretation of data will be required.

MOLECULAR GENETIC DEFECTS AND RECURRENT PREGNANCY LOSS

Parental karyotype abnormalities are one of the best accepted causes of RPL, yet they are found in less than 5% of couples presenting with a chief complaint of RPL[31]. Advances in molecular genetics strongly suggest that cytogenetic analysis underestimates the possible contribution of genetic abnormalities to many diseases. The authors believe that molecular genetic abnormalities may be a relatively common cause of RPL in humans. For example, there is an increased rate of embryonic loss in families with certain polygenic disorders, such as neural tube defects[32], suggesting a pre-embryonic or embryonic selection on a molecular level. In addition, an increased rate of female offspring in families with certain X-linked recessive disorders, such as incontinentia pigmenti syndrome or oral-facial-digital syndrome type I[33] has been observed, again suggesting pre-embryonic or embryonic selection against male conceptuses due to molecular mutations. Finally, the sheer number of childhood and adult diseases now known to be caused or linked to a molecular cause points overwhelmingly in favor of molecular genetic causes of at least some proportion of RPL.

To date, the evidence for molecular genetic abnormalities causing or being associated with RPL in humans is scant. Investigators have found a difference in CD 46 gene polymorphisms between healthy couples and those with unexplained RPL[34]. This gene codes for a glycoprotein that is now recognized as being identical to the membrane cofactor protein (MCP) of the complement system and to the trophoblast leukocyte common (TLX) antigen. MCP controls complement activity by altering the structure of C3b and C4b to allow inactivation by proteinases. Thus, cell surface expression of MCP offers protection from complement-mediated cytolysis. Individuals with specific mutations in the MCP gene may lack this protection against the complement system and be susceptible to complement-mediated tissue destruction in various tissues and subsequent RPL.

Over 200 gene loci known to be associated with human hereditary disease have been mapped to both human and mouse chromosomes[35], suggesting that murine models may be useful in the study of RPL in humans. Evidence in rodent models indicates that molecular genetic abnormalities can cause recurrent embryonic and fetal loss[36]. In the mouse, the t-locus is on chromosome 17, 15 centimorgans from the major histocompatibility complex (MHC)[37]. The t-complex encodes cell- and stage-specific proteins which have effects on embryonic development and genetic recombination. This locus is characterized by genes that encode antigens present on sperm and on embryos[37]. Dominant and recessive mutations have profound effects on embryonic development. Recessive t alleles may be lethal, semilethal, or viable, and various mutations are responsible for embryonic demise at different stages of development. This first mutation discovered in the T/t region is known as the brachyury (T) mutation[38]. This mutation affects embryonic axial development and apparently leads to malformation of the allantois and subsequent failure of the formation of a chorioallantoic placenta. Embryos homozygous for this mutation die at 10–11 days' gestation, when umbilical circulation is established[39]. Other examples include, homozygotes for t^{12} consistently reach the morula stage but die before blastocyst formation, and homozygotes for t^{w73} fail to complete implantation normally[40]. Human homologs of the mouse t-complex have been cloned and localized to chromosome 6[41]. Exploration for possible mutations of the human homolog of the t-locus in couples with recurrent pregnancy loss should be a priority.

The murine t-complex is an imprinted region in the genome and is associated with a deletion that is lethal at day 17 of gestation when maternally inherited[42]. Genomic imprinting refers to the differential expression of maternal or paternal genetic material producing a particular phenotype. This effect is based on the parent of origin of the gene(s) involved. DNA methylation and subsequent inactivation has been suggested to be the mechanism by which gene imprinting is regulated[43–45]. Because genomic imprinting causes an area of DNA to be reversibly inactivated, a mutational event could either silence a gene vital to early development or cause an inappropriate gene(s) to be expressed. Much of the research has been accomplished in mice. Experiments transferring nuclei between fertilized eggs must contain one female and one male pronucleus. Mice, manipulated to have only maternal (gynogenetic) or paternal (androgenetic) genomes, were unable to proceed through embryogenesis[46]. Naturally occurring human analogs exist. The paternal genetic contribution appears to be essential for the development and function of placental and extraembryonic tissues, whereas the maternal contribution is required for embryonic development. Ovarian teratomas are embryonically derived and contain tissues from all three germ layers which are characterized by a diploid karyotype with all 46 chromosomes being maternal in origin. Conversely, complete hydatidiform molar gestations are diploid and have two paternal haploid chromosomes and no maternally derived chromosomes[47].

Three of the dozen or so recognized murine imprinted genes map to the distal end of chromosome 7. Conceptuses with two maternal copies of the distal end of this chromosome die late in pregnancy and show evidence of fetal growth impairment[48,49]. Conceptuses with two paternal copies die at about 10 days of gestation. A maternally inherited copy of one of the specific genes on the distal end of chromosome 7, the *mash 2* gene, must be present for trophoblast development[50]. This imprinted gene encodes a transcription factor expressed in trophoblast progenitors.

Information on mutations potentially important in human recurrent abortion comes from experience with transgenic mouse models in which the experimental mutation results in murine embryonic or fetal loss. In these cases, either the insertion of a transgene or a gene knockout interferes with an essential endogenous gene. Copp[36] has reviewed 54 lethal mutations for which the morphology of affected embryos is described. For some housekeeping gene mutations, the nature of the normal gene product is fundamental to cellular functions or interrelationships. However, mutations in genes variably expressed can also be lethal. For example, conceptuses with an E-cadherin knockout, lacking this calcium-dependent cell adhesion molecule, fail to form trophectoderm epithelium[51]. In other mutations, the nature of the normal gene product is uncertain, but the morphology of the pregnancy losses provides certain evidence of when, and some evidence of how, the normal gene functions in embryo–fetal development.

PROPOSED STUDIES

It seems likely that molecular genetic abnormalities occur in humans as a relatively common cause of miscarriage, though no specific mutations have as yet been identified. Increased HLA sharing among couples with RPL does not explain whether HLA antigens are directly responsible for recurrent miscarriage or whether other recessive lethal alleles linked to the MHC are the cause. Lethal alleles linked to the MHC in humans may explain why some investigators have found that male and female partners with a history of RPL are more likely to share one or two HLA DQ α alleles than couples without such a history[52]. Using the now widely available methods of polymerase chain reaction, mutation detection and DNA sequencing, exploration into the human homologs of the t-complex is now possible.

Abortus tissue collected as soon as possible after suction curettage followed by isolation of both RNA and DNA provide valuable materials for future experiments in search of an etiology for RPL. Both fresh tissue and paraffin blocks from abortus tissue may be used for DNA extraction. Initially the DNA extracted may be screened for mutations or polymorphisms in candidate genes. The candidate gene approach has the merit of testing specific hypotheses, namely 'does a certain gene exert a major effect in the etiology of RPL in individuals under investigation?' Candidate genes to be screened early include those encoding proteins vital to cell interactions and immune responses.

Alternatively, one could perform a genome-wide search for DNA marker linked to RPL.

Positional cloning is the isolation of a disease gene starting from the knowledge of its genetic physical location in the genome. Polymorphic short tandem repeat (STR) markers can be used to screen the entire genome for RPL. Lacking an experimental control, genetic studies in humans rely on the ascertainment of related individuals (sibling pairs, nuclear families or extended pedigrees). Sib-pair tests are based on comparison of polymorphic DNA markers in sisters who both have the trait being studied under the null hypothesis of independent segregation between the disease allele and marker loci. If affected siblings show increased sharing of marker genotypes it can be inferred that a disease maps close to the marker's chromosomal location. A prior knowledge of the mode of inheritance is not required.

What other genes might be involved in RPL? A potentially useful approach to this question without prior knowledge of sequence or function is the creation of subtractive cDNA libraries. With the use of DNA sequencing, previously unrecognized genes unique to RPL may be found.

The advance in DNA technology has led investigators to a new frontier in medical science. Cytogenetics is no longer the only examination technique for a genetic cause of recurrent pregnancy loss. Using new techniques, genetic mechanisms may be found to be responsible for the majority of recurrent pregnancy loss.

LUTEAL PHASE DEFECT (LPD)

Progesterone and the proper physiological effect of progesterone on the endometrium is an absolute requirement for blastycyst implantation and early embryonic survival. Not surprisingly, therefore, many physicians believe that defects in the luteal phase or early pregnancy progesterone production or an endometrial effect may be a cause of RPL. Investigators have reported that up to 60% of women with RPL have endometrial histology compatible with LPD[53–55]. However, the association between LPD and RPL is far less than convincing, and whether there is a progesterone deficiency or inadequate response to progesterone causing repetitive pregnancy loss remain controversial. The most glaring problem is that a properly designed study has never been done to determine the prevalence of a LPD in women with RPL compared to matched women with normal fertility. This task is not merely perfunctory. Up to one-half of normal fertile women have a single out-of-phase endometrial histology (lag of 2 or more days)[56,57], and a histological lag of 2 or more days may be found in fully 25% of normal fertile women[57]. Thus, reports of 20–30% of women with RPL having LPD may represent normalcy. The interobserver variation in interpretation of endometrial biopsies is also a major problem. Scott et al.[58] concluded that a mean interobserver variation of just under one day would alter clinical management in 22–39% of infertile women.

Though the major focus has been on progesterone, a large number of other biochemical factors play a role in female reproductive tract preparation for oocyte fertilization, implantation and embryonic growth. Several groups of investigators have observed that women who abort have either polycystic ovaries or hypersecretion of luteinizing hormone (LH)[59–61]. Regan et al.[61] found that women with high follicular phase LH levels had a fivefold increase in the rate of spontaneous abortion. They hypothesized that the raised LH concentration might adversely effect the proper maturation of the oocytes.

From a basic science standpoint, the pertinent effects of progesterone and other hormones on the endometrium are just beginning to be understood. Like other epithelial cells, endometrial cells express collagen/laminin receptors throughout the menstrual cycle[62]. However, luteal endometrium expresses certain integrins not present in the follicular phase, such as the α_1 subunit, under the influence of progesterone. Correlations with clinical features are currently being studied.

Infertile women with endometrial biopsies that lag more than 2 days have delayed expression of certain integrins, such as the vitronectin receptor, on luteal luminal and glandular epithelial cells[62]. Proper expression of the vitronectin receptor may be crucial to nidation and implantation. A recent blinded study shows that at least some infertile women have abnormal integrin expression in the luteal phase[63].

Less is known about the expression of cell adhesion molecules in early pregnancy. Stromal decidual cells from early first trimester-induced abortion tissue express receptors that bind laminin, fibronectin, vitronectin, ICAM-1 and collagen I and IV[64,65]. Not only do these molecules likely play a role in the attachment and outgrowth of the trophoblast to the decidua, they also may play a role in the recruitment of important maternal cells to the region.

PROPOSED STUDIES

The relationship between luteal phase hormones and development of luteal phase endometrium and decidua of early pregnancy is fundamental to the study of RPL. With little difficulty, one could propose dozens of experiments taking many years to complete. A first question to answer is what is the sequence of cellular adhesion molecule expression in normal luteal endometrium. Studies in humans could be performed on serially obtained endometrial biopsy specimens. Early pregnancy tissues would have to be studied using accurately dated animal tissues or induced abortion material from humans.

An important second question to ask is how and when gestational hormones (or other molecules) influence cell-cell interaction. One approach to this area is through the use of hormonal manipulation in castrated female experimental models. It may even be possible to recruit women who have undergone bilateral oophorectomy to participate in such experiments. The chronology of the expression of cellular adhesion molecules in developing decidua could be studied using different regimens of progesterone or estradiol or both.

Even without endometrial histology consistent with LPD, many physicians routinely administer progesterone to patients with RPL. Though not apparently harmful to mother or embryo, the medication is modestly expensive and long-term effects on the conceptus have not been determined. Despite claims by some that progesterone is efficacious in preventing spontaneous abortion in women with RPL[66], no properly designed, randomized, controlled trials have been performed. Such a trial must:

1. Include women with recurrent early first trimester loss as their chief complaint;
2. Document the presence or absence of LPD by sequential luteal phase biopsies;
3. Begin treatment with progesterone immediately after ovulation;
4. Be placebo controlled and blinded;
5. Have spontaneous abortion and live birth as the primary endpoints of the study.

The trialists might randomize all patients with either a documented LPD or no explanation for their RPL and correlate endometrial histology with treatment and outcome in both groups.

'ALLOIMMUNE-MEDIATED' RECURRENT PREGNANCY LOSS AND IMMUNOTHERAPIES

Perhaps no area in the field of RPL is more controversial than that of alleged alloimmune-mediated RPL and its treatment. Those who believe that an alloimmune-mediated cause for RPL exists point to murine models of apparent embryo rejection through natural killer cell mechanisms[67]. However, there is no direct scientific evidence that alloimmune factors play a role in human pregnancy loss, largely because the immunological mechanisms of normal human pregnancy acceptance remain poorly understood.

In spite of this, some reproductive immunologists believe that allogeneic similarities between the male and female reproductive partners might be associated with recurrent pregnancy loss. In keeping with this paradoxical hypothesis, several groups of investigators have reported a tendency for reproductive partners with unexplained recurrent pregnancy loss to share human leukocyte antigens (HLA), for the female partners to fail to produce serum 'blocking factors', or for the female partner to fail to produce antileukocytotoxic antibodies against paternal leukocytes. Other investigators have refuted the significance of each of these factors, and none of these tests provide results that predict the next pregnancy outcome in treated or untreated recurrent miscarriage patients[11,12].

Even though no alloimmune mechanism has been unequivocally shown to cause recurrent pregnancy loss in humans, a number of immunotherapeutic regimens are being empirically utilized in couples with otherwise unexplained pregnancy loss. The most widely used regimen involves immunizing the female partner with the male partner's leukocytes. There is, however, no consensus regarding patient selection or the dose, route or timing of immunizations. Complications have been infrequently reported, but reactions at the injection site, fever, myalgias, platelet and erythrocyte alloimmunization, and a cutaneous graft-versus-host-like reaction, have occurred. Immunization using viable leukocytes carries risks similar to those of blood transfusion, including the transmission of viral diseases.

The live birth rate following maternal immunization with paternal leukocytes in uncontrolled series ranges from 50 to 83%[68]. Four properly designed, randomized, prospective studies have been published, but each included less than 60 patients[69–72]. One found that maternal immunization with paternal leukocytes was beneficial in preventing recurrent pregnancy loss[69], but the other three found no difference in the abortion or live-birth rates between immunized patients or controls.

In an effort to determine whether paternal leukocyte immunotherapy might be efficacious in a proportion of patients with unexplained recurrent pregnancy loss, the American Society of Reproductive Immunology organized two independent meta-analyses[73]. The same data from prior studies were available to both meta-analysis groups. Results from both analyses suggested a statistically significant benefit to immunotherapy. However, the clinical impact was limited in that approximately 10 patients would have to be immunized for every attributable live birth. Critics of the meta-analytic approach have pointed out that the slight clinical benefit may have been due to such factors as patient selection bias in the original studies.

Given the controversial nature of immunotherapy for recurrent pregnancy loss, a brief review of recent developments regarding the basic immunology of pregnancy is needed to place the studies on immunotherapy in context. One hypothesis advanced by Wegmann[74] suggests that growth factors and lymphokines produced by T cells in decidua provides important nutritional support for the embryo. Termed 'immunotrophism', this hypothesis is supported by the finding that T cell-derived growth factors, such as GM-CSF, supports trophoblast growth and differentiation[75]. Also, abortion-prone mice (CBA × DBA/2) administered exogenous growth factors have decreased abortion rates and larger birthweights[76]. However, animals without a functioning T cell system, the scid/scid mouse, reproduces normally with pups of normal birthweight[77]. In addition, transgenic mice without functional GM-CSF have normal fertility[78]. These data suggest that T cells and T cell products play a permissive but non-essential role allowing for maintenance of normal pregnancy. Hence, the immunoregulatory environment in which they become activated must be a critical component for 'normal' T cell function in normal pregnancy, as uncontrolled or unregulated T cell activation could potentially lead to pregnancy loss.

One of the more exciting developments in the past five years is a new theory on how T cells respond to specific antigen[79]. The specific response of T cells depends on the amount and nature of lymphokines produced after the T cells have been specifically activated. In the Mossman hypothesis, there are two phenotypic subtypes of CD4+ T cells based on the lymphokines they produce after activation, termed Th1 and Th2. Activated Th1 CD4+ T cells produce primarily IL-2 and IFN-γ and mediate delayed-type hypersensitivity and cell-mediated immune responses via activation of CD8+ T cells. Conversely, Th2 CD4+ T cells produce primarily IL-4, IL-5, IL-6 and IL-10 after activation and stimulate B cells to become plasma cells hypersecreting specific antibody. Additionally, IL-10 acts to inhibit Th1 CD4+ T cells and production of almost all cytokines by almost any cell[80]. Although Mossman and Coffman's[79] original work was performed using murine T cell clones, other investigations indicate that this functional dichotomy of CD4+ T cells plays an important role in determining T cell responses to foreign antigen *in vivo*[81–83].

In murine pregnancy, T cells and other decidual immune effector cells appear to produce cytokine profiles typical of a Th2-type response. Splenocytes obtained from murine pregnancy produce, after activation, progressively less IL-2 and more IL-4 with advancing gestation[84]. Moreover, T cells obtained from murine decidua produced only growth factors, including IL-3, GM-CSF and IL-6 after activation. Decidual cells produced IL-4, IL-5, and IL-10 during all stages of mouse gestation[85]. The immune response in human pregnancy is less clear. A report by Hill *et al.*[86] shows that peripheral blood mononuclear cells obtained from women with recurrent pregnancy loss produce cytokines typical of a Th1-type response after stimulation with trophoblast antigens, whereas cells from normal women produce primarily Th2-type cytokines. These provocative studies indicate that women with and without recurrent pregnancy loss have different immune responses as reflected by cytokine production, but more importantly that there is a fundamental aberration in the immunoregulation of immune effector cells in women with recurrent pregnancy loss.

PROPOSED STUDIES

There is no question that the effectiveness of paternal leukocyte immunotherapy continues to be highly debated. Most authorities agree that a well-designed prospective trial is crucial; such a trial, sponsored by the National Institutes of Health, is currently underway in the United States.

There are many important basic scientific avenues of investigation. Although the data from Hill *et al.*'s study[86] are preliminary, they do provide some rationale to the study of the effects of immunotherapy on cytokine production by immune effector cells resident in the decidua. One possible consequence of immunotherapy could be to alter a maternal immune response from a Th1-type response, wherein embryotoxic cytokines are elicited, to a Th2-type response such that embryotoxic cytokine production is limited or eliminated. Indeed, there is experimental evidence to suggest that this shift in cytokine production may occur after transfusions[87]. Studies to address this possibility are needed, since such work would provide the rationale for further investigation or provide evidence to abandon this treatment modality. Similarly, experiments to study the effects of other immunotherapies postulated to have beneficial effects on pregnancy outcome, such as intravenous immunoglobulin (IVIG), on immune regulation should be elucidating.

Our understanding of the events of early human pregnancy with regard to cytokine elaboration and the regulation of T cell proliferation is poorly understood. Studies are needed to explore the roles of different immune effector cell populations during implantation and early pregnancy. An important aspect of these studies should be not only to describe the location, amount and ontogeny of cytokines expressed in the area, but also to understand how different cytokine gene expression is regulated. If human pregnancy is a Th2-type immunologic microenvironment, what factors account for establishing this unique environment? If these immunoregulatory influences are disturbed, does this result in pregnancy loss?

For example, what is the immunoregulatory role of endogenous eicosanoids in decidua? Prostaglandin E_2 (PGE_2) has been detected in the early pregnancy tissue[88] and has been postulated to have important T cell inhibitory properties in this context. Betz and Fox[89] have found that T cells activated in high concentrations of PGE_2 (10^{-8} M) produce lymphokine profiles typical of a Th2 T cell, with inhibition of IL-2 production and enhancement of IL-4 production. Thus, the presence of arachidonic acid metabolites in the dedicua may be one contributing immunoregulatory factor leading to the Th2-type response of pregnancy. Studies using cyclo-oxygenase inhibitors should provide some insight into the role of arachidonic acid metabolites in regulating cytokine production by immune effector cells.

Steroid hormones have potent immunoregulatory properties. Glucocorticoids in pharmacologic concentrations have long been known to inhibit the production of IL-2 by T cells[90] but T cells activated in the presence of physiologic concentrations of glucocorticoids (10^{-9} M) have also been found to inhibit IL-2 while enhancing IL-4 production[91]. 1,25-Dihydroxyvitamin D_3 inhibits IL-2, GM-CSF and IFN-γ production by activated T cells[92–94]. Although these two steroids act to decrease the IL-2 producing capacity of T cells, dehydroepiandrosterone (DHEA) has been shown to be a natural enhancer of IL-2 production by activated T cells and the ability to enhance IL-2 production *in vivo* is dependent on available precursor (DHEA-S) and is correlated with the activity of steroid sulfatase in the lymphoid tissue[95]. Although the precise immunologic effects of progesterone

are not entirely clear and progesterone has no direct effect on lymphokine production, this hormone induces a secondary 34 kDa protein which has inhibitory effects on T cells, and progesterone receptors have been identified on T cells in pregnant women[96]. How does the local steroid hormonal microenvironment of early pregnancy regulate cytokine production by immune effector cells in decidua?

One approach to answer this question would involve modulating the steroidogenic enzymes in the decidua and blastocyst. For example, one enzyme which appears to be essential to establish normal pregnancy is 3β-hydroxysteroid dehydrogenase (3β-HSD). 3β-HSD has two enzymatic sites, a dehydrogenase and an isomerase[97]. This enzyme simultaneously converts pregnenolone into progesterone and DHEA to androstenedione. Thus, 3β-HSD mediates a steroid metabolic chain which results in a steroid environment which establishes a T cell 'suppressive' milieu. 3β-HSD activity is expressed in the preimplantation mammalian blastocyst[98] and pregnenolone and DHEA are the two steroids at highest concentration in uterine luminal fluid[99]. Any T cell activated in the normal hormonal milieu of the endometrium would be predicted, based on the steroid immunoregulatory environment, to produce lymphokines characteristic of a Th2-type response. If inhibitors of 3-hydroxysteroid dehydrogenase (e.g. epostane), which are known to induce pregnancy loss[100], also cause alterations in cytokine production by T cells, then this finding suggests that 3β-HSD plays a critical role in providing a steroid hormonal environment which dictates a Th2-type immune response.

Another excellent candidate to study is the role of progesterone in regulating T cell and immune effector cell cytokine production and activities. To date, the immunoregulatory properties of progesterone are poorly understood, surprisingly so given the critical role of progesterone in early pregnancy survival. Similarly, experiments designed to test the role of 1α-hydroxylase in determining T cell responses in decidua via production of 1,25-dihydrioxyvitamin D_3 would be most interesting. Studies designed to understand the basic mechanism of the immunologic and endocrinologic interactions of early pregnancy are critically needed to understand more fully the role of steroid hormones, peptide hormones and other intercellular messengers which can potentially regulate the function and activity of T cells and other immune effector cells.

REFERENCES

1. Ramsden, G.H., Manasse, P.R. and Johnson, P.M. (1990) Recurrent miscarriage (letter). *Lancet*, **336**, 1191.
2. Simpson, J.L., Mills, J.L., Holmes, L.B. *et al.* (1987) Low fetal loss rate after ultrasound-proved viability in early pregnancy. *JAMA*, **258**, 2555–7.
3. Goldstein, S.R. (1994) Embryonic death in early pregnancy: a new look at the first trimester. *Obstet. Gynecol.*, **84**, 294–7.
4. Byrne, J., Warburton, D., Kline, J. *et al.* (1985) Morphology of early fetal deaths and their chromosomal characteristics. *Teratology*, **32**, 297–315.
5. Fantel, A.G. and Shepard, T.H. (1987) Morphological analysis of spontaneous abortuses, in *Spontaneous and Recurrent Abortion* (eds M.J. Bennett and D.K. Edmonds), Blackwell Scientific Publications, Oxford, pp. 8–28.
6. Warburton, D. (1987) Chromosomal causes of fetal death. *Clin. Obstet. Gynecol.*, **30**, 268–77.
7. Stern, J.J. and Coulam, C.B. (1992) Mechanism of recurrent spontaneous abortion. I. Ultrasonographic findings. *Am. J. Obstet. Gynecol.*, **166**, 1844–52.
8. van Leeuwen, I., Branch, D.W. and Scott, J.R. (1993) First trimester ultrasonography findings in women with a history of recurrent pregnancy loss. *Am. J. Obstet. Gynecol.*, **168**, 111–14.
9. Coulam, C.B., Stern, J.J. and Bustillo, M. (1994) Ultrasonographic findings of pregnancy losses after treatment for recurrent pregnancy loss: intravenous immunoglobulin versus placebo. *Fertil. Steril.*, **61**, 248–51.
10. Poland, B.J. and Yuen, B.H. (1978) Embryonic development in consecutive specimens from recurrent spontaneous abortions. *Am. J. Obstet. Gynecol.*, **130**, 512–15.
11. Coulam, C.B. (1992) Immunologic tests in the evaluation of reproductive disorders: a critical review. *Am. J. Obstet. Gynecol.*, **167**, 1844–51.
12. Cowchock, F.S. and Smith, J.B. (1992) Predictors of live birth after unexplained spontaneous abortions: correlations between immunologic test results, obstetric histories, and outcome of next pregnancy without treatment. *Am. J. Obstet. Gynecol.*, **167**, 1208–12.
13. Centers for Disease Control (1993) Recommendations for use of folic acid to reduce number of spina bifida cases and other neural tube defects. *JAMA*, **269**, 1233–8.
14. Triplett, D.A. (1993) Antiphospholipid antibodies and thrombosis. A consequence, coincidence, or cause? *Arch. Pathol. Lab. Med.*, **117**, 78–88.
15. Asherson, R.A. and Hughes, G.R. (1992) Vascular disease and thrombosis: relationship to the antiphospholipid antibodies. *Contrib. Nephrol.*, **99**, 17–25.
16. Branch, D.W. (1987) Immunologic disease and fetal death. *Clin. Obstet. Gynecol.*, **30**, 295–311.
17. Branch, D.W., Silver, R.M., Blackwell, J.L. *et al.* (1992) Outcome of treated pregnancies in women with antiphospholipid syndrome: an update of the Utah experience. *Obstet. Gynecol.*, **80**, 614–20.
18. Oshiro, B.T., Silver, R.M., Scott, J.R. *et al.* (1996) Fetal death is a more specific clinical feature for antiphospholipid syndrome than embryonic loss. *Obstet. Gynecol.*, **87**, 489–93.
19. De Wolf, F., Carreras, L.O., Moerman, P. *et al.* (1982) Decidual vasculopathy and extensive placental infarction in a patient with repeated thromboembolic accidents, recurrent fetal loss, and a lupus anticoagulant. *Am. J. Obstet. Gynecol.*, **142**, 829–34.
20. Out, H.J., Kooijman, C.D., Bruinse, H.W. and Derksen, R.H.W.M. (1991) Histopathological findings in placentae from patients with intrauterine fetal death and anti-phospholipid antibodies. *Eur. J. Obstet. Gynaecol. Reprod. Biol.*, **41**, 179–86.
21. Lockwood, C.J., Romero, R., Feinberg, R.F. *et al.* (1989) The prevalence and biologic significance of lupus anticoagulant and anticardiolipin antibodies in a general obstetric population. *Am. J. Obstet. Gynecol.*, **161**, 369–73.
22. Harris, E.N. and Spinnato, J.A. (1991) Should anticardiolipin tests be performed in otherwise

healthy pregnant women? *Am. J. Obstet. Gynecol.*, **165**, 1272–7.

23. Peaceman, A.M., Silver, R.K., MacGregor, S.N. and Socol, M.L. (1992) Interlaboratory variation in antiphospholipid antibody testing. *Am. J. Obstet. Gynecol.*, **166**, 1780–7.

24. Silver, R.M., Porter, T.F., van Leeuwen, I. *et al.*, (1996) Anticardiolipin antibodies: clinical consequences of 'low-titers'. *Obstet. Gynecol.*, **87**, 495–500.

25. Branch, D.W. (1994) Thoughts on the mechanism of pregnancy loss associated with the antiphospholipid syndrome. *Lupus*, **3**, 275–30.

26. Damsky, C.H., Fitzgerald, M.L. and Fisher, S.J. (1992) Distribution patterns of extracellular matrix components and adhesion receptors are intricately modulated during first trimester cytotrophoblast differentiation along the invasive pathway *in vivo. J. Clin. Invest.*, **89**. 210–22.

27. Fisher, S.J. and Damsky, C.H. (1993) Human trophoblast invasion. *Semin. Cell Biol.*, **4**, 183–8.

28. Branch, D.W., Dudley, D.J., Mitchell, M.D. *et al.* (1990) Immunoglobulin G fractions from patients with antiphospholipid antibodies cause fetal death in Balb/c mice: a model for autoimmune fetal loss. *Am. J. Obstet. Gynecol.*, **163**, 210–16.

29. Blank, M., Cohen, J., Toder, V. and Shoenfeld, Y. (1991) Induction of anti-phospholipid syndrome in naive mice with mouse lupus monoclonal and human polyclonal anti-cardiolipin antibodies. *Proc. Natl. Acad. Sci. USA*, **88**, 3069–73.

30. Silver, R.M., Pierangeli, S., Gharavi, A.E. *et al.* (1995) Induction of high levels of anticardiolipin antibodies in mice by immunization with β₂-glycoprotein I does not cause fetal death. *Am. J. Obstet. Gynecol.*, **173**, 1410–15.

31. Scott, J.R.S. and Branch, D.W. (1995) Evaluation and treatment of recurrent miscarriage, in *Infertility, Evaluation and Treatment* (eds W.R. Keye, R.J. Chang, R.W. Rebar and M.R. Soules), W.B. Saunders, Philadelphia, pp. 230–49.

32. Alberman, E., Creasy, M. and Polani, P.E. (1973) Spontaneous abortion and neural tube defects. *Br. Med. J.*, **4**, 230–1.

33. Jones, K.L. (1988) Smith's recognizable patterns of human malformation, 4th edn. W.B. Saunders, Philadelphia.

34. Risk, J.M.,. Flanagan, B.F. and Johnson, P.M. (1991) Polymorphism of the human CD 46 gene in normal individuals and in recurrent

spontaneous abortion. *Hum. Immunol.*, **30**, 162–7.

35. Searle, A.G., Edwards, J.H. and Hall, J.G. (1994) Mouse homologues of human hereditary disease. *J. Med. Genet.*, **31**, 1–19.

36. Copp, A.J. (1995) Death before birth: clues from gene knockouts and mutations. *Trends Genet.*, **11**, 87–95.

37. Bennett, D. (1975) The T-locus of the mouse. *Cell*, **6**, 441–54.

38. Dobrovolskaia-Zavadskaia, N. (1927) Sur la mortification spontanee de la queue chez la souris nouveau-zee et sur l'existence d'un caractere (facteur) hereditaire. *C. R. Soc. Biol.*, **97**, 114–19.

39. Chesley, P. (1935) Development of the short-tailed mutant in the house mouse. *J. Exp. Zool.*, **70**, 429–59.

40. Spiegleman, M., Artzt, K. and Bennett, D. (1976) Embryological study of a P/t locus mutation (t^{w73}) affecting trophectoderm development. *J. Embryol. Exp. Morphol.*, **36**, 373–81.

41. Blanche, H., Wright, L.G., Vergnaud, G. *et al.* (1992) Genetic mapping of three human homologues of murine t-complex genes localizes TCP 10 to 6q27, 15 cM distal to TCP 1 and PLG. *Genomics*, **12**, 826–8.

42. Winking, H. and Silver, L. (1984) Characterisation of a recombinant mouse t-haplotype that expresses a dominant lethal maternal effect. *Genetics*, **108**, 1013–20.

43. Swain, J.L., Stewart, T.A. and Leder, P. (1987) Parental legacy determines methylation and expression of an autosomal transgene: a molecular mechanism for parental imprinting. *Cell*, **50**, 719–27.

44. Hall, J.G. (1990) Genomic imprinting: review and relevance to human disease. *Am. J. Hum. Genet.*, **46**, 857–73.

45. Howlett, S.K. (1991) Genomic imprinting and nuclear totipotency during embryonic development. *Int. Rev. Cytol.*, **127**, 175–92.

46. Watson, D., Gilman, M., Witkowski, J. and Zoller, M. (1992) The introduction of foreign genes into mice, in *Recombinant DNA*, 2nd edn. Scientific American Books, New York, pp. 267–70.

47. Lawler, S.D., Porey, S., Fisher, R.A. and Pickthall, V.J. (1982) Genetic studies on hydatidiform moles. *Ann. Hum. Genet.*, **46**, 209–22.

48. Searle, A.G. and Beechey, C.V. (1990) Genome imprinting phenomena on mouse chromosome 7. *Genet. Res.*, **56**, 237–44.

49. Ferguson-Smith, A.C., Carranach, B.M., Barton, S.C. *et al.* (1991) Embryological and molecular investigations of parental imprinting on mouse chromosome 7. *Nature*, **351**, 667–70.

50. Guillemot, F., Caspary, T., Tilghman, S.M. *et al.* (1995) Genomic imprinting of *Mash 2*, a mouse gene required for trophoblast development. *Nature Genet.*, **9**, 235–42.

51. Larue, L., Ohsugi, M., Hirchenhain, J. and Kemler, R. (1994) E-cadherin null mutant embryos fail to form a trophectoderm epithelium. *Proc. Natl. Acad. Sci. USA*, **91**, 8263–7.

52. Ober, C., Steck, T., van der Ven, K. *et al.* (1993) MHC class 2 compatibility in aborted fetuses and term infants of couples with recurrent spontaneous abortion. *J. Reprod. Immunol.*, **25**, 195–207.

53. Grant, A., McBride, W.G. and Moyes, J.M. (1959) Luteal phase defects in abortion. *Int. J. Fertil.*, **4**, 323–9.

54. Botella-Llusia, J. (1962) The endometrium in repeated abortion. *Int. J. Fertil.*, **7**, 147–54.

55. Tho, P.T., Byrd, J.R. and McDonough, P.G. (1979) Etiologies and subsequent reproductive performance of 100 couples with recurrent abortion. *Fertil. Steril.*, **32**, 389–95.

56. Shoupe, D., Mishell, D.R. Jr, Lacarra, M. *et al.* (1989) Correlation of endometrial maturation with four methods of estimating day of ovulation. *Obstet. Gynecol.*, **73**, 88–92.

57. Davis, O.K., Berkeley, A.S., Naus, G.J. *et al.* (1989) The incidence of luteal phase defect in normal, fertile women, determined by serial endometrial biopsies. *Fertil. Steril.*, **51**, 582–6.

58. Scott, R.T., Snyder, R.R., Stickland, D.M. *et al.* (1988) The effect of interobserver variation in dating endometrial histology on the diagnosis of luteal phase defects. *Fertil. Steril.*, **50**, 888–92.

59. Sagle, M., Bishop, K., Ridley, N. *et al.* (1988) Recurrent early miscarriage and polyscystic ovaries. *Br. Med. J.*, **297**, 1027–8.

60. Homburg, R., Armar, N.A., Eshel, A. *et al.* (1988) Influence of scrum luteinising hormone concentrations on ovulation, conception and early pregnancy loss in polycystic ovary syndrome. *Br. Med. J.*, **297**, 1024–6.

61. Regan, L., Owen, E.J. and Jacobs, H.S. (1990) Hypersecretion of luteinising hormone, infertility, and miscarriage. *Lancet*, **336**, 1141–4.

62. Lessey, B.A., Damjanovich, L., Coutifaris, C. *et al.* (1992) Integrin adhesion molecules in the human endometrium. Correlation with the normal and abnormal menstrual cycle. *J. Clin. Invest.*, **90**, 188–95.

63. Lessey, B.A., Castelbaum, A.J., Sawin, S.W. and Sun, J. (1995) Integrins as markers of uterine receptivity in women with primary unexplained infertility. *Fertil. Steril.*, **63**, 535–42.

64. Salafia, C.M., Haynes, N., Merluzzi, V.J. and Rothlein, R. (1991) Distribution of ICAM-1 within decidua and placenta and its gestational age-associated changes. *Pediatr. Pathol.*, **11**, 381–8.

65. Ruck, P., Marzusch, K., Kaiserling, E. *et al.* (1994) Distribution of cell adhesion molecules in decidua of early human pregnancy. An immunohistochemical study. *Lab. Invest.*, **71**, 94–101.

66. Daya, S. (1989) Efficacy of progesterone support for pregnancy in women with recurrent miscarriage. A meta-analysis of controlled trials. *Br. J. Obstet. Gynaecol.*, **96**, 275–80.

67. Clark, D.A., Chaouat, G., Mogil, R. and Wegmann, T.G. (1994) Prevention of spontaneous abortion in DBA/2-mated CBA/J mice by GM-CSF involves CD8+ T cell-dependent suppression of natural effector cell cytotoxicity against trophoblast target cells. *Cell Immunol.*, **154**, 143–52.

68. Branch, D.W. (1992) Immunologic aspects of pregnancy loss: alloimmune and autoimmune considerations, in *Medicine of the Fetus and Mother* (eds E.A. Reece, J.C. Hobbins, M.J. Mahoney and R.H. Petrie), J.B. Lippincott, Philadelphia, pp. 217–33.

69. Mowbray, S.F., Gibbons, C., Liddell, H. *et al.* (1985) Controlled trial of treatment of recurrent spontaneous abortion by immunization with paternal cells. *Lancet*, **i**, 941–3.

70. Cauchi, M.N., Lim, D., Young, D.E. *et al.* (1991) Treatment of recurrent aborters by immunization with paternal cells – controlled trial. *Am. J. Reprod. Immunol.*, **25**, 16–17.

71. Ho, H.N., Gill, T.H., Hsieh, H.J. *et al.* (1991) Immunotherapy for recurrent spontaneous abortions in a Chinese population. *Am. J. Reprod. Immunol.*, **25**, 10–15.

72. Gatenby, P.A. Cameron, K., Simes, R.J. *et al.* (1993) Treatment of recurrent spontaneous abortion by immunization with paternal lymphocytes: results of a control trial. *Am. J. Reprod. Immunol.*, **29**, 88–94.

73. Coulam, C.B., Clark, D.A., Collins, J. and Scott, J.R. (1994) Worldwide collaborative observational study and meta-analysis of allogenic

leukocyte immunotherapy for recurrent spontaneous abortion. *Am. J. Reprod. Immunol.*, **32**, 55–72.

74. Wegmann, T.G. (1988) Maternal T cells promote placental growth and prevent spontaneous abortion. *Immunol. Lett.*, **17**, 297–302.

75. Athanassakis, I., Bleackley, R.E., Paetkay, V. *et al.* (1987) The immunostimulatory effect of T cells and T cell lymphokines on murine fetally derived placental cells. *J. Immunol.*, **138**, 37–44.

76. Chaouat, G., Menu, E., Clark, D.A. *et al.* (1990) Control of fetal survival in CBA × DBA/2 mice by lymphokine therapy. *J. Reprod. Fertil.*, **89**, 447–58.

77. Croy, B.A. and Chapeau, C. (1990) Evaluation of the pregnancy immunotrophism hypothesis by assessment of the reproductive performance of young adult mice of genotype *scid/scid.bg/bg*. *J. Reprod. Fertil.*, **88**, 231–9.

78. Dranoff, G., Crawford, A.D., Sadelain, M. *et al.* (1994) Involvement of granulocyte–macrophage colony-stimulating factor in pulmonary homeostatis. *Science*, **264**, 713–16.

79 Mossman, T.R. and Coffman, R.L. (1989) TH1 and TH2 cells: different patterns of lymphokine secretion lead to different functional properties. *Annu. Rev. Immunol.*, **7**, 145–73.

80. Moore, K.W., O'Garra, A., de W., Malefyt, R. *et al.* (1993) Interleukin 10. *Annu. Rev. Immunol.*, **11**, 165–90.

81. Romagnani, S. (1994) Lymphokine production by human T cells in disease states. *Annu. Rev. Immunol.*, **12**, 227–57.

82. Del Prete, G.F., De Carli, M., Mastromauro, C. *et al.* (1991) Purified protein derivative of *Mycobacterium tuberculosis* and excretory-secretory antigen(s) of *Toxicara canis* expand in vitro human T cells with stable and opposite (type 1 T helper or type 2 T helper) profile of cytokine production. *J. Clin. Invest.*, **88**, 346–50.

83. Fitzgerald, T.J. (1992) The Th1/Th2-like switch in syphilitic infection: is it detrimental? *Infect. Immun.*, **60**, 3475–9.

84. Dudley, D.J., Chen, C.L., Mitchell, M.D. *et al.* (1993) Adaptive immune responses during murine pregnancy: pregnancy-induced regulation of lymphokine production by activated T lymphocytes. *Am. J. Obstet. Gynecol.*, **168**, 1155–63.

85. Lin, H., Mosmann, T.R., Guilbert, L., Tuntipopipat, S. and Wegmann, T.G. (1993) Synthesis of T helper 2-type cytokines at the maternal-fetal interface. *J. Immunol.*, **151**, 4562–73.

86. Hill, J.A., Polgar, K. and Anderson, D.J. (1995) T-helper 1-type immunity to trophoblast in women with recurrent spontaneous abortion. *JAMA*, **273**, 1933–6.

87. Kirkley, S.A., Cowles, J., Pellegrini, V.D. *et al.* (1995) Cytokine secretion after allogeneic and autologous blood transfusion. *Lancet*, **345**, 527.

88. Scodras, J.M., Parhar, R.S., Kennedy, T.G. and Lala, P.K. (1990) Prostaglandin-mediated inactivation of natural killer cells in the murine decidua. *Cell Immunol.*, **127**, 352–67.

89. Betz, M. and Fox, B.S. (1991) Prostaglandin E_2 inhibits production of Th1 lymphokines but not of Th2 lymphokines. *J. Immunol.*, **146**, 108–13.

90. Cupps, T.R. and Fauci, A.S. (1982) Corticosteroid-mediated immunoregulation in man. *Immunol. Rev.*, **65**, 133–45.

91. Daynes, R.A., Dudley, D.J. and Araneo, B.A. (1990) Regulation of murine lymphokine production in vivo. II. Dehydroepiandrosterone is a natural enhancer of interleukin 2 synthesis by helper T cells. *Eur. J. Immunol.*, **20**, 793–802.

92. Tsoukas, C.D., Provvedini, D.M. and Manolagas, S.C. (1984) 1,25-dihydroxyvitamin D_3. a novel immunoregulatory hormone. *Science*, **224**, 1438–40.

93. Reichel, H., Koeffler, H.P. Tobler, A. and Norman, A.W. (1987) 1alpha,25-dihydroxyvitamin D_3 inhibits gamma-interferon synthesis by human peripheral blood lymphocytes. *Proc. Natl. Acad. Sci. USA*, **84**, 3385–9.

94. Tobler, A., Miller, C.W., Norman, A.W. and Koeffler, H.P. (1988) 1,25-dihydroxyvitamin D_3 modulates the expression of a lymphokine (granulocyte-macrophage colony-stimulating factor) posttranscriptionally. *J. Clin. Invest.*, **81**, 1819–23.

95. Daynes, R.A. and Araneo, B.A. (1989) Contrasting effects of glucocorticoids on the capacity of T cells to produce the growth factors interleukin 2 and interleukin 4. *Eur. J. Immunol.*, **19**, 3219–25.

96. Szekeres-Bartho, J., Kilar, F., Falkay, G. *et al,.* (1985) Progesterone-treated lymphocytes of healthy pregnant women release a factor inhibiting cytotoxicity and prostaglandin synthesis. *Am. J. Reprod. Immunol. Microbiol.*, **9**, 15–24.

97. Luu-The, V., Takahashi, M., de Launoit, Y. *et al.* (1991) Evidence for distinct dehydrogenase and isomerase sites within a single 3β-hydroxysteroid dehydrogenase/5-ene-4-ene isomerase protein. *Biochemistry*, **30**, 8861–5.

98. Dickmann, Z., Dey, S.K. and Gupta, J.S. (1976) A new concept: control of early pregnancy by steroid hormones originating in the preimplantation embryo. *Vitam. Horm.*, **34**, 215–42.

99. Stone, B.A., Petrucco, O.M., Seamark, R.F. and Godfrey, B.M. (1986) Concentrations of steroid hormones, and of prolactin, in washings of the human uterus during the menstrual cycle. *J. Reprod. Fertil.*, **78**, 21–5.

100. Crooji, M.J., De Nooyer, C.C., Rao, B.R. *et al.* (1988) Termination of early pregnancy by the 3β-hydroxysteroid dehydrogenase inhibitor epostane. *N. Engl. J. Med.*, **319**, 813–17.

INDEX

Page numbers in *italics* refer to tables, those in **bold** refer to figures.

Clinical Management of Early Pregnancy. Edited by Walter Prendiville and James R. Scott.
Published in 1999 by Arnold, ISBN 0 340 74100 7